Rehabilitation Medicine

THE MANAGEMENT OF PHYSICAL DISABILITIES

By the same author:

REHABILITATION OF THE SEVERELY DISABLED

1—Evaluation of a Disabled
Living Unit

2—Management

Rehabilitation Medicine

THE MANAGEMENT OF PHYSICAL DISABILITIES

P. J. R. NICHOLS
M.A., D.M. (Oxon.), F.R.C.P., D.Phys.Med. (Lond.)
Director of Mary Marlborough Lodge, Disabled Living Research Unit, Nuffield Orthopaedic Centre, Headington, Oxford; Director of the Oxford Rehabilitation Research Unit, Nuffield Department of Orthopaedic Surgery, University of Oxford

with the assistance of

E. A. HAMILTON
M.A., B.M., B.Ch., D.Phys.Med.
Mary Marlborough Lodge, Nuffield Orthopaedic Centre, Headington, Oxford; Assistant Medical Officer, Oxford Artificial Limb and Appliance Centre, Nuffield Orthopaedic Centre, Headington, Oxford

with a contribution by

B. L. HAZLEMAN
M.B., M.R.C.P.
Addenbrooke's Hospital, Cambridge

BUTTERWORTHS
LONDON · BOSTON
Sydney · Wellington · Durban · Toronto

THE BUTTERWORTH GROUP

ENGLAND

Butterworth & Co. (Publishers) Ltd
London: 88 Kingsway, WC2B 6AB

AUSTRALIA

Butterworths Pty Ltd
Sydney: 586 Pacific Highway,
NSW 2067
Also at Melbourne, Brisbane, Adelaide and Perth

SOUTH AFRICA

Butterworth & Co (South Africa) (Pty) Ltd
Durban: 152–154 Gale Street

NEW ZEALAND

Butterworths of New Zealand Ltd
Wellington: 26–28 Waring Taylor Street, 1

CANADA

Butterworth & Co (Canada) Ltd
Toronto: 2265 Midland Avenue,
Scarborough, Ontario, M1P 4S1

USA

Butterworths (Publishers) Inc
Boston: 161 Ash Street, Reading,
Mass. 01867

First published 1976

ISBN 0 407 00120 4

Library of Congress Cataloging in Publication Data

Nichols, Philip John Russell.
Rehabilitation medicine.

Includes bibliographies and index.
1. Physically handicapped—Rehabilitation.
I. Hamilton, Elizabeth Ann, joint author. II. Title.
[DNLM: 1. Physical therapy. 2. Occupational therapy.
3. Rehabilitation. WB460 N621r]

RM930.N5 617 75–40041

ISBN 0–407–00120–4

Filmset and printed in England by
The Camelot Press, Ltd, Southampton

. . . that which is everybody's business is nobody's business

Izaak Walton
Compleat Angler

Contents

Preface

During the past few years, general interest in rehabilitation has been awakened and as a subject it has been seen to be one of the growing points of medicine. It is difficult to define as a subject in itself, as it is an integral part of much of clinical medicine and most of rehabilitation is applied commonsense and an understanding of people who have become ill or disabled. All clinicians should be concerned with the rehabilitation of their patients, but there are many who will not have had the opportunity as students, nor in their post-graduate years, to develop an understanding of the wider aspects of patient care called 'rehabilitation'. This book is an attempt to describe the 'rehabilitation approach' to common clinical problems and to describe the contribution of the physiotherapist and occupational therapist to the management of these patients.

Perhaps an apposite title would be *The Management of the Moderately Disabled,* indicating its place as a companion volume to *Rehabilitation of the Severely Disabled.*

The secret of rehabilitation is the giving of the right help at the right time. The help needed may be simple advice or reassurance, or it may be intensive physiotherapy, or it may be the supply of a complex appliance and training in its use, or it may be vocational guidance and retraining.

This book is written for all those who have an interest in their patients beyond the immediate problems of diagnosis and therapeutics. It is hoped that general practitioners in particular will find it of interest and value for they must often be the co-ordinators of the health and care services, and many patients needing rehabilitation are never referred to hospital.

Above all, we hope that this book will convince its reader of the need for integration between hospital and community services if rehabilitation is going to become a reality for those who need it.

In order to avoid a lot of repetition, we have used rheumatoid arthritis as a model to describe the 'totality' of the rehabilitation approach. In the chapter on rheumatoid arthritis we have described in considerable detail the procedures and advice relating to domestic arrangement and activities of daily living. A similar amount of detail would have been appropriate in other chapters but would have involved unnecessary repetition. Readers are therefore asked to refer back to the chapter on rheumatoid arthritis when considering other disabilities, for the details of advice are appropriate whatever the physical disability.

P. J. R. N.
E. A. H.

Acknowledgements

We would like to express our sincere gratitude to all who have helped by sharing their knowledge and experiences of rehabilitation with us. Our views and attitudes are continually changing under the influence of our colleagues through the patients they refer to us, by consultations, by case conferences and by private discussions. In this sense we owe a considerable debt of gratitude to all the medical staff of the Nuffield Orthopaedic Centre and the Nuffield Department of Orthopaedic Surgery, and in particular Dr. A. G. Mowat.

We are also indebted to Dr. D. J. Lane and Dr. W. S. Hamilton of the United Oxford Hospitals for help with the chapter on chronic bronchitis.

Dr. E. Williams read the manuscript and contributed many helpful suggestions which have been incorporated.

We would like to pay tribute to Mrs. C. Newman, Mrs. E. Payne and Mrs. N. Wright who undertook the typing.

1—Organization of Rehabilitation Services

INTRODUCTION

In the early years of this century, the spa towns were centres for much of the physical treatment used in the management of patients. They specialized for the most part in the treatment of 'rheumatism' and other medical disorders of the locomotor system. In addition to hydrotherapy (or balneotherapy) the physical treatments employed included electrotherapy (heat, light and electrical stimulation), movements, manipulation and massage. In 1931, the Section of Balneology and Climatology of the Royal Society of Medicine fused with the Section of Electrotherapeutics and formed the Section of Physical Medicine, and the specialty of 'Physical Medicine' was created.

The majority of patients for whom physical treatment is prescribed are those suffering from 'rheumatic conditions' which are subject to natural remissions and exacerbations. The response to treatment will depend on the patient's motivation as well as the personality of the therapist.

Thus, the scientific evaluation of physical therapy is very difficult, and much physical therapy remains empirical in nature and unproven in value.

Partly because of the inexactness of diagnosis and treatment, and partly because physical therapy is only a part of the total management of patients, the term 'physical medicine' has fallen into disrepute. 'Rheumatology' has emerged as a clinical specialty with close links to General (Internal) Medicine. *Rehabilitation* is an appropriate term to embrace the many physical, social and organizational aspects of the after-care of most patients who require more than acute, short-term definitive care.

REHABILITATION

Principles

Although the term 'rehabilitation' has taken on many different meanings, in its widest sense it 'signifies the whole process of restoring a disabled person to a condition in which he is able, as early as possible, to resume a normal life'.* There can therefore be no doubt that it is the concern of all clinicians but with a differing emphasis in different specialties.

There is a relative lack of interest among the medical professions in the problems of convalescence. Publications on the subject are scanty, little research has been undertaken, and little attention has been devoted to the medical aspects of recovery. The main interests of clinicians often lie only in diagnosis and acute definitive treatment. The doctor's role in the convalescent period is often considered of minimal importance, and the patient's attitude during this period is traditionally passive.

Rehabilitation is 'creative convalescence', and as such, represents that active contribution made by medical, paramedical staff and patient to the restoration of health during the recovery phase which follows the intensive definitive treatment.

The rehabilitation principles laid down by Robert Jones in his 'curative workshops' during the First World War were not widely taken up during the 20 years of peace, but in the Second World War, specialists of various clinical disciplines in the armed forces and emergency medical services combined to establish the modern approach of full-time intensive orthopaedic rehabilitation and converted 'convalescence' into 'rehabilitation'. The pattern was developed by grouping patients with similar disabilities, narrowing the remedial aims of each group, increasing the number of groups or classes and grading their activity to enable patients to make a graduated progression through the classes as functional improvement occurred. Each class had an activity programme based on a few simple, remedial exercises, e.g. 'quadriceps setting exercises' or 'walking exercises' or 'shoulder mobilizing exercises' or 'spinal extension exercises'. Management was augmented by specific physiotherapy, occupational therapy, and hydrotherapy where necessary.

* From Report of the Committee of Enquiry on the Rehabilitation, Training and Resettlement of Disabled Persons (1956), par. 5. Chaired by the Rt. Hon. Lord Piercy, Cmd. 987. London; H.M.S.O.

Most patients admitted to hospital require little in the way of complex rehabilitation, *providing the supervising clinician clearly communicates to the patient, relatives and family doctor, the expected progress of the disease and the outcome of treatment.* The will to recover, which is inherent in most patients, is intensified where confidence in those who give medical care is shown to be justified by good treatment and manifest understanding of their problems.

Some patients, however, do benefit considerably from periods of intensive rehabilitation and a more closely supervised convalescence. Such patients need admission to a centre which is structurally and functionally orientated towards recovery; where a purposive atmosphere instils confidence; and where the individual skills of a rehabilitation team are integrated and co-ordinated to assist each patient to achieve maximal functional efficiency. Within the category of patients needing these special rehabilitation facilities are those with multiple injuries; those with complex lesions—such as crush injuries of the hands or injuries of the head or spine; and those requiring a high standard of physical fitness before return to work is possible.

The intensive full-time regime, and the later integration of retraining for work with the initial rehabilitative exercise programme are of the utmost benefit.

The majority of patients with illnesses and injuries which have had efficient primary definitive treatment can be rehabilitated within the organization of the District General Hospital as in-patients, as out-patients on a Day Hospital basis, or as residents in a hostel. With adequate rehabilitation, the incidence of prolonged morbidity can be significantly reduced, and the duration of disability can be shortened, providing patients start their planned rehabilitation soon after the onset of disability.

There is considerable evidence that delay in *making* decisions and delay in *communicating* decisions can increase morbidity and delay return to work.

The advantage of organized rehabilitation lies in its ability to combine an integrated medical and functional assessment with the co-ordination of the activities of the many agencies (medical, social, educational and industrial) concerned with a patient's return to work. There is a particular advantage to be gained by combining the medical and industrial sections into a single rehabilitation unit, so enabling the patient's rehabilitation to progress smoothly without unnecessary delays.

Probably 1 in 3 patients discharged from hospital would benefit considerably from a period of 'rehabilitation' to speed recovery of function and confidence, and to allow for realistic planning of return to work. The benefits to the individual patient from such a rehabilitative period are complemented by the economic advantage to the community.

Rehabilitation after injury

If the patient has a residual disability, discussion between the doctor (either hospital or general practitioner) and the employer, directly or through a medical social worker or Disablement Resettlement Officer, is often sufficient to enable the patient to return to work. But too often, the appropriate decisions are not taken, or decisions depend too much upon personal idiosyncrasies or variations in organization of the local medical services.

Uncomplicated appendicitis is characterized by rapid and smooth recovery, but traditions, the patient's domestic convenience, the whim of the individual surgeon and the hospital bed state are the determining factors influencing the length of the patient's stay in hospital. For example, the period before returning to normal activities after uncomplicated appendicitis varies considerably: 10 days for housewives, 14 days for schoolchildren, and up to 70 days for insured men.

Fractures of the wrist or hand are relatively minor injuries, rarely associated with complications, requiring only a short period of immobilization of the hand and wrist and resulting in little interference with function. After such fractures, patients in manual work usually have considerably more time off work than those in sedentary occupations, and although litigation may be involved in about one third of the cases, there may be little evidence of impairment of motivation to return to work.

Although some patients could manage while in plaster, they often do not return to work as they may feel, not unreasonably, that the wearing of a plaster might interfere with work and render them unacceptable to an employer. Indeed, it seems clear that it is part of the hospital doctor's duty to dispel these doubts and make an authoritative recommendation as regards the patient's fitness for work. When such action is taken, there is a need for close and rapid communication between hospital and general practitioner so that the G.P. can back up the hospital's recommendation for return to work.

If rehabilitation is taken to mean the promotion of maximal possible recovery, then wherever there is a patient with a physical disability, appropriate physical rehabilitation service must be provided. In this context, one must not forget that recovery depends on the patient's mental concentration, endurance and motivation almost as much as his physical capability, and it is usually necessary to stream patients so that the elderly, frail and those with chronic disability are separated from the young and vigorous with temporary disability.

Rehabilitation and medical conditions

Patients with rheumatic disorders and strokes make up a high proportion of those with chronic physical disability. The physical management of these patients is not very different from the rehabilitation of patients with injury, but the tempo and pattern of activity are different in the two groups. Because the numbers are so large, there has been a marked change in the emphasis of all physiotherapy and rehabilitation departments.

In the case of rheumatoid arthritis, it has been shown that with early diagnosis and treatment and regular follow-up and intensive care during remissions and exacerbations, a high proportion of patients can be kept independent at home and at work.

In a retrospective survey of results of treatment in one Rheumatology Centre, over 60 per cent of the patients remained fit for full or restricted work over a follow-up period of 6 years. The majority of the patients with rheumatoid arthritis could be improved functionally by planned rehabilitation, although the men were often unable to continue in either heavy manual work or very skilled work. With increasing advances in surgical techniques for the management of rheumatoid arthritis, the proportion of patients remaining at work should increase (*see* Chapter 4).

Stroke is one of the commonest disabilities of the locomotor system. With adequate rehabilitation, about 20 per cent of stroke patients will return to full work and a further 30 per cent will make a useful contribution about the home. Thus, approximately 50 per cent of those affected can achieve a working status. It is the impairment of intellectual function and speech defects which are usually the stumbling blocks to resettlement, and these are related (as with head injuries) to the extent of the original lesion and the subsequent brain damage (*see* Chapter 9).

Rehabilitation of amputees

The young amputee rarely presents problems of rehabilitation (*see* Chapter 10) but nowadays over 60 per cent of all amputees are over 60 years old and suffering from peripheral vascular disease; unfortunately, amputation is often carried out as an ablative procedure after many other procedures directed towards saving a gradually dying limb. The patient, being elderly, often responds poorly and is resigned to a severe physical handicap. A better approach would be to accept amputation as the first stage in regaining active function and as a necessary preliminary to satisfactory limb-fitting in all but the very senile.

The use of 'early walking aids' enables many lower limb amputees to be mobilized as early as possible while still in the surgical ward. With such aids, many patients can be returned home walking a few weeks after amputation.

A well-organized, integrated limb-fitting service, backed by the rehabilitation services, can ensure the provision of the appropriate appliance or prosthesis at the right place at the right time (*see* Chapter 11).

A similar dynamic approach can be applied to upper limb amputation. Intensive rehabilitation instituted soon after amputation, together with the use of temporary training devices, leads to early return to work and a greater acceptance of functional artificial arms.

Rehabilitation of spinal injuries

Spinal injury units were established because of the need to assess, treat, rehabilitate and initiate resettlement of patients suffering from paraplegia. The clinical and rehabilitation needs of these patients were such that an integrated spinal injury organization was a natural solution.

Since the institution of Spinal Injury Centres, the results of treatment and rehabilitation have steadily improved, and now some Centres claim that 40–60 per cent of paraplegics return to work or domestic independence. Achieving these results depends on a high standard of initial definitive treatment and a co-ordinated and intensive period of rehabilitation; this involves training in bladder care, skin care and a wheelchair existence, and usually extends over a period of 6–9 months.

Ideally these Centres should be sited at District General Hospitals with adequate supportive facilities, and should form a focus for much of the rehabilitation services of that particular District General Hospital.

Head injuries

The majority of patients with head injury suffer a minor injury requiring only simple treatment. Good initial assessment followed quickly by a period of attendance at the rehabilitation department of the District General Hospital is all that post-concussion syndrome requires.

The more severe head injury patient requires a sophisticated system of progressive care involving physical rehabilitation together with educational, speech and behaviour therapy. Intellectual impairment with loss of memory, loss of concentration, loss of sense of responsibility, and emotional lability and depression are the main adverse features.

There is considerable pressure for the provision of special Head

Injury Rehabilitation Centres in association with Neurological and Neurosurgery Centres. Such Centres require residential accommodation and a high ratio of staff to patients.

Some patients with head injury tend to be aggressive and require close collaboration between neurological, psychiatric and rehabilitation staff. In severe cases, the process of rehabilitation may extend over many years; but with good facilities for physical, psychiatric and industrial rehabilitation and follow-up, many patients with head injury can be returned to work in the community.

RESETTLEMENT IN WORK

Resettlement may be defined as the process of returning the patient to the most appropriate social situation. Planning resettlement must start as soon as the immediate definitive treatment is under way, with the aim of returning the patient to his original work and way of life, while overcoming any residual disability as far as possible and reducing the handicap to a minimum.

Resettling a disabled patient in work depends on many factors besides the severity of the disability. Among such factors are: the age of the patient, the nature of the work, the patient's education and domestic background, together with social and economic factors. One of the most relevant points affecting the success of resettlement is the time elapsing from the onset of disability until the definitive plans for return to work or training are brought into effect.

For some patients, return to their original work is not possible, and a detailed reappraisal of their working capability is necessary as a preliminary to retraining and re-employment.

At the present time, the responsibility for industrial assessment and training lies with the Department of Employment (formerly the Ministry of Labour), and one of the major hurdles of return to work has been the need for the patient to complete 'medical rehabilitation' before starting industrial rehabilitation. If industrial assessment and retraining is available alongside medical rehabilitation, the total disability time can be reduced. Rehabilitation should be a continuous process from hospital to workbench, and this path cannot be smooth and efficient if administrative barriers are allowed to persist. Ideally, hospital rehabilitation departments should be able to initiate industrial rehabilitation and have direct access to the excellent assessment and training facilities of the industrial units, while still supervising the patient's overall management.

There is considerable value to be gained from the appointment of Hospital Disablement Resettlement Officers (D.R.Os) to help assess patients' resettlement problems, and to provide the critical link between hospital, work and industrial retraining facilities. A hospital D.R.O. should be a man well versed in local industry, with personal contacts, who can talk to patients, soon after admission—in their own language—and help to allay their fears, act as a go-between for hospital and employer, and advise both sides on the patient's likely working capabilities. He is able to identify resettlement problems early and to plan for return to work and retraining. A system of checking on every hospital admission by the Hospital D.R.O., as well as the Social Workers, can have undoubted advantages.

REHABILITATION DEPARTMENTS

Good rehabilitation requires careful organizing, and each District General Hospital should provide a rehabilitation service.

Patients will initially be the responsibility of consultants of many different disciplines, but when the immediate (definitive) care is over, facilities for long-term management are often best handled by the co-ordinated efforts of the general practitioner and his team of paramedical workers in co-operation with the social services.

A Department of Rehabilitation should:

(1) Be an organization for the provision and co-ordination of the physical therapy services of the hospital and its dependent clinics.

(2) Be an advisory service on all problems of rehabilitation and resettlement:

(a) By direct clinical referral of patients to the consultant in charge of the Department.

(b) By referral to clinics devoted to special aspects of rehabilitation, e.g.

Functional assessment unit.

Wheelchair (and other appliances) clinics.

Resettlement clinics for advising and co-ordinating medical, social, industrial and training aspects of a patient's return to work.

(3) Co-ordinate and correlate all services concerned with rehabilitation and resettlement in the community.

(4) Provide a continuous programme of teaching and research into problems of rehabilitation and physical handicap.

Such a Department requires some beds, at least of a hostel nature, if it is to serve its purpose adequately.

SPECIAL REHABILITATION UNITS

There will always be a need for some specialized units for managing the more severely disabled (for example, patients with head injuries, spinal cord lesions, or the very severely disabled); and these are likely to be organized on a regional basis, drawing patients from a group of District General Hospitals. At these units, there will usually be a consultant who devotes all or most of his time to medical rehabilitation.

Apart from providing special facilities for management of the more severely disabled patients, a regional residential rehabilitation unit might be expected to provide all or some of the following facilities:

(1) Short-term in-patient rehabilitation for patients unable to return home immediately because of social problems or travel difficulties.

(2) Detailed functional assessment and long-term supervisory care of the severely disabled.

(3) Development and manufacture of special appliances and equipment for the severely disabled.

(4) Accommodation of patients needing prosthetic services, including amputees for limb-fitting and rehabilitation.

(5) Facilities for assessment and training of disabled patients and their relatives.

(6) Wheelchair appliance service.

(7) Information service dealing with all aspects of equipment and facilities for the disabled.

(8) Advice, help and training for professional workers on rehabilitation or resettlement.

(9) Facilities for early industrial assessment and retraining.

THE CONSULTANT IN CHARGE OF REHABILITATION SERVICES

The clinician directing rehabilitation services must be first and foremost a physician. He must be able to unravel the complexities of physical disorders of the locomotor system whether neurological, rheumatological, orthopaedic or psychological. Whilst not required to be a diagnostic virtuoso, he must have a working understanding of these specialties which can only come from a thorough grounding in internal medicine and orthopaedic medicine. Without such a grounding, his collaboration and consultation with colleagues, and his ability to derive the optimum return from the rehabilitation services will be restricted. In these circumstances, he will tend to become an administrative technologist rather than a consultant adviser with wide-ranging interests; for the management of patients must always be comprehensive and include the use of drugs, physical treatment and appliances. Full rehabilitation implies clinical, functional, social and welfare assessment and a co-ordinated approach to the patient's total management.

A consultant with responsibilities for directing the rehabilitation services of a District General Hospital should have his own particular clinical interests. Often he will be concerned with the diagnosis and treatment of rheumatic disorders, but he may well have other clinical interests such as neurology or orthopaedics. He may also collaborate very closely with colleagues in geriatric medicine and mental subnormality, where there is a pressing need for rehabilitation services.

The prescribing of physical therapy can be as precise as the prescribing of drugs, but detailed prescribing pre-supposes detailed knowledge of the agencies employed, and a willingness to monitor the patient's progress very closely and to re-prescribe at very frequent intervals, for response to physical treatment can vary considerably and rapidly. This entails frequent attendances by the patient at out-patient clinics or frequent visits by the doctor to the physiotherapy department in the hospital and is time-consuming to both.

A possible and probably more logical alternative is to encourage the physical therapists to develop a deeper understanding of their subject and so to become more able to assume a greater responsibility for the day-to-day variations in therapy, and for the management of the departments in which they work. The training and experience of physical therapists varies considerably, and indeed the training given in different countries also varies considerably, particularly in the proportion of practical to theoretical knowledge imparted. In the United Kingdom, the training is orientated towards the practical aspects of physical therapy, and the qualifications to practice this are granted in a Diploma. In many other countries, although the therapists complete a Degree Course, their practical experience may be very much less.

As a general principle, physical therapists should be primarily practical in their approach and their training, and their work should be directed towards practical assessment and practical treatment. The patient's individual response to the therapist determines the therapist's choice of treatment and the response she expects from the patient. The clinician's function is to establish the overall guidance and direction of the patient's management.

The consultant in charge of rehabilitation can give the therapist the best chance of achieving the results he wants by:

(1) giving an accurate diagnosis;
(2) giving clear indications of the aims of treatment;
(3) giving a clear indication of the likely outcome;

(4) specifying where drug therapy or disease characteristics may necessitate particular care in the administration of various treatments.

He should remember that short, intensive periods of therapy are more likely to have a therapeutic value than the prolonged intermittent attendances for palliative treatment which rapidly become more of a social outing than a therapeutic activity.

He should encourage the therapist to record details of the nature and effect of treatment so that feed-back information from her trained observations may substantially influence future management and enable her to contribute fully to its outcome.

SUMMARY

The foundations of good rehabilitation lie in good medicine—accurate diagnosis, careful prognosis, and early, appropriate and adequate definitive care. The superstructure of rehabilitation depends considerably upon the bricks of physical therapy: physiotherapy (including remedial exercises); occupational therapy; industrial rehabilitation; and the various aspects of the social services.

Unfortunately, responsibilities tend to become separated, and it is often necessary to have one consultant who can bring about the integration of the provisions of the Department of Health, the Department of Education, the Department of Employment and Productivity, the Local Authorities and any other organizations involved. This integration calls for good organization and management and clearly defined lines of communication and areas of responsibility.

There is a need in every hospital for one consultant to be responsible for co-ordinating these services. In some instances, he will undertake this only in a supervisory role, but in other instances, particularly where the rehabilitation service plays a large part in the hospital activities, he may make this his special interest. As a corollary to this approach, the paramedical professions should be more closely concerned with the management of rehabilitation services and take a greater part in the co-ordination of various aspects of rehabilitation.

BIBLIOGRAPHY AND REFERENCES

Buckinghamshire County Council (1970). Report of the Working Group on Services for the Physically Handicapped and Rehabilitation in Milton Keynes

Department of Health and Social Security (1972). Statement by the Committee on the Remedial Professions. London; H.M.S.O.

Department of Health and Social Security (1973). 'The remedial professions.' A report of a Working Party set up in March 1973 by the Secretary of State for social services. London; H.M.S.O.

Ministry of Labour and National Service (1956). Report of an enquiry on the rehabilitation, training and resettlement of disabled persons. London; H.M.S.O.

McKenzie, M., Weir, R. D., Richardson, I. M., Mair, A., Harnett, R. W. F., Curran, A. P. and Ferguson, T. (1962). *Further Studies in Hospital and Community*. Oxford; Nuffield Provincial Hospitals Trust

Nichols, P. J. R. (1969). 'Physical medicine.' *Br. J. Hosp. Med.* **2**, 1152

Nichols, P. J. R. (1974). 'Rehabilitation in the reorganised National Health Service.' *Occupational Therapy* **37**. No. 7

Oxford Regional Hospitals Board (1973). *Community Hospitals Research Programme: Day Care in the Community Hospital*

Scottish Home and Health Department: Scottish Health Services Council (1972). *Medical Rehabilitation: The Pattern of the Future*. London; H.M.S.O.

2—*Physiotherapy*

INTRODUCTION

The origins of physical therapy are shrouded in antiquity, and many forms of treatment referred to in the earliest medical records include the use of heat and hydrotherapy for the alleviation of discomfort from diseases of the locomotor system. Over the years, the pattern of medical practice has changed considerably, as more and more specific treatments have been discovered. Before the discovery of specific treatments such as antibiotics, the only available therapy for many patients was palliative and supportive. As the effectiveness of therapy has advanced, so early mobilization and early discharge of patients have become the rule, and the pattern of hospital in-patient physiotherapy has changed, with less treatment of patients in bed and a wider use of mobilizing techniques and general rehabilitation.

Treatment evaluation

Most physical treatments involve dramatic situations—electric currents, heat, light and direct personal contact of patients with the therapists. Such conditions favour the placebo reactor, and the role of the physical therapist is partly to exploit the empirical placebo response and partly to apply rational remedial therapy.

Many of the conditions traditionally treated by physical methods are degenerative, chronic and episodic. They are also subject to unpredictable remissions and exacerbations. No treatment is likely to produce dramatic results in the chronic degenerative locomotor disorders, but most of the patients respond to care and attention. This is what so many physiotherapy departments provide. Unfortunately, there has been remarkably little scientific evaluation of either the disorders or the treatments. It has been well shown in other fields that it is only when clinical problems are correlated with their underlying pathological mechanisms that therapeutic advice can be given on a rational basis. At the present time, there is still too much that is taught and practised in physiotherapy departments which is based upon an amalgam of tradition, personal experience and subjective patient response. Consequently, physiotherapy in the chronic locomotor disorders remains a part of medical practice which has built up its own folklore and which is veiled in pseudo-science. The situation is aggravated by an entrenched, empirical and self-perpetuating training system which is wary of any change.

Trends in physiotherapy

Gradually, the mysticism surrounding physiotherapy is being cleared away, and the rehabilitation concept of progressive patient care is being more widely introduced. Many physiotherapists are challenging traditional methods and are seeking to widen their theoretical understanding of the techniques they use and to become partners in planning and organizing therapy with clinicians of all specialties.

Physiotherapists are concerned with the maintenance of total body function during acute illness, as well as the maintenance of joint range and muscle power of the limbs. They are also concerned with early mobilization and short-term rehabilitation after illness or injury. For long-term patients, physiotherapy is concerned with the assessment for many aids and appliances associated with locomotor function, such as splints, calipers, artificial limbs, wheelchairs, hoists and so on, and with training in their use.

More and more clinicians and therapists believe that if a patient needs physiotherapy he needs it frequently (i.e. daily), at least in the early stages of treatment. Intermittent, palliative, passive treatments are expensive in the time of the department and in the cost and time spent in travelling to and from hospital. Such treatments contribute little to the patient's management.

Physiotherapy and occupational therapy

Occupational therapists are, in general, more concerned with functional activities than with locomotor capability, but their interests will, of necessity, frequently overlap those of the physiotherapists, and a combined approach will achieve the optimal result.

From time to time there may appear to be a conflict of interest between the physiotherapist and the occupational therapist. For example, the physiotherapist may train the patient with rheumatoid arthritis to walk with sticks or crutches, but the patient may be unable simultaneously to undertake any domestic activity such as carrying a saucepan or teapot. The occupational therapist can teach the patient to be independent in the kitchen by using a wheelchair which she can propel with her hands while carrying domestic equipment on a tray; or 'paddle' with her feet, leaving the hands free. The conflict between the use of crutches or wheelchair is apparent rather than real and is easily resolved when *optimal* rather than *maximal* total functional efficiency is sought.

Collaboration, based on a full clinical, functional and social assessment, will enable the clinician to direct the most appropriate balance of activities to give the best functional recovery consistent with the patient's clinical condition.

Within the rehabilitation team there must also be close collaboration with the speech therapists, social workers, clinical psychologists, and all the other professions supplementary to medicine which are involved in the total management of a patient in the community. Without close collaboration under clinical direction, individual effort can often be dissipated, with consequent frustration to all concerned, including the patient.

Types of physiotherapy

It is conventional to describe the physical techniques under the separate headings of *active* and *passive* procedures. Passive physical treatments are mainly based upon the administration of soothing, pain-relieving applications of heat and the use of massage in various modes and mixtures. Active physical treatment is largely based upon exercises, ranging from minimal movements of single muscles to encourage recovery after paralysis or injury, to intensive exercise routines akin to the circuit training practised by athletes.

This classification is useful for the construction of an academic syllabus and for descriptive purposes but is virtually meaningless in the treatment of patients, as we hope to show in subsequent chapters.

The physiotherapist

The physical rehabilitation of a patient is a continuous process, from the onset of disability to the achievement of optimal rehabilitative potential, and the physiotherapist may employ many different techniques to achieve the end result. Frequently, it will be necessary to use different methods to achieve similar results. The art of physiotherapy lies in selecting the appropriate technique for a particular patient at a particular time. Furthermore, the quality of the physiotherapy depends almost entirely upon the quality of the physiotherapist. The quality of the physiotherapist depends upon her personality, her understanding of the patient and his disability, and her ability to contribute to the overall rehabilitation of the patient. In addition to having a detailed knowledge of all available techniques of physiotherapy, the physiotherapist must have a sound understanding of general medical and surgical care, of the availability and use of aids and appliances, and of the available resettlement facilities provided by the statutory and voluntary bodies. The physiotherapist must be trained to play an important role in the assessment of physical disability and in the instruction of techniques by which a patient can overcome or adjust to that disability. It is only by using this overall approach to rehabilitation that she can make an optimal contribution.

PASSIVE PROCEDURES

Heat

Heat has been used as a treatment for musculo-skeletal pain since time immemorial. There is no doubt that for many conditions giving rise to pain within the locomotor system, heat does have a palliative effect.

Heat may be applied to the body by changes in the environmental temperature, by contact with warmed substances, e.g. warm water, hot water bottles or wax baths, or by the radiation of energy into the body.

Hot water is probably the most widely used agent for conductive heating either as warm baths, hot soaks or compresses, but this is too commonplace a form of therapy to be acceptable to many patients (and their physicians) as a treatment in a hospital physiotherapy department, however often and effectively it is used in the home.

'Wax baths' are a convenient form of applying direct heat to the extremities. Paraffin wax used for treatment is solid at room temperature and melts at 130°F (54°C). Once melted, it remains liquid at a temperature of about 120°F. Melting is achieved in an electrically heated bath. The wax is then applied to the skin—either by immersion of the part or by application with a brush at 118°–120°F (48°–49°C). The wax is easily peeled off after a treatment period (usually 20–30 minutes with 6–7 coatings of wax) and is returned to the stock for re-use. The heating effect is mainly due to the latent heat of solidification and to the specific heat of the wax. There is no evidence that immersion in wax is of any more benefit than immersion in warm water.

Electromagnetic radiations have two main properties which may be significant:

(1) The wavelength.
(2) The intensity.

In general, the hotter the source, the greater the proportion of shorter wavelength emission, and the shorter the wavelength the more easily the radiation is absorbed by water or dispersed. Radiant heat lamps are a convenient and relatively cheap source of heat in a dispensable form. The heat provided is no different from that of an electric fire. Electric pads and infra-red lamps provide heat mainly of a longer wavelength. They have a disadvantage in that they take longer to heat up—in fact some infra-red lamps need about 10 minutes to heat up and to reach an even temperature—and thus can be time-wasters in a busy department.

From the therapeutic point of view, the value of these lamps is probably two-fold. First, there is local warming. The emissions penetrate through the skin and into the subcutaneous tissue with consequent peripheral vascular dilation. Second, the patient has time to rest and relax before the next part of the treatment.

Temperatures developed in the tissues are the product of the pattern of heating, the characteristics of the tissues being treated, and biological factors associated with the organism as a whole.

The patterns of relative heating are an expression of the energy available for heating, determined by dielectric constants and conductivities of the tissues traversed by microwaves. The value of the specific heat of each tissue layer determines the temperature increments over a period of time; therefore, 'instantaneous' temperature distribution might be very different from one resulting from exposure over a period, depending upon biological factors such as blood flow and muscle contraction.

Skin and fat are poor conductors of heat. The skin temperature rises rapidly when in contact with the heat source, but the underlying tissues show a temperature rise of a lesser degree depending partly on the heat dissipated on the skin surface (by sweat and convection) and partly on the conductivity of the subcutaneous tissue (thickness of fat) and the amount of heat dissipated by the circulating blood. Muscle and joint temperature is not altered by heat conduction; but both tissues may show a delayed rise in temperature if a large area of the body is heated for 20–30 minutes, and this is associated with an overall rise of body temperature of 1–2°C.

The subcutaneous blood flow follows the skin blood flow, and when the skin temperature is raised, the skin blood flow increases by several hundred per cent. Thus both are increased by local or general heating of the body. However, surface heating is limited by the direct effect of heat on the skin tissue. A skin temperature of over 109°F (43°C) is associated with pain and a temperature of over 113°F (45°C) will rapidly produce arteriolar flare and a wheal.

Because of the problems of 'conducting' heat to deeper tissues, many techniques have been devised in an attempt to produce 'deep heat'. This work assumes that deep heat will have a therapeutic effect—as yet an unproven theory. In particular, it is assumed that heat will increase the flow of blood in the deeper structures.

The only published investigations on this subject indicate that although local and general heat will increase the blood flow through the skin and subcutaneous tissue, there is a much less impressive and often unreliable response in the deeper tissues. An increase in the muscle temperature may be associated with an increase in blood flow, but this is only of a limited amount compared with the increased flow through the skin. Any increase which does occur is quite insignificant compared with that which occurs in association with voluntary muscular contractions.

Short-wave diathermy

Much has been written about short-wave diathermy and there is a widespread belief that this form of electrical treatment will produce deep heat (the word 'diathermy' means 'heating through').

The heating effect is produced by placing the patient within an electric field created by a high frequency, alternating current. In effect, the patient forms part of the secondary circuit of a high frequency generator. It is impossible to measure the input into the patient, and the only control of the field's intensity depends on the patient's skin sensation of heat and its level of heat tolerance. If the tissues were homogeneous, short-wave diathermy would heat through them. If there were no conduction to untreated parts, then heat loss would eventually be determined by the temperature at the surface and the boundaries between treated and untreated tissue. In practice this does not often occur, for tissues are not homogeneous. Therefore it is impossible to achieve an even heating effect in the body. The highest current density will be at the surfaces, and heat will be dissipated by circulating blood and by conduction to surrounding tissues.

These effects are minimized by crossfire techniques or combining plate electrodes with conduction cables. However, it is impossible to record the true effects of the various techniques of administering this form of treatment, since the introduction of any form of thermocouple or recording device deforms the existing electrical field. Studies on blood flow and radioactive isotope clearance have failed to demonstrate that short-wave diathermy has an appreciable advantage over conventional heat radiators.

Ultrasound

Sound waves with a frequency of over 20 000 cycles per second are undetectable by the human ear and are referred to as 'ultrasound'. High frequency ultrasound (800 000–1 000 000 cycles per second) produced by applying a high frequency current to a crystal is now used in many physiotherapy departments. The therapeutic machines produce vibrations of approximately 800 kHz with an output limited to 3 W/cm^2. The effects of the vibrations are mechanical, heating and chemical. The selection of the wavelength and the limitation of the power output restrict the effect to that of heating and there is no convincing evidence that ultrasound, in the form in which it is presently used, has any other effect on tissues. Animal experiments have shown, however, that ultrasound given in therapeutic doses can accelerate healing and regenerative processes. Under certain circumstances, ultrasound can produce 'standing waves' in blood vessels, with 'banding' and stasis of red cells, which have obvious theoretical dangers.

The physiological effect of therapeutic heat is by no means clear. It certainly brings about a temporary easement of pain in some patients. However, muscle spasm is not necessarily painful and muscle spasm is not necessarily relaxed by heat. Indeed, in some patients, spasm and pain may be exacerbated by heat.

As with all forms of physiotherapy, the therapist should be allowed to use heat at her discretion, as required, and to employ whichever techniques of heat administration she considers most appropriate.

Ice

Pain and stiffness of musculoskeletal origin may well respond to heat, as indicated above, but they are also often considerably reduced by the application of cold packs.

The relative value of applying heat or cold has been argued for centuries, and currently, cold applications (e.g. ice packs, iced baths and cold compresses) are gaining considerable vogue. There is mounting physiological and clinical evidence to show that the therapeutic use of ice by local application, or by immersion in ice and water, can decrease the spasm of spastic muscles and also produce a vasodilation in deep tissues.

Ice therapy is now widely used in the mobilization of two main groups of patients:

(1) Those patients with pain and oedema associated with recent trauma or surgery or an exacerbation of arthritis.
(2) Patients with spasticity (e.g. hemiplegia, or paraplegia).

This form of treatment has been reported as being particularly helpful in the management of the acute painful shoulder, whether idiopathic or associated with stroke or injury; for post-operative management of patients after patellectomy carried out for generalized osteo-arthritis of the knee; and for the painful spasm associated with spinal cord lesions.

Electrotherapy

Direct current—iontophoresis

Electrical currents applied directly to the tissues at low intensity have been used therapeutically to induce chemical changes resulting in an increase in skin blood flow, and also to introduce substances such as histamine into the skin so as to accentuate these vascular changes. This process is known as iontophoresis and is certainly effective as an irritant. Both histamine ionization and the application of direct current on its own are thought by many to cause increased circulation and therefore an improvement in the nutrition of the tissues in the path of the current. These techniques are therefore prescribed in physiotherapy to improve the circulation of deeper structures and to relieve muscle spasm.

Experiments using radioactive isotope clearance techniques show that both the application of a direct current and histamine iontophoresis bring about an increase in the skin circulation—histamine iontophoresis gives an increase of about 100 per cent over direct current alone. However, the changes in the muscle circulation are of a minor nature. Any increase in circulation in the deeper tissues only occurs as part of a generalized histamine reaction. Thus the main effect of both direct current and histamine iontophoresis is superficial, neither technique producing consistent circulatory effects deep to the skin. Both techniques are, however, capable of giving counter-irritation, a method of treatment practised since time immemorial, and more cheaply produced by flagellation with nettles or the application of histamine ointment.

Interrupted direct current will stimulate muscle fibres or nerve fibres depending upon the intensity of the current and its duration. Muscles can only be stimulated directly by long-acting current (100 ms).

Short duration and long duration currents can be applied in many ways with various patterns of rhythm and superimposed surging and diminution. The currents therefore impose a variety of sensory effects and patterns of muscle contraction.

Such techniques have been employed as a means of maintaining active muscular contraction of denervated muscles. Some orthopaedic surgeons insist that recovery after denervation is improved by regular stimulation with 'galvanic' currents, whereas others believe that regular, frequent mobilization of the flail joints and the rigorous prevention of postural oedema is as effective a method of preventing contractures and a poor end result.

Short duration direct current (less than 1 ms duration) or 'Faradic stimulation' has two effects:

(1) Stimulation of sensory nerves.
(2) Stimulation of muscle via the motor nerves.

The discomfort produced by the stimulus is such that the contraction produced is rarely more than 30 per cent of that which can be produced voluntarily. There is no satisfactory evidence that muscle power can be improved by electrical stimulation and certainly any reported effect is insignificant compared with the increase in power which appropriate exercises can produce.

However, electrical stimulation can be of considerable value in those conditions in which voluntary contraction is apparently 'inhibited'. For example, when a joint is acutely inflamed, either as in a traumatic synovitis or an acute arthritis, the muscles acting on that joint will waste. This is certainly true as far as the knee is concerned, in which increased tension in the joint may be produced by an effusion and will induce a positive inhibition and rapid wasting of the quadriceps muscle. Similar inhibitor mechanisms may well exist for other muscles and joints.

A similar, effective use of electrical stimulation of muscle is in the treatment of flat feet, when the patient is unable to demonstrate active contraction of the intrinsic muscles of the feet. Once again, a short course of frequent electrical treatment (2 to 3 times daily for several days, using small individual electrodes and stimulating the intrinsic muscles alone) will often enable the patient to gain adequate voluntary control to continue with the essential 'foot shortening' intrinsic muscle exercises.

A third area of use for electrical stimulation lies in the retraining of muscles after surgical transplantation. Sometimes patients have difficulty in achieving adequate contraction in the newly sited muscles, and electrical stimulation helps to improve an activity pattern leading eventually to the establishment of satisfactory voluntary control.

EXERCISE THERAPY

Exercise therapy occupies about 60 per cent of the physiotherapist's training time and nearly 70 per cent of her working time.

Of all the physical methods of treatment available, exercises have probably been subjected to more statistical evaluation than any other, but the true value of the various techniques of exercise application is still by no means clear. There are almost as many exercise routines as there are physiotherapists and remedial gymnasts.

There are innumerable reports in the medical and physiotherapeutic literature extolling the virtues of specific techniques, routines and types of apparatus. As yet no report has failed to prove that a particular technique of routine gives good results, but as yet there is no *controlled* clinical trial in which various techniques and routines are compared under adequate controls. Until an authoritative comparison is produced, each practitioner will tend to develop a routine from her own experience, and providing she believes in her routine and can inspire the patient to follow it, her results will usually be to her own satisfaction. One of the reasons for this unclear state of affairs is that 'muscle strength' is the usual criterion for assessment and measurement, but this is only part of the story, for a muscle's function depends on its strength, endurance, speed of action and co-ordination with other muscles.

Muscle strength can be defined in two ways:

(1) The power which a muscle can develop instantaneously in an attempt to overcome an imposed load, either in lifting a weight (isotonic) or during static (isometric) contraction against a fixed resistance.

(2) The power which a muscle can develop in resisting an applied load. (This will usually be assessed by a 'break' or 'yield' test which will give consistently higher values than the isometric contraction.)

Muscle endurance is the capacity to maintain or repeatedly develop a certain degree of tension. Strong muscles are at an advantage if expected to perform prolonged exercises at a low level of activity as inevitably their endurance will be greater than that of weak muscles.

Speed of contraction is a function of the rate of increase in tension of muscle fibres, the resistance to be overcome, the number of times the fibres contract, and the range of motion which each contraction imposes.

Co-ordination is the ability of the muscles to act together in correct sequence at the appropriate speed and tension, and is more a function of neurophysiology than muscle physiology.

It is generally agreed that the only way to increase muscle strength and endurance is by active voluntary exercise. Furthermore, when the strength and bulk of a healthy muscle is increased by active exercise, other muscle groups—particularly the antagonists and the contralateral muscles—also become stronger.

Exercise has local effects on the joints and muscles exercised, and it also has secondary effects upon the body as a whole. Thus, exercise therapy may be directed towards the local effect—increasing the function of a specific muscle group—or it may be directed towards the effects upon the body as a whole in terms of general fitness, including the improvement of cardiac function.

The local effects of muscular exercise and thus the functions of exercise therapy may be prophylactic or therapeutic. They are to:

(1) Preserve muscular function during a period of immobilization of any joint, preventing atrophy, fibrosis, venous and lymphatic stasis, and maintaining joint mobility above and below those joints immobilized.
(2) Strengthen weak muscles and mobilize stiff joints.
(3) Re-establish neuromuscular co-ordination.
(4) Prepare for functional activity (practice of skills).
(5) Encourage the patient by the regular demonstration of his increasing ability to perform the exercises demanded of him.

Assisted movements

These involve the active collaboration of the patient, who contracts certain muscles, while the therapist assists his movement. This type of exercise is particularly useful during early recovery after paralysis, and also in early mobilization of joints after injury or operation when movements are inhibited by pain as well as weakness. As the patient progresses, movement may be achieved without assistance from the therapist.

Free movements

Such exercises may be undertaken with the assistance of slings or in water, to eliminate the effects of gravity. As joint range and muscle power increase, so the resistance may be increased in an effort to further increase muscle power. There are many techniques for introducing and increasing resistance to muscle action. The resistance may be supplied by the physiotherapist's direct manual resistance, by gravity, by weights, by springs, by simple or complex combinations of resistances imposed by many different types of apparatus, or by using the physical properties of water as in the practice of hydrotherapy.

Isometric and isotonic exercises

Physiologically, muscle contractions can be classified as: (1) isometric—increasing muscle tension without altering the muscle length; or (2) isotonic—exercises performed against a steady load with joint movement occurring.

Isometric exercises

Simple isometric exercises are usefully performed when a joint is immobilized. This type of exercise is particularly applicable to limbs immobilized in plaster casts, whether because of fractures, orthopaedic procedures, or joint inflammation, e.g. quadriceps setting exercises with a fully extended knee when a leg is in long leg plaster. There is good evidence that even in acute arthritis from whatever cause, e.g. trauma, rheumatoid arthritis or haemo-arthrosis, muscle bulk can be maintained and wasted muscle encouraged to increase in bulk by isometric exercises, provided the joint is adequately splinted and acute muscle inhibition is overcome initially by a few treatments of electrical stimulation. It is important to stress that acute arthritis may well be aggravated by isometric exercises even if the joint is adequately splinted, and the management of such cases requires considerable skill and experience.

Isometric exercises can also be given to any muscle groups acting across a joint which is not splinted by applying supramaximal load, but care must be taken to ensure that the load is not able to act and suddenly produce joint movement when the muscle is relaxed.

Isotonic exercises

Isotonic exercise is often used for building up muscle power after injury by applying predetermined weights and requiring the patient to perform a predetermined number of resisted movements. There are many differing techniques, some with the same load, some with increasing loads, some with decreasing loads. There are many rules for determining the load and the number of contractions, but no real guide as to the method of determining the most effective technique of exercising.

Considerable evidence exists to show that the isometric exercises can induce as much, and probably more, improvement in muscle power as isotonic exercises, and that active isotonic movement should be directed towards gaining joint movement rather than increasing muscle power.

In practice, resisted exercise routines involve combinations and modifications of these two main types of muscle contractions.

Exercises with apparatus

The use of apparatus has two advantages: it enables a physiotherapist to supervise several patients at a time and thus get through more work, and when weights or spring balances are used, it enables accurate records to be maintained.

Weights are often cumbersome, noisy, and uncontrolled. Because free exercises involve movement, exercises with weights are neither isometric nor isotonic.

Spring balances, provided they are well designed and allow little movement, are of much more use than weights in providing either a true isotonic or a measured isometric contraction. Recording has a further value in that it gives the patient an incentive with *every* contraction.

However, there are many disadvantages. Patients left to their own devices often cheat or develop trick movements. Some pieces of apparatus are positively dangerous if inadequately supervised, for the apparatus is not immediately adaptable when troubles arise and uncontrolled weight-resisted activities may well give rise to exacerbations of synovitis or injure already damaged ligaments.

Spring balances form the basis of most 'dynamometers'. With a few spring balances and a set of wall bars for their fixation, any physiotherapy department can have a 'dynamometer' for exercising and recording the contraction strength of any muscle group.

However, there are disadvantages in using springs, for the resistance increases as the movement proceeds, and the muscle becomes less able to overcome the resistance. Similar criticism can be levelled against exercises carried out on slings with gravity only as the resistance.

Techniques can be devised where the spring balance is used to assist rather than resist. For example, in re-education of the calf muscles after fracture of the tibia and fibula, an overhead spring balance can be used to assist the patient to 'lift' on the weak plantar flexors. As the muscle power increases, the poundage recorded on the spring balance decreases.

As a basis for planning exercise therapy, the following points can be assumed:

(1) Strength is built up in a muscle most effectively by resisting the movement the muscle produces—maximum resistance allows no movement, and the contraction becomes isometric.

(2) Repeated resistance exercises are believed to improve muscle endurance.

However, there are many other variations in the exercise routines commonly prescribed. Some authorities start with a high resistance, reducing throughout the exercise sessions. Others reverse this procedure, gradually increasing resistance. Others still believe in 'power exercising' with no variation in resistance, but there is no adequate comparative evaluation to guide the clinician or therapist.

Proprioceptive neuromuscular facilitation

Recently techniques have been introduced under the general classification of *proprioceptive neuromuscular facilitation*. First, it is believed that there are certain patterns of mass muscle movement, and that by performing multiple joint movements in these patterns, there is greater physiological facilitation of all muscles in the appropriate group; thus one or more small muscles may be 'called in' as part of the movement pattern when it would be impossible to obtain an isolated contraction, resistance being given to stronger muscles in the correct sequence of movement before 'pivoting' to the weak muscles. Second, by employing resistance, stretch reflexes and peripheral stimuli (i.e. by stimulating the proprioceptors in the muscles and joints), the demand made on the neuromuscular mechanism can be increased and its response facilitated.

The principles of proprioceptive neuromuscular facilitation are:

(1) Maximal resistance applied by the physiotherapist's hand.

(2) Proprioceptive stimuli induced before and during contractions by:

(a) Deep pressure.
(b) Stretch before contraction.
(c) Traction and compression of the joint.

} all supplied by the physiotherapist's hands.

(3) Set movements performed in diagonal or spiral patterns.

(4) The patient always just 'wins', that is to say movement in the pattern is always allowed.

There are two main advantages over other methods. First, the *movements* and *resistance* are at all times in the physiotherapist's control. Second, no apparatus is required. Unfortunately, these techniques are time consuming for physiotherapists because it is a case of one patient–one physiotherapist. Also, for the first time in the history of physiotherapy there is now a tendency for the physiotherapist to show greater signs of fatigue than the patient. However, those experienced in these techniques are convinced that they far exceed the effectiveness of all other techniques for the building up of strength in weak muscles.

Mobilizing exercises

Mobilizing exercises aim at increasing joint movement and are usually introduced when there is no evidence of active joint disease. They may have to be regulated by the recurrence of joint symptoms or by the evidence of adverse joint reaction. Pain or effusion or loss of range are immediate indications of the need to reduce the range of movement employed in the exercises.

These exercises are often preceded by the application of heat or ice packs, or they may be performed in water (hydrotherapy), in suspension apparatus, or using gymnasium apparatus (wall bars, parallel bars), the technique depending on the particular clinical situation, the facilities available, and the prejudices and predilections of the therapist or clinician. The physiotherapist responsible needs guidance regarding the restrictions necessary and the degree of response to activity which she may expect from the demands made of the patient.

As recovery proceeds, the specific exercises should give way to more purposive and functional activities. Walking, getting in and out of bed or on and off the lavatory, dressing and the gradual increase of activities up to the level of normal living and working are all purposive exercise activities and entail close collaboration between physiotherapist and occupational therapist.

Fitness training

For some patients, a high level of physical fitness is necessary, and rehabilitation should be taken to a level little short of the training programme necessary for sport. For others, there is no need for such intensive rehabilitation, and a rapid return to normal or near-normal living and working conditions will provide the necessary exercise.

For the first group, remedial games and athletic training are the relevant exercise activities; for the second group, functional activities are more appropriate.

The various systems of exercise introduced for specific muscle groups can be adapted to general physical training and incorporated into the technique known as 'circuit training'. Circuit training is a grouping together of a set of exercises designed to:

(1) Exercise the main muscle groups with consequent increase in strength and endurance.
(2) Obtain maximal general effect and improve general stamina.
(3) Improve certain skills by practice.

Circuit training is the logical final stage of any exercise programme. It not only aims at a functional end result, but also requires that the individual patient compete against his own capability initially and eventually adapts the exercise programme for non-specific exercising and the maintenance of general health.

The intensity and duration of exercise and activity routines employed vary considerably with the clinical problem. Many physiotherapists and remedial gymnasts will be more concerned with short-term effects of injury, and they will bear the particular responsibility of ensuring that patients return to maximal function in the shortest possible time. Regular, frequent, intensive exercise in the immediate post-injury period may well prevent prolonged morbidity. For example, most patients with simple fractures of the lower limbs can well return to work while still immobilized, provided they have first been taught to walk properly in plaster of paris and have been indoctrinated with the need to exercise immobilized muscles adequately, using isometric techniques.

Functional activities may encourage a patient to greater effort than repetitive exercises in the gymnasium and enable all concerned to obtain a realistic assessment of the patient's capabilities.

PASSIVE MOVEMENTS

Passive movements are the movements of joints and muscles produced by a therapist unaided by the voluntary contraction of the relevant muscles by the patient. They help to maintain proprioceptive sense in the excessively weak or paralysed muscles. Such movements also help to maintain joint mobility or to re-establish mobility in joints which have stiffened up. They are particularly useful in the early phases of management after paralysis from any cause, but the need for a prolonged programme of passive movements in conditions such as brachial plexus lesions has probably been exaggerated.

In the acute early stages of hemiplegia, passive movements of the arm as a whole, and the shoulder in particular, are important in preventing the common and disabling complication of 'frozen shoulder'. Passive movements of the leg help to prevent flexion deformities of the hip and knee and an equinus deformity of the foot. Similarly, during the period of early flaccid paralysis following spinal cord lesions, passive movements of the legs are important to prevent the development of deformities. However, when spasticity develops, great care and gentleness is needed to carry out adequate passive movements without causing any soft tissue damage. Patients may be unconscious or suffering from diminished or absent sensation, and the usual protective mechanisms are absent.

In a number of patients with strokes or spinal injury, periarticular calcific deposits appear, particularly around the hip joints. These deposits are sometimes judged to be akin to traumatic myositis ossificans and are associated with over-vigorous passive movements or injudicious attempts to achieve the full range of joint movement while muscles are in spasm. The fact that similar deposits are rarely encountered after flaccid paralysis indicates that the muscle spasm has a part to play in the aetiology. For these reasons, adequate relaxation achieved by hydrotherapy, hot packs, adequate anti-spasmodic drugs, or the appropriate injection of local anaesthetic (45 per cent alcohol or phenol) provides an important prelude to passive movements and the ensuing re-educative physiotherapy when recovery begins.

TRACTION

Limb traction

As a brief surgical manœuvre, traction is used to reduce a fracture or dislocation. Continuous traction applied to the limbs is used to relieve pain, secure rest and overcome painful muscle spasm, to gain and to maintain anatomical alignment, and to prevent or correct deformity.

Such forms of traction may be 'fixed' traction, e.g. Thomas' splint, 'balanced' or 'sliding traction', or a combination of fixed and balanced traction.

The physiotherapist's concern is to understand the principles of traction and to counter traction so that she can maintain joint mobility and muscle power within the restrictions of the traction and its consequent immobilization. In addition, the orthopaedic physiotherapist will be concerned with the pressure areas and the state of the skin, which is often at risk during prolonged traction. These techniques are, however, special ones, usually restricted to orthopaedic hospitals and accident departments, and are not a particular concern in this book.

Spinal traction

Traction has been used in the treatment of neck pain and backache for many years, and, as with many other forms of physiotherapy, there is a mass of reported personal experience, dogma and folklore. Unfortunately, there has been little scientific investigation and few authenticated therapeutic trials.

The only effects which traction can be expected to achieve are some distraction between vertebrae at the intervertebral disc and apophyseal joints, tensing the longitudinal ligaments of the spinal column (particularly the posterior common ligament), and some slight widening of the intervertebral foramina. These effects can only be expected to occur while the traction is being applied. Continuous traction might be employed also to achieve effective immobilization of a patient in bed. There is some evidence to suggest that acute lesions of the neck and back respond to more vigorous manipulative procedures whereas the less acute lesions tend to be self-limiting. Those that persist with considerable general limitation of movement appear likely to respond to traction or immobilization. Persistent pain, associated with restriction of specific movements, may also respond better to mobilizing techniques.

Some authors argue that traction is a form of manipulation or a *part* of manipulation, or a preliminary to manipulative procedures. Many authorities advise a combination of treatments, particularly the use of a support (cervical collar or lumbosacral belt) in association with traction. A well-fitting support often seems to prove beneficial after a short period (20–30 minutes) in traction, and to prolong the symptomatic improvement achieved by traction.

Manual traction is traction applied by the physiotherapist's hands, usually only for brief periods, often combined with lateral and rotational manœuvres (the entire procedure being under the therapist's direct control), and is really more properly classified as a manipulation. The best results are usually obtained in the presence of acute symptoms.

Continuous traction is applied through some form of harness and continued for 24 hours or longer. The forces used are relatively small and the treatment is used mainly as an in-patient procedure, and usually reserved for severe, intractable root pain.

Sustained traction is a technique of traction usually applied for 20–30 minutes.

Intermittent traction is similar to sustained traction but applied intermittently, the traction being alternately applied and withdrawn, the pulsation being applied by various mechanical devices.

Sustained and intermittent traction are applied through harnesses. In the case of cervical traction, the patient's body weight provides adequate counterweight. For lumbar traction two sets of harnesses are usually used, providing a symmetrical pull on the torso.

The force used may be large, from about 15–25 lb (6·8–11·3 kg) for cervical traction, to 40–50 lb (18·2–22·7 kg) for lumbar traction, but under careful control, cervical traction may be increased to 40–50 lb and lumbar traction to between 70 and 150 lb (31·7–68·1 kg).

The angle of traction, the position of the head and neck, and the weight applied are usually achieved by trial and error. Indeed, the position and weight which produce relief of pain vary from patient to patient, and for each patient they may vary considerably from day to day. Most patients with neck and arm pain respond to traction, but most also respond to simple positioning or to the application of a firm collar. However, most physiotherapists believe they can achieve best results by a combination of these techniques, varying their treatment according to the patient's response. Because of the variability of the response, it is unwise to be too specific when prescribing such treatments. Indeed, it is more appropriate to give the physiotherapist latitude of approach, and if the patient does not respond to traction, it should be discontinued and other measures tried until relief from pain is achieved. Often patients with an acute lesion respond badly to sustained traction as they are particularly prone to rebound pain when traction is relaxed.

There seems to be little theoretical reason for expecting traction to be effective in degenerative spondylosis of the cervical spine, any more than it is likely to be effective in osteo-arthritis of a limb joint. Traction will reduce the natural cervical lordosis (with a pull of 20–25 lb (9·1–11·4 kg)) and a separation from C2–C7 of 3–14 mm can be demonstrated to occur at a pull of about 45 lb (20·4 kg). However, there is evidence that the first radiological indication of cervical spondylosis is a loss of cervical lordosis, and thus traction might well be expected to reproduce and exacerbate the early changes and the accompanying symptoms in some instances.

In the lumbar spine, traction has been demonstrated to produce a separation of about 2 mm at each disc space; but such separations are unstable and reversible.

Therapeutic trials of traction have been inconclusive, and mostly without adequate controls, but there is adequate physiotherapeutic folklore to encourage physiotherapists to master the techniques; to use them for patients with persistent pain; to learn to assess the patients; and to retain an inquisitive, objective and sceptical attitude to both treatment and patient.

Perhaps the only absolute rule about the use of traction in the treatment of skeletal pain is that it should never be used unless an absence of bony metastases has first been demonstrated by radiological investigation.

MANIPULATIVE PROCEDURES

There is much controversy about manipulative procedures, most of which is engendered by lack of understanding, imprecision of diagnostic terms and valueless speculation about the pathology of undefined clinical syndromes. In the commonly held view, a manipulation is a passive movement restoring range of movement to a joint which is 'stuck' with intra- or periarticular adhesion, 'subluxated' or in some manner restricted in its movement. The procedure is usually regarded as being instantaneous in imparting relief, forceful in character and often accompanied by a 'snapping' sensation or sound. It is also widely believed that the technique is understood only by a small group of physicians, osteopaths and chiropracters.

During recent years, however, many of the techniques previously restricted to such practitioners have been rationalized and are being taught to large numbers of physiotherapists. In the professional sense, the term 'manipulation' can be used to describe any procedure applied passively to a relaxed part of the body for the purpose of restoring joint range and functional activity. Force and flamboyance are usually unnecessary, and sudden dramatic manœuvres are not always associated with dramatic recovery.

Certainly, the popular medical literature and the folklore of patients is full of personal histories of dramatic cures, but the scientific literature is surprisingly void of authenticated studies detailing diagnostic criteria, relapse rates and adequately controlled trials.

Physiotherapists are experienced in handling stiff and painful joints, and now that they are being more widely encouraged to learn and to practice manipulative techniques, these can be included in the normal physiotherapeutic repertoire and should also be introduced into the controlled clinical trials which are beginning to play an important part of physiotherapy training and practice.

Radiological examination of a joint is an essential preliminary to manipulation. Spinal manipulation should never be undertaken if there is evidence of vertebral fragility or instability, nor in the presence of neurological signs of cord compression or irritation.

Careful, passive examination of the joint is the beginning of the manipulative treatment. The full examination of a joint's passive range cannot be separated from the initial exploratory passive treatment by stretching and manipulation. Modern physiotherapeutic manipulation consists of a repeated sequence: examination, followed by exploratory passive increase in mobility range, then by re-examination and recording of the range attained. Forceful procedures only follow on after a similar procedure with less force has achieved an increase in mobility range, which is retained. Such gentle techniques require considerable practice and sensitivity. They are gaining considerable support from physiotherapists. They are more properly referred to as 'mobilizing techniques', whereas 'manipulation' is probably more correctly restricted to those manœuvres involving a sudden, high-velocity movement. These latter techniques also require much skill and practice, yet their complexity is not necessarily reflected in their usefulness.

To summarize, both 'manipulations' and 'mobilizations' are techniques of increasing joint range by passive movements. The former are based on single quick movements and are often less controlled than the latter repetitive, gentler movements. It is claimed that because mobilization is more 'controlled' it can therefore be more localized, particularly in relation to spinal joints.

Although there is a considerable volume of anecdotal case law, there are as yet no acceptable clinical trials, nor long-term follow-up studies. Both these forms of physiotherapy deserve a more detailed scientific and unemotional appraisal than they have so far been subjected to.

BREATHING EXERCISES

Medical conditions

Depending upon the needs of the individual patient, the physiotherapist treating a medical condition may seek, by breathing exercises, to:

(1) Maintain chest wall mobility, e.g. ankylosing spondylitis.

(2) Compensate for weakness of muscles of respiration, e.g. tetraplegia, anterior poliomyelitis, myasthenia gravis.

(3) To assist patients to expectorate sputum.

(4) To alleviate the effects of bronchial obstruction or spasmodic constriction, e.g. chronic bronchitis, bronchial asthma.

(5) To counteract the increase in P_{CO_2} which occurs with inadequate alveolar ventilation.

There is some evidence that breathing exercises can be helpful in the agitated patient. They seem to allay anxiety and they can be a useful adjunct to the treatment of cardiogenic dyspnoea or insomnia.

Surgical conditions

In treating patients undergoing surgical procedures, the physiotherapist teaches breathing exercises pre-operatively when possible, so that in the early post-operative days, which are not conducive to learning new procedures, the exercises may be remembered and used as needed.

The value of breathing exercises has never been clearly established, but they have become traditional in many hospitals. Indeed, such techniques may occupy the attention of 10–20 per cent of the available physiotherapy staff of a District General Hospital. Recent studies indicate that much of this activity is of little value, and the physiotherapist would be better employed in undertaking the energetic treatment of 'at risk' patients before surgery, and in contributing to the care and management of the chronic bronchitic (*see* Chapter 12), rather than attempting to give breathing exercises to all pre-operative and post-operative patients.

Respiratory complications of surgery

The common post-operative chest complications are likely to derive from blockage of the smaller branches of the bronchial tree by secretions. This leads to infection and local areas of collapse. Expulsion of the secretion by coughing and drainage is the most effective method of prophylaxis and treatment. The overall incidence of these complications has remained virtually unchanged in spite of advances in surgery, anaesthesia and chemotherapy. Patients undergoing abdominal operations are more at risk than patients having operations on the limbs, and upper abdominal operations are more prone to such complications than lower abdominal operations. Such complications appear to be associated with the almost invariable sharp reduction in ventilatory function which follows upper abdominal surgery and which is probably due to temporary diaphragmatic inhibition.

The inhibition of ventilatory function in itself may not be particularly dangerous, but patients who are elderly, who have a history of chronic bronchitis, and who are cigarette smokers are particularly at risk. Pre-operative physiotherapy, associated with an intensive 'no smoking' campaign, can reduce the likelihood of clinically significant post-operative complications.

Patients with chronic bronchitis are considered at special risk, whatever the operation they are undergoing, if a general anaesthetic is given or if post-operative bed rest is necessary. For them, pre- and post-operative breathing exercises are mandatory, and apart from daily or twice daily sessions with the physiotherapist, such patients should be instructed pre-operatively in relaxation and controlled diaphragmatic breathing and required to take a number of deep breaths every hour. It is customary to recommend a minimum of 10 deep breaths, but there is no scientific basis for this specific recommendation.

Patients undergoing thoracic surgery, upper abdominal and major spinal surgery are also at special risk of developing post-operative pulmonary collapse. For them, too, regular deep breathing at hourly intervals with the operation wound supported, when possible, by pressure from the hand of the physiotherapist, the nurse or the patient himself, is essential. Assisted coughing, regular postural drainage and regular suction may also be necessary post-operative measures to ensure efficient pulmonary ventilation, encourage expectoration and promote venous return, and in this way discourage the development of pulmonary collapse and infarction.

If such complications arise, then physiotherapy directed towards assisted expulsion of bronchial secretions (while supporting the surgical wound) is often dramatic in its effect. Thus, the problem of the post-operative chest is mainly one of selecting 'at risk' patients before surgery, and treating them vigorously.

Circulatory complications

Post-operative physiotherapy is also directed towards improving venous return from the legs in order to prevent the development of deep venous thrombosis. Considerable scepticism now exists concerning the development of post-operative deep vein thrombosis. Indeed, it is now evident that, in many instances, the thrombosis occurs during a long period on the operating table. In some centres, active measures are in use to prevent the development of thrombosis during this time. These may involve electrical or mechanical stimulation of the calf muscles while the patient is unconscious during the operation. The mechanical measures consist of devices which move the foot through a range of movements at the ankle joint, alternately stretching and relaxing the calf muscles. Electrical techniques consist of the application of an interrupted electrical stimulus to produce intermittent calf-muscle contraction. The calves are usually encased in a bandage or gaiter, for passive movement of the calf without such a constrictive gaiter would be less effective in promoting venous return. Such devices may be left on the patients until they are able to co-operate by performing frequent active movements of the legs. This approach to the prevention of deep vein thrombosis is apparently much more successful than conventional post-operative physiotherapy, which may well be unnecessary for those without a deep vein thrombosis and too late for those who have developed it.

Physiotherapy in intensive care units

In an intensive care unit, it is necessary to distinguish between the need for elective prophylactic and therapeutic procedures, which are properly the role of the physiotherapist, and the emergency care of an 'acute chest', which all personnel in the unit should be trained to treat. Some patients in intensive care units will be paralysed and will require passive movements for the limbs; others will be recovering from cardiac conditions and will require gentle encouragement to move their limbs under the guidance of the cardiologist; others will be recovering from multiple injuries or major surgery, and their recovery will be a matter of graduated activity determined by their general clinical status. A proportion of patients in intensive care units require intensive respiratory care, and it is these to whom physiotherapeutic techniques—in particular the 'bag-squeezing' technique combining assisted coughing, drainage, and suction—can be life-saving.

Patients in respirators because of severe paralysis, and patients with chest injuries, present special problems of acute physical care, which are not properly the concern of this book.

Breathing exercises as a relaxation technique

During the recent re-awakening of Western interest in Eastern customs, exponents of Yoga and Karate have demonstrated anew the importance of effective voluntary breathing control in exercise performance and in mental and physical relaxation. Surveys currently being carried out appear further to indicate that voluntary control may also be learned and temporarily applied to certain processes normally controlled by the autonomic system, such as heart rate and blood pressure.

Despite these indications of the far-reaching effects which learned voluntary control can have on essential body functions, the term 'breathing exercises' is still used in a mildly derogatory fashion by those doctors who have not needed them for themselves or their patients. Even so, if breathing exercises are correctly taught, and correctly used, they appear to be of value.

When teaching relaxation technique, each physiotherapist uses the method of tuition which she has developed to suit her own personality and modifies it to suit the personality of each individual patient whom she teaches.

Most physiotherapists check that the patient is lying comfortably, and ask him first to contract the muscles of the upper limb and then relax them, then to tense the muscles and relax them, and finally to relax the muscles completely without preliminary contraction. This sequence is repeated for the muscles of the lower limbs and abdomen and the thorax, in this order. To help them relax, many patients need the assistance of evocative images—such as lying in a warm bath or bed on the first day of the holiday, or lying on hot sands listening to the sound of the surf—derived first from the physiotherapist's voice, and then from their own minds. It is important that once the technique of relaxation at will has been mastered, it should be practised regularly in the several positions in which any particular patient is likely to experience respiratory distress, and that such practice should become an important part of the programme of daily living for patients with chronic respiratory dysfunction.

When the patient can relax at will, he then learns first the 'awareness' of the various muscles, particularly those of respiration, and then the 'control' of the duration and power of their contraction. Against the resistance of the therapist's hand, and progressively against the resistance of his own fist, pillows or belts, he develops increasing strength in these muscles. He then learns how to control the timing and depth of breathing until the duration and volume of expiration and inspiration can be varied at will.

The need for the acquisition of breathing control is common to all conditions involving respiratory dysfunction. It is the optimal timing and mode of application of this control which is highly individual to each patient and his particular situation.

HYDROTHERAPY

Hydrotherapy has been a standard form of treatment for many diseases for many years. However, it is usually regarded as mainly being of value for rheumatic disorders and for patients with paralysis following poliomyelitis. For this reason, treatment pools were installed in the physiotherapy departments of hospitals specializing in these problems. Because most of the patients were severely disabled, the classical approach was to install a *small* pool, and hydrotherapy apparatus, such as a Hubbard tank, became the standard fitting. The emphasis in all this type of work was on individual passive treatment.

In the rehabilitation of lower limb injuries, following limb operations and in the general care of the arthritic patient, this 'classical' approach is exactly the opposite of that which gives the best results. A large heated pool, although an expensive item of equipment, provides a wide range of active therapy for a wide range of patients, and is a very adaptable piece of apparatus which should repay its cost in its general usefulness.

It is usual to regard hydrotherapy as providing buoyancy and thus assisting movement for weak muscles and damaged joints. It was this particular attribute which aided in the management of poliomyelitis and gained a high reputation for hydrotherapy. In fact, however, it can provide many other forms of activity, ranging from total suspension of the severely disabled to strong resistance exercises for those approaching the final stages of rehabilitation. This variation is provided by simple techniques involving either working with the water or against the water.

The assistance provided by the buoyancy of the water and the resistance which it offers can be enhanced by the use of flotation devices. These may be in the form of inflated cushions or rubber rings attached to the arms and legs. They can also be made from buoyant materials such as polystyrene.

Flat walking areas in the pool can provide the simplest form of graduated partial weight-bearing for re-education in walking after injuries or surgery of the lower limbs. The patient starts off in relatively deep water, where most of his weight will be taken by buoyancy, and graduates to shallow water as his condition improves, finally progressing to full weight-bearing outside the pool.

In some centres, the areas of different depth are separated by internal walls or rails, whereas at others, small pools of different depths are provided as 'annexes' of the main pool.

The warmth and the effect of the water are an excellent basis for mobilization of stiff joints. The only contra-indications to intermittent hydrotherapy, apart from patients encased in plaster of paris, must be incontinence and open or infected wounds. It is evident that this form of treatment could be used to advantage for a large number of patients of any rehabilitation unit.

In general, the best size for a treatment pool suitable for a major rehabilitation unit or department would be 40 ft by 20 ft (12·2 m×6·1 m) (18 ft × 14 ft is the recommended minimum size). It should be maintained at a temperature of 90°–95°F. There must be easy access into the water via shallow steps, and for the more severely disabled, appropriate hoists should be installed. Preferably, there should be graduated levels of depth from 3 ft to 4 ft 6 ins (91·5–137·2 m) or if it is not possible to provide graduation, a pool of constant depth of about 2 ft 6 ins to 3 ft (76–91·5 m). If the edge of the pool is raised above the floor of the department by 2 ft to 2 ft 6 ins (61–76 m), it facilitates transfers to and from wheelchairs and it is more easily supervised by instructors outside the pool.

Finally, there must be adequate changing room accommodation to allow for continuous use of the pool while patients are preparing to enter the pool and, later, drying and dressing after treatment. Indeed, the surroundings and necessary associated services are almost as important as the pool itself, and although they certainly add considerably to the space and cost involved, they contribute significantly to the efficiency of the department as a whole.

There are many practitioners experienced in rehabilitation who would be prepared to forgo almost all the other facilities normally present in a physiotheraphy department if they could retain a good, well-appointed hydrotherapy department.

The Spas in particular have flourished upon the reputation of hydrotherapy, although this is by no means the full extent of the medical service which these centres customarily supply.

Natural hot springs are reputed to have a number of properties associated with medical effects which are not present in heated mains water. There is, however, no scientific evidence that there is any effect other than warmth and buoyancy. The effectiveness of spa hydrotherapy treatment cannot be separated from the people who dispense and prescribe it, nor can it be considered apart from its surroundings. There is undoubtedly a very large placebo effect from physical treatment, which is enhanced by the traditional setting of the spa, but what probably contributes most to the efficiency of spa therapy is the overall regimen (the rehabilitation approach) which is imposed upon the patient. Those spas with a positive approach and good overall medical supervision can provide an excellent rehabilitation service for patients with locomotor disorders.

BIBLIOGRAPHY AND REFERENCES

General

The Physical Medicine Library (1969). S. Licht (Ed.). Connecticut; E. Licht

Volume 1: Electrodiagnosis and Electromyography.
Volume 2: Therapeutic Heat and Cold.
Volume 3: Therapeutic Exercise.
Volume 4: Therapeutic Electricity and Ultraviolet Radiation.
Volume 5: Massage, Manipulation and Traction.
Volume 7: Medical Hydrology.
Volume 8: Medical Climatology.
Volume 9: Orthotics, etcetera.
Volume 10: Rehabilitation and Medicine.
Volume 11: Arthritis and Physical Medicine.

Ultrasonics

Bierman, W. (1954). 'Ultrasound in the treatment of scars.' *Archs phys. Med. Rehabil.* **35**, 210

Dyson, M. and Pond, J. M. (1970). 'Effect of pulsed ultrasound on tissue regeneration.' *Physiotherapy* **56**, 136

Dyson, M. and Pond, J. M. (1973). 'The effects of ultrasound in the circulation.' *Physiotherapy* **59**, 284

Summer, W. and Patrick, M. K. (1964). *Ultrasonic Therapy*. Amsterdam; Elsevier

Exercise therapy

De Andrade, J. R., Grant, C. and Dixon, A. St. J. (1965). 'Joint distension and reflex muscle inhibition.' *J. Bone Jt Surg.* **47A**, 313

Gough, J. V. and Hadley, G. (1971). 'An investigation into effectiveness of various forms of quadriceps exercise.' *Physiotherapy* **57**, 356

Leach, R. E., Skyker, W. S. and Zohn, D. A. (1965). 'A comparative study of isometric and isotonic quadriceps exercise programmes.' *J. Bone Jt Surg.* **47A**, 1421

Lenman, J. A. R. (1959). 'A clinical and experimental study of the effects of exercise on motor weakness in neurological disease.' *J. Neurol. Neurosurg. Psychiat.* **22**, 182

Salter, N. (1967). 'Exercise therapy.' *Ann. phys. Med.* **4**, 81

Hydrotherapy

Bolton, E. and Goodwin, D. (1967). *Introduction to Pool Exercises* (3rd edn). Edinburgh and London; Livingstone

Davis, B. C. (1967). 'A technique of rehabilitation in the treatment pool.' *Physiotherapy* **53**, 2, 57

Duffield, M. H. T. (1969). *Exercise and Water*. London; Balliere, Tindall and Cassell

'Planning of hydrotherapy departments' (1965). Report of a Conference at the Hospital Centre, London. *Br. Hosp. J. Soc. Serv. Rev.* **75**, 2289

Manipulative procedures

British Association of Physical Medicine (1966). 'Pain in the neck and arm: a multicentre trial of the effect of physiotherapy.' *Br. med. J.* **1**, 253

Cyriax, J. H. (1971). *Textbook of Orthopaedic Medicine.* Vols 1 and 2 (5th edn). London; Balliere, Tindall and Cassell

Maitland, G. D. (1964). *Vertebral Manipulation.* London; Butterworths

Maitland, G. D. (1970). *Peripheral Manipulation.* London; Butterworths

Stoddard, A. (1959). *Manual of Osteopathic Techniques.* London; Hutchinson

Traction

Matthews, J. A. (1968). 'Dynamic discography. A study of lumbar traction.' *Ann phys. Med.* **9**, 275

Powell, M. (1970). *Orthopaedic Nursing* (6th edn). London; Livingstone

Yates, D. A. H. (1972). 'Indications and contraindications for spinal traction.' *Physiotherapy* **58**, 2, 55

Breathing exercises

Nichols, P. J. R. and Howell, B. (1968). 'Routine pre- and post-operative physiotherapy: results of a questionnaire.' *Ann. phys. Med.* **9**, 264

Nichols, P. J. R. and Howell, B. (1970). 'Routine pre- and post-operative physiotherapy: results of a trial.' *Rheum. phys. Med.* **10**, 321

3—Occupational Therapy

INTRODUCTION

Occupational therapy offers a service designed to help the patient to return to his former occupation, or, when necessary, to help the patient to adjust to an adapted or new occupation.

The term 'occupation' implies more than a person's actual work, whether that of a bricklayer, bank manager, housewife, student or schoolchild. It implies the role normally associated with the person's work in the person's own environment. It must also imply a sufficient degree of mobility, personal independence and psychological maturity to maintain that role.

Thus, occupational therapy may be defined as a paramedical service with the function of assisting the patient's return to the fullest possible physical, psychological and social competence both in his former occupation and in his customary role in life.

To this end, the occupational therapist is increasingly concerned with the assessment of the patient's physical capabilities, the exploitation of his residual skills, and the planning of the retraining of patients with a permanent disability. Practical assessment should precede the final stages of rehabilitation and resettlement, and repeated assessment can provide objective records of a patient's progress. There is no other profession supplementary to medicine so aptly suited to help the patient bridge the gap between physical disability and functional capability.

Occupational therapy training includes considerable study of psychology and at least 6 months' work in psychiatric hospitals prior to registration. The therapist therefore has an awareness of the closely interwoven psychological and physical factors in illness and disablement and of the impact of these factors upon the patient, his family and his social environment. The therapist's training enables her to offer some assessment of the patient's attitudes and social background, as well as his residual physical capability, and thus equips her to contribute to the planning of his rehabilitation programme and return to work.

Occupational therapists are taught the basic skills of home economics, wood and metal work, and heavy workshop techniques, together with creative work of all kinds, from painting and pottery to cooking and gardening, from typing and fretwork to bricklaying and house decorating.

When a patient is of normal retirement age, or is so severely disabled that it is impossible for him to resume work, the emphasis will be on finding positive and creative leisure interests that will bring him into contact with other people, so reducing the isolation which severe handicap inevitably brings.

Consequently, occupational therapy still carries with it the relics of the 'arts and crafts' image, and some of the practitioners and teachers unfortunately still place undue emphasis on training in traditional but superficial aspects of the work. These activities were never intended to be an end in themselves, but a means whereby the therapist could assess and train a patient's manual skill, range of joint movement, learning ability and work tolerance. Diversional and recreational activities have their place in the overall management of long-stay patients and patients with chronic disability, but in present-day rehabilitation, the emphasis on the importance of these aspects of occupational therapy has changed.

The most important contribution that the modern occupational therapist makes is in the assessment of a patient's actual and potential functional capability with or without aids and appliances. The design, manufacture and prescription of these aids and appliances is influenced by the informed opinion of the therapists who train patients in their use.

Although the complete functional assessment of a patient must include the social, clinical, educational and domestic implications, the functional capabilities must be expressed in a practical fashion in terms of normal activities, and this translation should be the occupational therapists' particular contribution. For these reasons, an increasing number of occupational therapists are employed in domiciliary work or are based in community services rather than hospital services. The occupational therapists working in a domiciliary setting are often attached to general practitioners and work in close co-operation with the Social Services at Health Centres and Community Hospitals and among patients in their own homes. The future trend would appear to be the further development of this aspect of the service as a link and extension of progressive patient care through hospital and out into the community.

PSYCHIATRIC PATIENTS

Although not the concern of this book, it is important to note that nearly half of all qualified occupational therapists work in psychiatric departments. As well as aiding diagnosis and helping to control symptoms through purposeful activity, a variety of situations are used whereby work, domestic, social and personal competence can be assessed. If necessary, modifications can be advised to prepare for return to normal life or at least to maintain as high a standard of functional integrity as is possible in those who suffer chronic and irreversible conditions.

Activities are carried out individually or in groups, according to each patient's needs. The therapy prescribed has several possible advantages—it may be of individual, group or social value and can also be designed to improve the patient's ability to form social relationships.

Creative activities give the patient means of expressing an emotion which would otherwise remain unrealized, or relieving an inhibition. Pottery and painting or musical and dancing activities are of particular value in this context. Apart from providing a means of self-expression, working with one's hands is a welcome diversion during a period of psychiatric treatment.

Similarly, the patient's capabilities for performing jobs and tasks can be evaluated. Initially this may be in clinical surroundings but may progress to assessment for employment in sheltered or open workshops. Coping at home may be difficult. Problems may arise in day-to-day activities such as cooking, cleaning and serving. These and other skills must be retaught, where appropriate; if possible, relatives and friends should be involved so as to encourage a cohesive family unit.

Contact with others may lead to control of expression or to an ability to express reasoned thought. It may also lead to an improvement in self-confidence and behaviour. It is important at this stage to maintain, encourage and improve the standards of personal care, fitness and hygiene. This will be by means of advice on diet, clothes, and care of the skin and hair, coupled with appropriate amounts of physical exercise.

OCCUPATIONAL THERAPY AND PHYSICAL DISABILITY

The occupational therapist has a role to play at many stages during the patient's development of and recovery from physical disability. By her assessment of his psychological and physical disability and handicap, she makes a major contribution to the initial understanding of his problems.

During treatment, she can contribute to the development of maximal functional capability through appropriate activities in relevant situations. At a later stage she can prepare the patient for return home to his particular social and economic situation.

The tools of the occupational therapist are the everyday activities of life:

Self-care activities Dressing, washing, feeding, toiletting and grooming.

Domestic and child-care activities Mainly for women but many can be usefully taught to men and should include house maintenance.

Work activities Clerical work, wood and metal work, and light industrial work.

Leisure activities Games, hobbies and gardening.

If the activity chosen has significance to the patient by relating to his intellectual level and social environment, it will gain and hold his co-operation, e.g. a repetitive packing job will have no significance to the middle-aged teacher, but will be a 'real' situation to a factory girl of 18.

The activity is chosen not to 'keep the patient busy' but because:

(1) It provides a medium for the occupational therapist's observation of functional performance and emotional reaction.

(2) It provides suitable physical exercise to build up precision skills, co-ordination and work tolerance.

(3) It provides suitable activities for training in the use of appliances, such as artificial limbs.

(4) It provides a means of assessing the patient's learning ability.

(5) It provides creative and expressive activities, e.g. art, music and drama, used in the diagnosis and treatment of mental illness.

Functional assessment

An essential preliminary activity and a necessary part of training is the assessment of the patient's functional capability; such a functional assessment forms the framework within which rehabilitation plans can be realistically shaped. It is therefore as important to the patient's future activity as the assessment of *disability* has been to an understanding of his present state.

Functional assessment:

(1) Gives a base line, at any given time, from which future progress or deterioration in function may be measured.

(2) Gives a guide to any changes which need to be made in the patient's routine and functional techniques or to the need for provision of appliances, aids and equipment.

(3) Adds to the diagnostic data, e.g. in a patient with brain damage the area of visuo-spatial defect or the nature of a dysphasia may be defined by observing the patient's performance throughout a series of activity patterns.

(4) Gives some prognostic guide as to physical function, e.g. comparative functional assessment of a hand with and without a simple corrective splint will give an indication to a surgeon whether surgical reconstruction will give his patient fuller hand function.

(5) Gives some prognostic guide as to the patient's motivation and ability to benefit from a programme of rehabilitation.

Assessment is an ongoing process and repeated reappraisal is necessary to define the patient's current problems and to indicate necessary adjustments in the rehabilitation programme. The activities which it entails may be carried out in hospitals, special rehabilitation units, work centres, sheltered workshops or the patient's own home.

In the rehabilitation of the physically handicapped, the main function of the occupational therapist is to help the patient to reach and maintain his optimal physical, psychological and social competence.

The patient's activities with which she is mainly concerned are:

(1) Mobility.
(2) Personal care.
(3) Domestic activities.
(4) Work potential.
  (a) Manual skills.
  (b) Ability to use educational skills.
  (c) Work tolerance.
(5) Educational and recreational activities.

The activities involved in personal care (including feeding, washing, dressing), domestic activities, such as cooking and housework, and mobility in relation to domestic and work situations are referred to collectively as activities of daily living (A.D.L.).

It is thus the occupational therapist who, by planned salvage operation, helps the patient to adjust to his new role occasioned by disability and who helps him to accept both the new role and a new environment, should this be necessary. Where disability exists, the occupational therapist first seeks methods and techniques to overcome the difficulty. Reorganization of daily routine and minor adjustment of habitual methods either at home or at work are often all that is necessary. Some aids or equipment may be of help, but the fewer and simpler the better. Additional services, such as home helps and meals-on-wheels, are available and are recommended, when needed, by the assessing occupational therapist. Finally, particularly for the more severely disabled, complex devices or adaptations to house and home may be the only way of retaining some level of independence.

General principles

The basis of all modern occupational therapy is the functional assessment of the patient. Whereas the physiotherapist will be concerned with recording the range or strength of the movement, the occupational therapist is more concerned with the applied range, strength and co-ordination in the performance of essential activities. Following their individual assessments, e.g. on a patient who has had a hip operation, the physiotherapist will be primarily concerned with devising an exercise programme to re-establish hip mobility and the patient's ability to sit, stand and walk. The occupational therapist will be more concerned with improving his ability to dress and use the toilet independently (activities which involve sitting, standing and walking). This assessment of the patient's functional capacity cannot be considered in isolation. It must be part of a total assessment, including the clinical evaluation of status and prognosis and a study of the patient's domestic and environmental background. Other factors, such as the patient's age, attitude of mind and social circumstances, must be taken into account.

The occupational therapist's functional assessment can be of many different varieties, depending upon the clinical situation and the assessment situation. Usually she will start with a structured enquiry directed towards delineating particular areas of difficulty. The initial enquiry entails questioning the patient about activities of daily living, work and hobbies. This is followed by more detailed checks and cross-checks but always it is necessary to observe the patient undertaking certain selected tasks. Answers to questions are notoriously misleading, and many patients give answers calculated to avoid complications. For example, few patients readily acknowledge difficulties in coping with personal toilet, for such an admission may lead inevitably to authoritative decisions being made about their ability to continue living independently at home. Thus, close observation of dressing and toilet activities in hospital or in the occupational therapy department will give more realistic information than simple questionnaires.

The next stage of functional assessment is the use of clearly structured tests. These tests can be repeated at intervals and used as a measure of the patient's progress. When the structured tests are activities of daily living, then the tests themselves become a training exercise and lead, therefore, to the solution of some problems which present difficulty, finally enabling the patient to 'pass the test'. This sequence of exposing the problems, trying to overcome them and then retesting, forms the basis of the occupational therapist's functional assessment.

However, if the problem-solving is to be realistic, it is necessary to extend the assessment procedure to gain maximal information about the patient's real problems in his own environment. For example, assessing a patient's ability to bath herself is unrealistic if the house in which she lives has no bath. Although most occupational therapy departments have their own assessment forms, which vary in detail, the information required to highlight the main problem areas follows a common pattern:

(1) Home conditions
  Type of residence.
  Accessibility (steps, etc.).
  Family and relatives or friends available for help.
(2) Mobility
  Walking, use of aids and appliances.
  Steps, etc., to be negotiated.
  Use of wheelchair.
  Need for and availability of outdoor transport.
(3) Personal care
  Washing, dressing, toilet and bath.
  Eating and drinking.
(4) Communication
  Speech, telephone, writing and typing.
  Reading.
  Transport available.
  Shopping.
(5) Domestic activities
  Meal preparation.
  Housework.
(6) Work
  Problems of job.
  Problems at work (including housework).
  Schooling and education of children or training school for older children.
(7) Leisure activities
  Past and present interests and problems.

As part of her work, the therapist will learn much about the patient's attitude, reactions, dependence, co-operation and adaptability to disability. This contributes considerably to the overall assessment. Many departments use different check lists for different clinical conditions. Thus, a patient with a temporary disability only needs a short check list, related to the specific problem which his temporary disablement incurs, whereas patients with more severe and more chronic disability require more extensive assessment procedures.

The elderly patient who falls and breaks a wrist may need some help and advice while her wrist is in plaster. The assessment will consist of a few key questions, a simple test and a short explanation. Patients recovering after total hip replacement need a different approach: encouragement in regaining confidence and confirmation that they can manage normal activities, such as sitting on a toilet. Amputees present a much greater problem, particularly if they are elderly. They need a considerable amount of help which should include training in dressing, bathing and the use of a wheelchair (for those occasions when they are unable to use their artificial limbs).

For the more severely disabled, it is important for the occupational therapist to carry out her practical assessment in related sequence. While a patient may achieve washing, dressing, cooking and feeding when assessed separately, the full sequence, from starting in bed to eating a cooked meal, may require a level of activity beyond the patient's endurance or may consist of a sequence of manœuvres which cannot be achieved in his particular domestic context. The determination of capability to achieve a continuous sequence of activities is particularly important in assessing the likelihood of the patient's return to work.

Thus, the occupational therapist working in hospital or rehabilitation unit requires considerable ingenuity in achieving realistic assessment and in inventing 'real life' situations corresponding to the patient's home or work. Without these practical tests, she is likely to make mistakes which can have considerable repercussions. For this reason, many forms of structured tests have been devised which duplicate domestic and work conditions. Many departments have an assessment kitchen or even a complete living area with bedroom, bathroom, kitchen or living room. Other departments have light and heavy workshops to provide realistic testing and training for industrial activity. All occupational therapy assessment and training, including leisure activities, should be related to activities useful to the patient.

Records and reports

It is upon the recorded information about the patient's disability that many complex, expensive and important decisions may be based. It is therefore incumbent upon the therapist to maintain careful and accurate records and to be able to present them in a clear and precise fashion. Verbal reporting is often called for within the team, but written records are essential for communication with others (e.g. from hospital to domiciliary staff) and for following progress over long periods of time. Here it cannot be over-emphasized that documentation of unsuccessful attempts and unsuccessful therapy can be more important in the long-term record than details of successful activities. Furthermore, it is essential to record *reasons* for decisions that are taken. If advice is given without explanations or notes do not record lack of success, other therapists may waste many hours covering the same ground. Had such written information been available, changes in the situation might have been revealed on review or recourse to the records, which would otherwise have remained unnoticed. With carefully planned check lists and details of performance, the occupational therapist's records can be as precise and as valuable to the clinician as the muscle chart and joint range records maintained by the physiotherapist. Whenever possible, the tests should be presented in a form which is immediately intelligible and, when repeated, should indicate clearly whether improvement or deterioration is occurring. Furthermore, the tests should, whenever possible, be selected so that the results can be recorded accurately, even if carried out by different therapists.

OCCUPATIONAL THERAPY IN SPECIAL UNITS

District General Hospital

The occupational therapy department of a District General Hospital usually comprises heavy and light workshops, a clerical section, a quiet area for study, and a domestic unit including kitchen, bedroom and bathroom, for assessing and training in activities of daily living.

A comprehensive, modern occupational therapy department is able to provide an atmosphere closely approaching that in a normal home or work situation. The assessment and testing is almost surreptitious. The occupational therapist will note whether the patient is anxious, depressed, co-operative, alert, moody, aggressive, euphoric or unrealistic. Over a period of time she will be able to note changes in behaviour (improvement or deterioration). Through simple activities she will be able to note the patient's power of concentration and his 'distractability'. Indeed, the surrounding distraction can be graded by altering the place in which simple activities such as playing games are carried out and by altering the complexity of the recreational activity.

Many simple leisure activities can be used to test memory and the ability to carry out both verbal and written instructions. Gardening, cooking and model building are all examples of apparently diversional activities which provide material for very reliable assessments. The patient's initiative (verbal and physical), his reliance upon others, his 'fatiguability' and his personality can all be gauged by the therapist while the assessment is undetected by the patient. Indeed, the occupational therapist can assess the response to adverse situations by spoiling the patient's chances in a game or apparently failing to provide correct or adequate materials.

The therapist's personality clearly plays a large part in this type of assessment, particularly with brain-damaged patients. About one half of all occupational therapists work in psychiatric hospitals, and a considerable proportion of their training is directed towards this field. This gives them a wider knowledge and understanding of behaviour, behaviour problems and abnormalities than many other workers in the field of physical handicap.

On the physical side, the occupational therapist can provide graded activity designed to increase muscle power, joint range, co-ordination and balance. Her work complements that of the physiotherapist, and extends the use of the patient's limbs to functional activities relevant to daily living. She is able to provide additional stimulus and interest through constructive and creative activities, employing different aspects of motivation to achieve similar objectives. In specific instances, functional or diversional activities can be adapted to supplement exercise regimes already introduced by the physiotherapist. Patients with hand injuries may, for example, spend time in the physiotherapy department exercising their hands in hot water or after wax treatment. This can be followed by a period in the occupational therapy department playing 'draughts' with specially designed heavy draughtsmen or playing a form of blow football using hand-squeezed pumps to blow the ball.

It is often argued that muscle strength, co-ordination and independence all improve simultaneously without specific therapy, but most patients do better and feel better if these activities are encouraged both by specific exercises (physiotherapy) and general or specific functional activities (occupational therapy).

Medical Rehabilitation Unit

When the emphasis in a Medical Rehabilitation Unit, whether outpatient or residential, is on active restoration of function and progression to a full day's work for the patient with a temporary disability, the occupational therapist's role will be mainly therapeutic. This will be achieved through her selection for each patient of appropriate activities calling for a repetitive movement of the injured part, and through the programme she devises in which a working activity involves progressively longer periods of standing, walking and co-ordination. Much of this activity will be supplementary and complementary to the general and specific exercises and activity given by the physiotherapist.

Prior to initiating the treatment programme, the occupational therapist investigates the patient's work potential and any relevant problems of mobility. The aim must be, if possible, to return the patient to his or her employment. If this is unrealistic, consideration must be given to transfer to an industrial training centre or to sheltered employment.

The occupational therapist will provide an assessment of the need for help and training with personal care and activities of daily living, and such training may well prevent further deterioration in the patient's condition.

Industrial Centres, Sheltered Workshops and Work Centres

An Industrial Centre usually consists of a Sheltered Workshop and a therapeutic Work Centre. Where possible, these are situated in an industrial trading estate, where a variety of small contract work is available from local firms, and the handicapped workers have daily contact with workers in adjoining industries.

A Sheltered Workshop is subsidized by the Department of Employment and Productivity and referral is usually through the Disablement Resettlement Officer. In these Workshops, the permanently handicapped who can cope with an 8-hour day, 5 days a week, but who are too disabled to compete in open employment, are able to earn a living wage. They are usually expected to travel to work independently.

Many disabled people cannot work at this level, and they may be referred to a Work Centre catering for the severely disabled who can benefit from regular work and who may progress to sheltered open employment. Such patients receive National Health Insurance or Unemployment Benefit, and are usually permitted to earn up to £2 per week. When necessary, transport is provided. Attendance may be for part or all of the working week, according to the patient's capacity.

The occupational therapist can contribute much to the Work Centre in co-operation with the Industrial Manager. She can assess the handicapped person's ability by a series of aptitude and work potential tests, advise the most suitable Centre for him, and adjust the work to his needs.

An atmosphere of realistic work and progress should be built up within such Centres and by frequent reassessment the opportunity should be open for a patient to progress to a Sheltered Workshop, though it is appreciated that there are administrative and financial difficulties involved in such a transfer.

A therapy area within the Work Centre can provide a quieter situation in which more help is available for the physically severely disabled and for mentally handicapped patients who need more supervision. Facilities for activities of daily living and social training should also be available within the therapy area, providing for individual help or work in small groups. Any workers needing this training would come out of the Workshops for short periods during the day.

All work facilities for the disabled should be closely associated with the clinical rehabilitation facilities and should be geared to allow the easy transfer of patients as and when their clinical and functional capabilities indicate that this is possible. This implies a level of collaboration, integration and interest between all departments concerned with the disabled which is not yet available, but which could develop with the reorganization of the National Health Service. Should regional 'rehabilitation' teams develop, they should include doctors concerned with occupational health and rehabilitation, the Workshop Manager, therapists, social workers, the Careers Advisory Officer and the Disablement Resettlement Officer.

Day Centres

In contrast to Day Hospitals which are therapeutic organizations, Day Centres are recreational and social and serve four main purposes:

(1) To 'maintain' the severely disabled and provide them with positive interests.

(2) To relieve the family of their care for short, regular periods.

(3) To provide social contacts and activities for the residents of Old People's Homes and Homes for the Young Severely Disabled.

(4) To provide a hot, nutritious meal (particularly important for those who live alone).

Ideally, patients would be referred to these Centres by the general practitioner and would be regularly reviewed by a visiting rehabilitation team. At present, Day Centres are run by the Social Services Departments of the Local Authorities, but after the integration of the Health Services in 1974, it is hoped that there will be closer collaboration between all the rehabilitation services concerned.

It is estimated that there should be one Day Centre for every 30 000 people. Each Centre should have a professionally trained supervisor, preferably from a paramedical profession, but would be largely staffed by assistants with lesser training and by volunteers.

An occupational therapist spending two or more sessions a week at the Day Centre can provide an extra service by advising on daily living problems and helping to organize a wide range of leisure activities catering for all intellectual levels.

Domiciliary occupational therapy

Visits by the occupational therapist to the handicapped person in his own home are necessary to assess his functional capability and to identify his problems in his own environment of house, family and community.

She should pass on relevant findings to the:

(1) General practitioner.

(2) Hospital—before the patient's admission or in preparation for his return home.

(3) Local Authority Departments concerned, including the housing department.

The occupational therapist will be able to:

(a) Continue activities of daily living training started in hospital and supply aids needed.

(b) Deal with difficulties of access and mobility.

(c) Assist the family and other helpers with difficulties in the care of the patient, and the social adjustment.

(d) Provide educational and recreational activities for those unable to attend the Day Centre.

In practice, the occupational therapist will often carry out the initial assessment and provide advice; the detailed activities are likely to be carried out by occupational therapy aids or Red Cross workers.

In practice, most patients are referred to the domiciliary occupational therapist by the general practitioner and do not reach a hospital department. The domiciliary occupational therapist of the future may be based in a Health Centre, which can facilitate communication with all members of the community care team.

A Disabled Students' Hostel, a Residential Home for the Young Disabled or an Old People's Home should all be considered in this context as the individual's home and should receive the services of a domiciliary occupational therapist.

The position of the occupational therapist in the team concerned with the rehabilitation of the severely disabled patient is well established. Less well recognized is the vital part which she can play in the rehabilitation of the temporarily or moderately disabled patient, whether this disability is physical or mental in origin.

Temporary disability often means a loss of cash and convenience to the average patient. He often understands too little about the interrelationship of time and motion to be able to reorganize either himself or his surroundings to minimize the disabling effects of his condition.

The occupational therapist assists such a patient by making an accurate assessment of his personal and environmental needs and his executive potential, both at home and at work, and by formulating a realistic programme by which the two may be satisfactorily integrated. For both mentally and physically disabled patients, she attempts to delineate areas of actual or probable functional difficulty and to compensate for any effects of disability by promoting a more efficient use of residual ability. For example, wearing an appliance may give rise to a serious loss of immediate functional efficiency, whether it is a replacement prosthesis such as an artificial limb or a corrective, compensatory or stabilizing device such as a caliper or a splint. Using her professional skills to identify the occupations which will give him the necessary practice in prosthetic use, an occupational therapist can teach the patient the necessary expertise by which he can regain manipulative skill.

To anyone with a locomotor lesion, daily life in the home, at work or in transit between the two, may be fraught with many hazards and discomforts. By simple alterations in body posture and movements, by minor but strategic changes in the arrangement and use of necessary home and work equipment, fittings and furniture, the occupational therapist seeks to alter the patient/milieu relationship until the patient's occupation and surroundings can play a useful role in the therapeutic programme.

Children's Assessment Unit

Children's Assessment Units are being planned in many areas in association with school facilities for the physically handicapped. These Units may be centred on an educational site rather than on a hospital site, but wherever the situation, an integrated course of occupational therapy and training can be planned as part of the child's total programme. A multidisciplinary team will assess and review the physically disabled children and those with behavioural, emotional, learning and speech difficulties who are referred by the school medical officer, the general practitioner or the paediatrician.

The Assessment Unit will also provide a continuing counselling service for parents and will have the responsibility for bridging the gap between education and employment.

In this type of organization, the occupational therapist with specialized knowledge and experience of children's disorders is able to:

(a) Organize play therapy for purposes of observation and assessment.

(b) Assist in the testing of developmental level and ability.

(c) Assist in assessment of perceptive loss.

(d) Give training to children and parents in activities of daily living and general independence.

(e) Advise on any aids needed for school or at home.

(f) Inform the domiciliary occupational therapist concerned of the progress and relevant recommendations.

ASSESSMENT OF SPECIAL PROBLEMS

For the majority of patients, a simple functional assessment covering the activities of daily living is all that is required prior to returning home from hospital. However, the occupational therapist may be required to be more specific in the assessment. She may have to deal with problems created by the particular clinical condition, e.g. stroke or rheumatoid arthritis, or with particular activities of employment, e.g. clerical work or light engineering.

Activities of daily living

On admission to hospital, many patients with temporary or permanent disability and most elderly people will be found to have some impairment of function. Although not essential for their care, a careful assessment of their functional capabilities will reveal some activity or activities which could be achieved more easily. Many activities of daily living—getting in and out of bed, getting on and off the toilet, dressing, housework and leisure activities such as gardening—involve complex manœuvres which become a burden for the elderly, arthritic or mildly infirm. A few simple changes of activity pattern or a few simple aids can often make life easier. The timely support of the social services through the provision of a home help or meals-on-wheels may enable the patient to retain independence at home for a longer period of time. Such an assessment service, coupled with provision of appropriate help, can contribute much to the quality of life. Assessment must begin as soon as possible. If the patient is in hospital, it should be initiated there but only with close co-operation with the community services. Provision and continuity of care must be fostered by means of good communications between hospital and community-based workers. The occupational therapist has a vital part to play in bridging the gap between the patient's clinical care and community care.

A major area of activity for many occupational therapists will therefore lie in assessing patients' aids to daily living, in providing these aids, and in training in their use.

The most frequently required aids are:

Walking aids—frames, sticks and crutches.
Bath and toilet aids.
Simple dressing aids.

The equipment most frequently required includes:

Hoists.
Wheelchairs.

All of these items need individual assessment and practical trials. Thus, occupational therapists need to assess patients in all activities of daily living, determining the need for alterations to be made in the home, demonstrating the safest routines in the kitchen, helping with dressing, effecting necessary adaptations to clothes, re-enforcing speech training, and helping with difficulties in shopping, social activities and so on.

Patients in hospital will start this training in the hospital occupational therapy department and then continue in the home situation, if possible with the same occupational therapist. The integration of the hospital and domiciliary service is a goal which might become possible when the Health Services are integrated, but is rarely possible at present.

Pre-vocational assessment

Ideally, the man with a disability should return to normal working conditions either full- or part-time. Apart from the financial benefits, he gains status, dignity and social contacts, together with the satisfaction which most men achieve from work. When this level of activity is not possible, a man may be able to earn a reasonable income by working in his own home or in a sheltered environment. This restricts his social contacts and limits his horizons but may nevertheless enable him to retain interest, dignity and status. For those who are unable to achieve a working status, a specific leisure activity may offer enough creative outlet—physical or intellectual—to enable a disabled person to lead a happy and surprisingly satisfactory life.

For a woman, a main aim is usually to be able to run her home and care for her children and husband, thus fulfilling her normal role in the life of the family. If this is not possible, the next level of achievement to be aimed at is the running of the home with help and assistance. Again, for the severely disabled, a specific creative activity should be the aim for everyone unable to achieve a level of domestic independence.

For children, the end result aimed at should be normal school life, even for the severely physically disabled. Only through as near-normal school life as possible is a satisfactory transition from school to work environment likely to occur. When normal schooling is impossible then special schooling may enable the severely physically disabled child to achieve a good education. However, integration into employment is likely to be more difficult, and the transition from school to community is often not achieved. For the very severely disabled, tuition at home may have to be instituted and can be very successful. Problems almost inevitably arise when schooling comes to an end or when family support is threatened by the parents' increasing age or ill-health.

Thus the early assessment of rehabilitative potential of a patient of any age may be a very important activity and may set in motion a chain of activities which can lead to success or failure in terms of a disabled person's ultimate integration or re-integration into the community.

An occupational therapist may frequently be the first person to broach the problem of a patient's possible return to work. This may be a simple matter calling only for a clinical decision to be made concerning the timing of return to work, or it may be a long and complex procedure involving a series of assessments and periods of training.

The initial pre-vocational assessment comprises a review of the clinical situation, the patient's general functional capabilities, previous employment, domestic situation, financial status and family responsibilities.

On a more specific basis, his attitude towards work, his learning ability and 'fatiguability' are important features which must be assessed. It is important to clarify the likely problems relating to domestic circumstances and the area in which he lives—the availability of employment and availability of suitable transport. With regard to physical disability, it is important to establish not only the patient's ability to work but his ability to cope independently with transport to and from work, and with feeding and toilet activities while at work.

Finally, a preliminary assessment of his level of physical activity in relation to past employment or other specific jobs can be established by a series of relatively simple tests.

Pre-vocational assessments of adults with a physical disability must always start from past experience in terms of education, training and work. Knowledge of local industries is of considerable help and here the Disablement Resettlement Officer (D.R.O.) should be of assistance. With the increasing establishment of hospital D.R.Os, the resettlement of adults in hospital will tend to become more of a routine activity of the hospital social worker and hospital D.R.O. Although the hospital occupational therapist and the D.R.O. will clearly need to collaborate very closely, it is the D.R.O. who is likely to take the initiative for the men with temporary and minor disabilities, whereas the occupational therapist is likely to take the initiative for the housewives and the more severely disabled men. Furthermore, she is likely to be concerned with providing some simulated activities at various levels of physical and intellectual activity which will enable the hospital D.R.O. to make a realistic appraisal of the man's working capabilities. The increasing collaboration between the occupational therapist, the D.R.O. and the assessment team of the Industrial Rehabilitation Unit gives considerable scope for development in the future. Unfortunately, at present these activities tend to be administratively and geographically isolated, but the modern trend is to bring the skills and expertise together, preferably in close proximity to the clinical situation. This ensures a rapid transition from hospital to industrial assessment and a unified collaborative approach towards return to work.

Clerical assessment

Aptitude and capability for clerical work can be readily assessed in an occupational therapy department. Preliminary tests involve writing, copy typing and typing from shorthand, graded spelling tests, reading lists and simple arithmetic. Progression from these involves reading aloud, discussion about the passages read and writing a letter on the subject discussed. The ability to use common reference books such as telephone directories or trade catalogues is also important. Simple office procedures, such as filing, answering the telephone and taking and passing on messages, can be simulated.

Tests of more advanced capability using adding machines, dictaphones or shorthand can often be found within the hospital, making it possible to achieve a realistic assessment.

Geriatric assessment

Elderly patients usually present a complex clinical problem, as they frequently suffer from a number of specific illnesses simultaneously. Many also suffer from some degree of intellectual deterioration, and this will have a significant effect on their capabilities.

Although many elderly patients will be able to accomplish many individual activities of daily living, their ability to return to some level of independence will depend more upon their memory, their ability to initiate action, their understanding of simple problems, their level of concentration and their degree of unimpaired judgement. These features can be assessed by simple tests involving memory, vocabulary, calculation and orientation in time and place. In addition, routine activities of daily living are designed to assess co-ordination, power and general physical capability.

Specific disabilities

Tests of general functional capability, by means of activities of daily living or pre-vocational assessment activities, are non-specific and are relevant to almost all physical disability. However, occupational therapists have a further part to play in devising and carrying out assessments relevant to specific disability. These assessments are used not only to clarify the degree of specific disability, but also to contribute to an objective evaluation of the patient as a whole, the effectiveness of treatment and the need for specific reconstructive surgery. Examples of such disabilities are rheumatoid arthritis, stroke and low back pain.

Rheumatoid arthritis

Rheumatoid arthritis provides a notable situation in which general assessment and specific assessment based upon occupational therapy are of considerable importance in determining the management of a patient.

The general assessment leads to a programme of instruction and training designed to help the patient understand and overcome his disabilities whilst yet preserving function, and to prevent unnecessary deterioration and deformity. Some stress on joints is inevitable during the activities of daily living, but by careful planning and reprogramming, many unnecessary harmful stresses can be eliminated or reduced. Aids and splints are used when it is not possible to overcome difficulties without them. For example, the use of drip-dry clothes and household linen eliminates the need for ironing, and a chair with a seat at an appropriate height minimizes the demands made on upper limbs for pushing up from a sitting to a standing position. Similarly, appropriate grab rails in the toilet and in the bathroom will reduce the repeated weight-thrusting stress sustained in the upper limbs during toilet and bathing activities. Naturally, there is considerable interest in and concentration upon the hands of the rheumatoid arthritic, and many occupational therapists have developed sophisticated tests for assessing hand function.

Hand function tests are usually constructed around the various types of grip:

Pin grip adequate opposition of thumb; good intrinsic control; good sensation.

Key grip strong intrinsic control; stable, terminal and proximal interphalangeal joints.

Knife grip as for key grip; good flexion of index finger.

Handle grip or power grip adequate abduction of thumb; good finger flexion; good power in long flexors of fingers and wrist dorsiflexors.

Tests can be devised to measure the individual grips and to record them in terms of power and precision. However, hand function only becomes of use if the hand can be placed accurately in space and is therefore dependent upon total upper limb function. Activities such as eating and writing must each be assessed as co-ordinated activity sequences and can also be graded in terms of applied strength and precision. In rheumatoid arthiritis, the severely involved hand rarely approaches the strength recorded in normal hands, but the precision and functional ability which can be attained are often remarkable.

Hand function tests are of considerable value to the experienced team, and they provide the clinician with valuable information and insight into the need for and likely response to reconstructive surgery.

Strokes

Almost every occupational therapy department will have its share of patients with strokes.

The pattern of recovery is determined by the severity of the cerebrovascular accident. Functional assessment is often helpful in delineating those patients who have persistent defects of balance and those whose activities are hindered by residual sensory defects. It is important to reveal these features since they signify a poor prognosis as far as functional recovery is concerned. Patients who are unaware of their paralysed limb are unlikely to co-operate in activities such as dressing, which demand acceptance of the disability. Much more investigation of hemiplegia needs to be undertaken to perfect techniques for teaching these patients to adapt to their disabilities.

Formal speech therapy for patients with dysphasia following a stroke is often only available for short, infrequent sessions. Within the occupational therapy department speech training can be extended into several hours a day. In addition to individual training, group activities can often help the dysphasic patient to relax and spontaneous speech sometimes occurs in such an atmosphere. Singing, in particular, is a great morale booster, and likewise the repetition of well-known things, such as the alphabet or nursery rhymes. Relatives may need help and may need to be taught how to talk to the patient, phrasing their questions so that a 'yes' or 'no' answer is possible. They and the patient often need reassurance that he is not insane or mentally retarded now that speech is lost.

If there is an overwhelming residual disability, an occupational therapist is often the person upon whom both relatives and patients can vent their feelings of oppression and depression.

Visual and sensory defects may lead to dangerous circumstances, and the patient and relatives need to be taught techniques which are safe in potentially dangerous situations, such as the bathroom, workshop or kitchen.

Back pain

Back pain is a symptom which is more often referred to a physiotherapy department than an occupational therapy department at the present time, but many hospitals are recognizing that the occupational therapist's approach has a lot to offer. The occupational therapist can often analyse an industrial patient's living activities more thoroughly than a physiotherapist because she is more experienced in this form of assessment. She can then go through these activities and retrain the patient, particularly the housewife, to avoid provocative situations. This may entail reorganizing the way in which she carries out any particular activity, or it may involve the use of simple aids. Dealing with awkward cupboards, lifting children or heavy objects, and carrying out many routine household activities involving lifting and bending can precipitate the return of backache unless they are approached correctly. This is a particular area where collaboration between occupational therapist and physiotherapist can be of great benefit.

OCCUPATIONAL THERAPIST AS A TEACHER

The occupational therapist spends a great deal of her time in teaching patients. The teaching is based on assessment, but the logical outcome of assessment is a period of training (teaching). She teaches the patients individually and in groups to regain activities which have been lost or impaired by disability; to wear and use appliances; to use aids and equipment; to prevent damage and injury to affected joints; and to readjust to a changed set of circumstances. For these reasons, the occupational therapist needs a wide understanding not only of the disabilities, but of the mechanisms of learning and the techniques of teaching. There is an increasing awareness that patients forget a great deal of what doctors and therapists tell them. Instructions and advice are more likely to be forgotten than other information. The more the patient is told at one time, the more he will forget. The relationship between anxiety and the retention of information is complex, and moderately anxious patients remember more than the highly anxious and more than those who are not anxious.

Therefore, the contribution of the occupational therapist is often a vital one in training the patient to put into everyday practice the advice which the doctor gives to the relative about the underlying clinical condition.

BIBLIOGRAPHY AND REFERENCES

Goble, R. E. A. (1967). 'The role of the occupational therapist in disabled living research.' *Am. J. occup. Ther.* **23**, 145

Macdonald, E. M., Maccough, G. and Murrey, L. (1970). *Occupational Therapy in Rehabilitation* (3rd edn). London; Balliere and Tindall

Milton Keynes Report of the Working Group on Services for the Physically Handicapped and Rehabilitation (1970). Buckinghamshire County Council

Mountford, S. W. (1965). *Towards Rehabilitation: A Study of Widening Horizons*. Edinburgh and London; Livingstone

Mountford, S. W. (1971). *Introduction to Occupational Therapy*. Edinburgh and London; Livingstone

Occupational Therapist Board (1972). 'Future education and training of occupational therapists.' London; Council for Professions Supplementary to Medicine.

White, A. S. (1972). *Easy Path to Gardening*. London; Readers Digest (in association with the Disabled Living Foundation)

4—Rheumatoid Arthritis

INTRODUCTION

Among patients who suffer from diseases of the locomotor system those with rheumatoid arthritis rank numerically second only to patients with degenerative joint disease.

In the United Kingdom, rheumatoid arthritis affects about one million women and nearly half a million men. The importance of the disease derives from its natural history, its high incidence among younger people, its associated systemic effects and its involvement of multiple joints in a progressive inflammatory, and later, degenerative condition. About half the patients seen in hospitals or special rheumatology units will improve with care and treatment and about half will deteriorate almost inexorably.

There is increasing evidence that with a period of intensive in-patient therapy followed by careful out-patient supervision and readmission when necessary, many patients can be maintained in a good state of health and may remain actively employed for many years. With close collaboration between rheumatologists, orthopaedic surgeons and rehabilitation services, both in the hospital and in the community, even the most severely disabled patients can be improved and the majority of them can be helped to retain a good functional level and to remain independent in their own homes.

The intensive management in special units with a high staff/patient ratio advocated by some workers is well justified by the long-term results. Some of the most important contributions of these units are the accurate assessment of the patient's disability and handicap and the establishment of clear indicators of disease activity and progress.

From these baselines it is possible to form realistic therapeutic aims and detailed, agreed plans of management in terms of drugs, surgery and rehabilitation.

It is therefore very important to understand the clear-cut distinction between the aims of rehabilitation in the early, acute stages of the disease and those in the later, chronic stages.

Rheumatoid arthritis presents a challenge in general and specific management and illustrates the need for close collaboration between physician, orthopaedic surgeon and all those concerned with rehabilitation. The general pattern of care has five main aims:

Relief of pain.
Prevention of deformity.
Correction of existing deformity.
Improvement of functional capability.
Control of systemic manifestations.

In order to achieve these aims, a balance needs always to be maintained between rest and activity, and no less fine a balance between medical care and surgical intervention. The supervision of medication must be continuous and close, and is the combined responsibility of general practitioners, rheumatologists and surgeons. Splints can be used to provide rest, to correct deformity and to aid function of permanently damaged joints. Conventional passive physiotherapy has little place in the rehabilitation of the rheumatoid patient, other than as a palliative treatment. Patients vary in their opinion as to whether heat or cold give most relief to their symptoms. Passive movements usually evoke pain and muscle spasm, but carefully controlled static and resisted exercises can build up the bulk and strength of wasted muscles.

Occupational therapy is of help in assessing the functional capacity of patients and in training them to cope with the difficulties of daily living. Reassessment prior to return home, and pre-vocational assessment prior to resettlement in employment are other valuable contributions of the occupational therapist.

Stress has a definite effect on this disease and social adjustments and welfare care play an essential part in the general rehabilitation.

It is most important that the interrelationship between medical treatment and the activities of daily living be clearly established at the first meeting of the clinician and patient. Rehabilitation is not a series of regimes, supplemented by a selection of appropriate mechanical aids, which an occupational therapist or a physiotherapist grafts on to the final stage of the medical treatment of a patient. It embraces the total therapy offered to a patient with rheumatoid arthritis and aims at restoring him to normal active daily life. In this process it must never lose sight of the importance of the relief of pain. A patient in pain is worn down mentally and physically. He may well become depressed, choosing inactivity, even though he is irked by it, in an effort to minimize his discomfort. Therefore, one of the earliest and most important steps in the rehabilitation of a patient with rheumatoid arthritis is the institution of an adequate regime of medication employing drugs which are both anti-inflammatory and analgesic. The use of simple analgesics alone does not produce relief of the inflammatory condition in the joint which gives rise to much of the pain, nor does it relieve joint stiffness. When the pain load is reduced to its lowest level by appropriate drugs, the real personality of the patient emerges, and he is able to co-operate in the struggle to attain maximal independence.

An explanation of the difficulties which exist in the constant attempts to reconcile long-term and short-term aims is also essential in the case of each patient. While the attainment of the maximal degree of pain-free mobility and independence in the fastest possible time is the main object of every patient, it is important for him to realize that the level of mobility attempted at any one stage of the disease must be influenced by the effect which it may have upon mobility in the future. Thus, a patient may be advised to avoid walking with the assistance of elbow crutches to the limit of his endurance, since he may well exacerbate pain and precipitate deformity in his shoulders, hands and wrists. Similarly, a patient with active arthritis of shoulders and hands may be advised to avoid hand propulsion of a wheelchair and to accept a powered chair as a substitute in order to conserve function of the joints of his upper limbs. An explanation of the 'substitution value' of upper and lower limbs will enable a patient to realize that his upper limbs can give him movement even when his lower limbs cannot, and will make him less likely to over-use or badly use his arms and hands in an effort to regain or retain mobility.

CARE IN THE EARLY ACUTE STAGES

The primary objectives of treatment are the reduction of inflammation and pain, the preservation of function, and the prevention of deformity.

The essentials of treatment of early acute rheumatoid arthritis are (1) supervised rest, (2) the administration of anti-inflammatory drugs, (3) gentle physical therapy.

How these components of treatment are blended must depend upon the needs of the individual patient and the opinion of the doctor who supervises his care.

Bed rest

Whereas most rheumatologists believe that almost all patients need bed rest during the early acute stages of rheumatoid arthritis, some prefer their patients to remain ambulatory during milder attacks. In severe illness, however, bed rest is essential and must be complete. For this reason, it is difficult to achieve in the home, and lack of response to domiciliary bed rest is a clear indication for admission to a hospital. Whenever possible, such admission should be to a rheumatological unit where specialized care and treatment is available. As has been said earlier, follow-up studies indicate that rheumatoid patients are best managed in an independent unit, where medical care is integrated with physiotherapeutic skills and where the slowness of the patient's rate of progress is not accentuated by the faster recovery of patients with less chronic medical conditions. Within a rheumatology unit, the concept of total patient care for these patients can be realized in a manner which is impossible either in a mixed acute ward or an out-patient department.

Combined with bed rest, complete splintage of all affected joints—usually excepting those of one arm below elbow level to permit self-feeding—produces a state of maximal inactivity. After a day or two of frustration at being unable to move about in their usual manner, patients find that the lack of need to move painful joints itself produces a general relaxation and a profound relief from stress.

Administration of drugs

Further pain relief is produced by adequate medication and achievement of an effective dosage of anti-inflammatory analgesics. An adequate blood salicylate level is the first objective. If this has been achieved without pain relief or if gastric intolerance has occurred, other anti-inflammatory drugs are indicated. Sometimes adding a nightly dose of indomethacin or a small dose of prednisolone to an adequate dose of salicylate will relieve the pain and morning stiffness.

Phenylbutazone, indomethacin, antimalarials, gold and steroids have their place and their proponents. More recently, penicillamine, immunosuppressive and cytotoxic therapy have been introduced. The aim must always be to suppress the disease activity within the limits imposed by drug side-effects. A detailed discussion of the drug therapy of rheumatoid arthritis is outside the scope of this book, but it must be emphasized that the appropriate drug therapy is frequently the corner-stone of medical management.

A salicylate preparation given in continuous, adequate dosage (3–6 g daily) is symptomatically the most effective drug treatment. The other drugs mentioned may be used in combination, depending upon the activity of the disease and its response to aspirin. A hypochromic, normocytic anaemia is a common feature of rheumatoid arthritis. It is generally refractory to treatment with oral iron but usually responds to parenteral iron. Unless adequately treated, the anaemia can be an added cause of apparent handicap.

Physiotherapy

The physiotherapist gives treatment in the acute stage by immobilizing the patient's affected joints with splints, supervising the performance of static exercises and encouraging gentle activity and postural changes within the restrictions imposed by the splintage.

The bed used should have a firm mattress or bed boards under the mattress. The patient should lie flat with only one pillow for his head and *no* pillows under the knees. He may sit up for short periods for meals or toilet, using a firm backrest. At other times he should lie flat with a bed-cage and padded footrest. He should be prone for 20–30 minutes, 2 or 3 times a day to prevent flexion contractures of the hips. Splintage of the involved joints for periods of up to 3 weeks is now strongly advocated by some centres. Skin-tight plaster of paris splints holding the joints in functional positions are surprisingly well tolerated. The common ones are:

(1) Posterior shells for the legs extending from gluteal crease to the heels with a right-angled foot plate and the knees in 3–5 degrees of flexion.

(2) Posterior arm splints from elbow to finger-tips with the wrist in mid-pronation and a few degrees of extension. A band is usually added to hold the fingers in a few degrees of flexion and the thumb is usually left free. For the more deformed wrists or hands, an anterior splint is probably more satisfactory.

During the acute stage physical therapy has little place, but as inflammation subsides, activity is gradually introduced. Static exercises can be taught to most patients even in their splints, and the only guides at this stage are the tolerance of the patient and the experience of the therapist. Passive movements are best avoided altogether. Once it is realized that immobilization for up to 3 to 4 weeks can be safely employed without risks of permanent loss of movement, the traditional urge to 'maintain mobility' can be ignored.

The stage at which static (isometric) exercises and gentle active exercises are introduced depends entirely on the patient's general and local response to the total treatment. Increasing pain and subsequent stiffness are important warning signs which must not be ignored but must cause the exercise programme to be reduced accordingly. In general, short (5 minutes or less) periods of activity spread at hourly or 2-hourly intervals are likely to be better tolerated and more effective than sessions of physical therapy of more traditional duration.

The performance of exercises can usually be facilitated by a preceding period of warmth, either from wax baths, heat lamps or warm water. For some joints, ice packs produce greater pain relief and better relaxation of the surrounding musculature, but individual response is so varied that it may be necessary to try several palliative measures for a patient before the most appropriate is found.

As the patient responds, physical activity can be gradually increased and the splints can be removed for increasing periods. Weight-bearing is introduced only when the muscles are clearly strong enough, and adequate appropriate walking aids are essential to provide graded weight relief. Other activities such as personal toilet and dressing are also part of the patient's graded exercise routine. At this stage, particularly close collaboration between physiotherapist, occupational therapist and nursing staff is essential to adjust a patient's activity level to his physical capability, while the patient himself gradually learns to undertake the responsibility of determining the pattern of exercise and activity necessary for his recovery.

This staged mobilization is an intensely individual procedure and may need to be revised from day to day.

RETURNING HOME

By the time the patient returns home, he has been taught to manage his life in such a way as to minimize his disabilities and to avoid aggravating his illness. The actual time at which he leaves hospital will be related to the suitability of his home conditions and his own ability to satisfy the demands made upon him by the architecture of his home and the behaviour of his family and friends.

The patient's overall care will then be the responsibility of his family doctor. Good liaison must exist between all concerned and clear recommendations as to future management should be passed on from rheumatologist to general practitioner. However comprehensive the recommendations may be, it is impossible to foretell the relapses and remissions which do occur in this disease. Unpredicted events may well take place and it would seem that, however competent the family doctor, the patient with a chronic, progressive and painful disorder is not satisfied unless he has access to specialist opinion.

All except the mildly affected should probably be reviewed occasionally by a rheumatologist, but it is important to avoid long ambulance journeys and lengthy out-patient waiting periods.

It must be emphasized that everyday care remains in the hands of the family doctor and his personnel.

From his rheumatologist and family doctor the patient will have learned the natural history of his illness and of the need to remove stress and fatigue from his life by careful planning of his daily programme; to fragment and vary his routine on any one day according to his condition; to take rests when he needs them; to use the exercise regimes and postural habits taught by the physiotherapist; to employ the methods and aids for his daily living activities advised by the occupational therapist. Before his regular routine of hand and foot exercises and quadriceps drill, supplemented by specific exercises for other affected joints, performed in several short sessions of 5–10 minutes each day, he may sometimes use heating or cooling techniques. The heat may be from a hot bath or shower, an electric fire or domestic infra-red lamp. Alternatively, the patient may apply ice-filled bags to cool a joint, or submerge hands or feet in water in which crushed ice from the refrigerator is floating.

Fatigue is to be avoided. The housewife should be encouraged to take a mid-day rest, to rest when joints are painful, and not to push resolutely on through pain. Hand and foot exercises and quadriceps drill must become a part of life.

The patient must come to terms with the practical aspects of his life at home and at work. Organization of daily life should be as simple as possible, following a programme of rest, work and exercise.

ASSESSMENT

The major aim of rehabilitation in chronic disorders is to attain a satisfactory state of equilibrium between the demands made on the patient by his work, his home and his family, and his physical ability to meet those demands. No equilibrium can be obtained without an accurate knowledge of the factors concerned in both, and this demands an accurate assessment of the patient and his milieu. Rheumatoid arthritis is a progressive disease, and the clinical condition of the patient tends constantly to change; thus, many repeated assessments of disease activity and functional capacity are needed if the medical, surgical and rehabilitative aspects of his management are to be appropriately blended. The chronicity of the disease is great, and its effects are so far-reaching that such assessments must be total, combining the specialized opinions of clinician, physiotherapist, occupational therapist, medical social worker, clinical psychologist and nursing staff. Repeated assessment enables a knowledge of a patient's physical state, intellectual and psychological make-up and present and future situations to have an appropriate influence on his overall management.

As some aspects of care call for a reversal of approach,

collaborative assessments and detailed consultations are necessary at all stages so that a change from conservative care to a more aggressive surgical approach, or a decision to reduce activity and rely more upon aids and appliances can be discussed frankly with the patient. At all times, the patient's complete understanding of his disease and realistic aims for his treatment are essential to his management.

Functional assessment

The total assessment of the rheumatoid arthritic patient provides information on a number of separate features:

(1) General disease activity.
(2) Local joint disease activity.
(3) Degree of deformity and consequent functional disability.
(4) Extra-articular features and complications.
(5) Concurrent illness, both physical and psychological.
(6) Family, work and social state, and ability to fulfil commitments at home, at work and in society, with delineation of specific difficulties.

These functional assessments provide pertinent summaries of a patient's disabilities. Clinical examination will provide details of muscle power and joint range, but what matters to the patient is the combination of joint and muscle action used in his everyday life. What he wants from those who give him care is the expertise which enables them to detect and rectify a breakdown or threatened breakdown in his personal equilibrium of real need and functional ability. Repeated assessments can do just this.

For the less disabled patient, whose management is largely in the hands of his family doctor, regular enquiry to ensure that daily living activities can be adequately performed will often suffice, although ideally, regular visits by a domiciliary occupational therapist to a patient in his own home would provide more accurate information about a patient's true functional balance. A patient in hospital, or at an out-patient clinic, often tends to put the best face on things—from a desire to please or to avoid 'fussing', from courtesy, or from embarrassment—and he may give a highly inaccurate account of himself. In his own home he ceases to 'put on an act' and discrepancies between his capabilities and his home circumstances become apparent. It is what he does do, rather than what he can do, which counts.

For the more severely disabled patient, repeated and detailed functional assessments are even more important. The employment of standardized methods of enquiry and recording enable estimations of improvement and deterioration to be made and accurate plans for future management to be outlined.

Method of functional assessment

Functional assessments rely partly on standardized questioning by the therapist and partly on her observation of the patient's performance of relevant daily living activities.

A preliminary scanning enquiry made by the occupational therapist into the activities of every patient attending a rheumatology out-patient clinic can focus the attention of the clinical team on the spheres of activity at risk. For in-patients a more detailed functional assessment is the usual practice.

In such an enquiry, the occupational therapist questions the patient about difficulties in:

(1) Personal care
  Washing.
  Toilet.
  Feeding.
  Dressing.
(2) Mobility
  Walking.
  Wheelchair.
  Transfers.
(3) Dexterity
  Reaching.
  Lifting.
  Carrying.
  Handling.
(4) Home conditions
  Structure of house.
  Housework.
  Shopping.
  Cooking.
  Cleaning.
  Clothes maintenance.
(5) Hobbies/recreation
(6) Outdoor activities
(7) Work
(8) Communication
(9) Personality and mental state
  Positive or negative attitude.
  Quick or slow reaction.
  Anxious or relaxed.
  Co-operative or resentful.
  Dependent or independent.

The more detailed enquiry analyses the patient's ability to perform specific actions and tasks. Assessments of mobility bear a relationship to trunk and lower limb function, whereas dexterity provides an estimate of upper limb power, co-ordination, range and speed of movement. Information of this sort is increasingly important as a prelude and a sequel to joint surgery.

MANAGEMENT AT HOME

The majority of patients with rheumatoid arthritis can live a relatively normal life in a normal environment, providing they observe certain general rules and remain under constant clinical review. In the domestic situation control is one of the key words in the patient's management of his disease, for it is only by controlling the precipitating factors that the exacerbations of rheumatoid arthritis may be minimized. Broadly speaking, anything producing physical, mental or emotional strain can precipitate an exacerbation, since rheumatoid arthritis, whatever its initial cause, behaves like a stress disease once it is established. Patients should therefore be counselled to live a balanced existence, aiming at:

(1) Sufficient sleep.

(2) Sufficient rest periods during the day, thus avoiding over-activity to the point of fatigue.

(3) Sufficient food of nourishing variety. Over-eating and obesity should be avoided and excess weight removed by dieting, when necessary.

(4) Sufficient fluid intake—bearing in mind the likelihood of renal damage from many of the drugs used in the therapeutic treatment of rheumatoid arthritis.

(5) Sufficient exercise of a moderate sort, which does not precipitate the pain in the joints but prevents them from stiffening.

(6) Suitable work where the physical and mental demands are within the patient's capabilities.

(7) Regulation of bowel action. It is possible that regular administration of analgesics may induce constipation, and if this is so, the introduction of increased roughage or a bulk-producing laxative may be necessary.

(8) Maintenance of good posture and good joint position at all times.

(9) Control of the tendency to anaemia deriving both from the rheumatoid process and from gastro-intestinal haemorrhages due to the drugs used in the disease. Women with rheumatoid arthritis who

suffer from heavy menstrual flow should have the severity of the periods controlled by regular hormonal therapy or be considered for hysterectomy.

Family relationships

Many patients with rheumatoid arthritis are 'crotchety' because of their persistent pain and frustration at the limitation it imposes. Naturally personal relationships tend to suffer both at home and at work. Adequate suppression of pain is important from every aspect of the patient's general management. All members of the family need to understand the nature of the disability.

When a man is affected, it may be necessary for him to change employment and to accept a somewhat reduced financial reward. This can lead to domestic stress, and the wife may have to take on a more dominant role in the partnership. When a woman is the patient, then her role in holding the family together may tend to suffer. Certainly rheumatoid arthritis, whoever the sufferer, will have a noticeable impact upon any family. Domestic routines will need to be adapted and the general standard of living may be reduced. Loyalties become divided, and both patient and partner may show real evidence of reactive depression. Such stresses should be guarded against, allowed for, and treated when present.

Need for aids and appliances

Patients with rheumatoid arthritis are faced with the limitation of function imposed by pain and physical disability. Most patients want to retain maximal independence and are reluctant to sacrifice this, even gradually. However, the struggle to retain independence often precipitates further pain and physical limitations. Rehabilitation aims at helping people to think and plan ahead with a realistic attitude to the situation involved. When possible, it forestalls the limitation of function. If restriction of bodily activity is unavoidable, or desirable, good rehabilitation should counsel its acceptance and its circumvention by means of aids and appliances.

A physiotherapist may be able to keep a man walking by exercising and splinting his legs and providing sticks, crutches and walking aids. But should she? An occupational therapist may be able to keep a man independent by teaching him how to dress himself. But should she? By accurate assessment, it becomes apparent at what point in time the physiotherapist is jeopardizing the function of the upper limbs by permitting them to over-compensate for the dysfunction of the lower. It is then that the need for a wheelchair existence is established. By accurate assessment, it becomes obvious when the exertion and pain of dressing becomes so great that it reduces total function by the extent of the fatigue which it induces. It is then evident that help must be accepted with this one activity to enable other activities of daily living to be accomplished.

In general, the majority of disabled patients manage to continue to live an active life without any aids, apparatus, appliances or special equipment and it is often more important to spend time advising them how to do without such aids, than prescribing them. Physical disability does not necessarily mean absolute handicap, for functional handicap is usually relative to architectural, mechanical, domestic, social and financial limitations.

In order to retain *optimal* rather than *maximal* independence, objective assessment and objective discussion with patient and family are essential.

It is necessary for the patient to learn that no lasting good can derive from endurance of a high level of unnecessary pain. For example, a rheumatoid arthritic with involvement of the hip joints can reduce his pain on walking by using crutches, but if he persists in walking the same distance on crutches as he did before he developed rheumatoid arthritis, he is courting disaster. By reducing the weight on his hips, he is increasing the weight on his hands and wrists, and by using them in an abnormal manner he is increasing their chance of becoming painful, inflamed and later deformed. Thus, when walking becomes painful, and it is appropriate to prescribe further analgesics or to recommend surgical procedures, the patient must come to accept one of the following alternatives:

(1) He can plan his daily living activities to avoid undue walking.

(2) He can use some walking assistance, such as crutches, sticks, quadrupeds, tripods or walking aids. If he does use these, however, and his hands, wrists and elbows are affected, he should use gutter crutches to reduce the strain taken by these joints. He should avoid axillary crutches, which have a detrimental effect on the shoulder joints, and also elbow crutches if their use exacerbates the pain in any of the joints of the upper limb or if there is active arthritis in these joints. Nor should he utilize the assistance so much that the structure and function of his arms and hands are prejudiced, and use of assistance *must* be coupled with an overall reduction of the day's activities.

(3) He can use a wheelchair. If the patient's hands are unaffected or relatively unaffected, then propulsion of the wheelchair by his hands is acceptable. If they are potentially or actually severely affected, he may propel with his feet or else resort to a powered chair. In this way, his hands and arms may be saved pain and later dysfunction.

Too many arthritics believe that they are 'giving in' if they resort to a wheelchair, but a wheelchair can so often be a prophylactic measure and could be more widely used with advantage to decrease the demands on a patient's limbs.

There are many simple aids and devices available from hospitals, local authorities and voluntary bodies which enable patients to use unmodified everyday articles. These are mainly personal aids, and those most commonly supplied are:

Bath aids bath seats, non-slip mats, safety handles.
Toilet aids raised W.C. seats, commodes.
Eating aids adapted cutlery, plates and cups.
Dressing aids elastic shoe laces, stocking aids and adapted clothing.
Walking aids sticks, frames.
Household gadgets pick-up sticks to increase reach, adapted kitchen and cooking gadgets to compensate for weak muscles and diminished range of movements, key and tap turners to increase the leverage applicable by weak and painful upper limbs.

For the more severely disabled, larger articles may be supplied to assist function. These pieces of equipment include:

Wheelchairs self-propelled, attendant propelled or electrically propelled.
Beds mechanical, electrical and tilting.
Hoists portable or ceiling tracked.
Chairs adapted or special design.
Kitchens adapted equipment and/or specially designed working surfaces.
Reading aids talking book library, bookrests, page turners.
Writing aids electric typewriters.
Intercommunication devices call systems, adapted telephones.

For the very severely disabled, there are complex sophisticated devices available (e.g. Patient Operated Selector Mechanism) to enable the patient to retain some control over his environment.

Walking aids

Many patients with rheumatoid arthritis will feel the need to resort to some form of weight-relieving assistance early on in the disease when lower limb joints are affected. Initially, a walking stick will help to relieve some of the weight passing through a painful swollen knee joint or hip joint. Many patients will ultimately need to use crutches, but as has been said earlier, axillary crutches should be avoided whenever possible because of their potentially harmful effect on the gleno-humeral joints. Elbow crutches and gutter crutches are more acceptable alternatives but the arm-pieces and forearm gutters often need padding, particularly to overlap sharp edges. Ideally, handgrips of crutches should be purpose-built for each patient from a mould of the patient's grip with his hand in a position of comfort. When facilities for making individual grips do not exist, the handles of the crutches may be bound with foam rubber to widen them or, alternatively, a foam rubber pad attached to a velcro strap may be worn around the palm of the hand. These manœuvres enable the crutches to be gripped firmly even when the hands are severely affected.

At a later stage it may become necessary to use a walking frame in preference to crutches. This should be of a height appropriate to the degree of involvement of the spine and upper limbs, with grips correspondingly sited in the vertical or horizontal plane. All walking aids, sticks, crutches or walking frames should be of the correct height. Sticks and frames usually should be held at the same height as the patient's greater trochanter when the patient is standing upright in shoes. All walking aids should have good broad-based ferrules which should be replaced as they become worn (*see* Chapter 13).

Wheelchairs

Wheelchairs can provide a means of independent progression for those with severe functional impairment of their lower limbs as well as a means of transport of considerable assistance to friends and relatives who manage the general care of the elderly and infirm.

The type of wheelchair required by any one patient needs careful assessment. The specifications may need to be different depending on whether the chair is for indoor or outdoor use, for self-propulsion, or for attendants to push. The final choice of chair depends as much on the home conditions as on the clinical needs. Often the needs cannot all be met in a single chair because of the difficulty in designing a wheelchair which is at once comfortable, light, robust and adaptable. Many of the more disabled wheelchair users will therefore require more than one wheelchair, e.g. one for work and one for home use, and these may be of different design. The design of most standard wheelchairs attempts to embody a compromise between the needs of the patient and his helpers and the demands of his home, his surroundings and his mode of outdoor transport in a composite structure of durable materials and reasonable cost. Since each patient has individual problems, modifications may occasionally be necessary, particularly for the more seriously disabled patients who may have involvement of all four limbs and trunk. Foot plates may need to be extended or built up; armrests, headrests or one or more padded, elevating legrests may be needed. However, as with all appliances, it is necessary for the patient to accept some restriction of his functional capabilities.

In recent years there has been an increasing use of electrically powered indoor wheelchairs for the more severely disabled; for some patients such a chair can prove to be the key to their resettlement.

Although the criteria for eligibility for a powered indoor wheelchair have been an inability to walk coupled with upper-limb disability so severe as to make hand-propulsion impossible, the conditions for supply are gradually changing. Long-term observation of disabled patients, particularly those with rheumatoid arthritis, strongly indicates that the stage of the disease at which they *should* not propel, comes long before the stage at which they *cannot* propel. The prescription of powered indoor chairs at this former stage is a prophylactic measure to prevent accelerated degeneration of the joints of the upper limbs through over-use. Not only does the issue of such a chair produce a considerable gain in functional efficiency in the immediate present by reducing pain and fatigue, but it also leads to prolongation of functional independence in personal care and daily living activities.

Often the conventional modes of controlling standard, powered indoor chairs will need modification to permit their use by the severe rheumatoid arthritic. However, head, chin and 'suck–blow' controls, as well as modified hand-controls, are now offered as alternatives for most standard powered chairs, and one of these is usually found to be suitable.

Usually a patient owning a powered wheelchair for indoor use is not also eligible for powered outdoor transport. From the rheumatoid arthritic patient's point of view, this may often be a matter for discussion. The patient who needs help indoors frequently also needs help outdoors, and the argument that a patient who is capable of controlling outdoor transport should not need a powered indoor chair is fallacious, since effort should be made to help him to conserve his upper and lower limb function.

Outdoor transport

Public transport in Britain is of a high standard of frequency and availability compared to that of many other countries. Such comparison is of no comfort to the rheumatoid arthritic patient who, on a bad day, cannot walk a hundred yards to the bus stop, cannot tolerate the wait in the cold, cannot grasp the grab rail to pull himself on to the bus platform. Even with help he may be unable to flex his hip and knee sufficiently to climb on to the bus. Even if he can manage this, he will probably find that ankylosed or arthrodesed knees are difficult to pack in between the seats. Even more acute is the problem when a further walk awaits a working man at the end of his bus ride before he can reach his place of work, or if a woman has to attempt to carry home a heavy shopping bag while supporting herself on elbow crutches.

To the patient who is moderately disabled, but must still earn his own living or do her own housework, and to the more severely disabled patient who would otherwise be confined to the house, suitable outdoor transport may well be the essential factor in maintaining outdoor independence.

There are several alternatives open to a patient who wants to drive, and those alternatives depend partly on the distribution and severity of his arthritic involvement, and partly on his income.

A mildly disabled patient with rheumatoid arthritis who drives his own car can increase his comfort and efficiency by installing in his car the following pieces of equipment:

(1) A panoramic mirror, an extra inside mirror and an extra wing mirror, to help minimize the amount of neck movement needed.
(2) A headrest integral with the car seat to reduce the chance of whiplash injury.
(3) An adequate heater to keep the car at an even temperature.
(4) A cloth or leather cover for the steering wheel to reduce the discomfort of gripping a rigid, cold, plastic surface with stiff fingers.
(5) Windshields for the windows, to decrease draughts.
(6) A special car seat or a special cushion to avoid backache.
(7) Extra large control knobs.
(8) Automatic transmission.

A more severely disabled patient with stiff, painful lower limb joints can have various hand controls fitted, depending on the nature of his disability. Thus, accelerator, brake and clutch may all be hand-operated with the brakes servo-assisted, so that a light touch can call forth an intensified response. The fitting of automatic transmission is also helpful to an arthritic patient with considerable involvement of the hands. The elimination of the effort of gear changing and clutch operation reduces the multiplicity of minor traumata to the fingers and left foot and prevents the infliction of pain which constant rapid changes of position and grip may precipitate.

As a patient becomes progressively more disabled, provided he has the money to pay for them, a large number of possible conversions can be fitted to the controls to compensate for specific disabilities. A disabled driver must, however, register his disability when applying for his next licence and should take the opportunity of belonging to the Disabled Drivers Association. Membership entitles a person to a sticker for his car and to the club magazine which publishes articles of interest to disabled drivers. Regular social events for members widen the horizons of the disabled driver and enable him to visit places and attempt activities which he might well avoid without the moral support of other disabled people. A disc which he can display will often enable him to park in places prohibited to the general public, so that he is within easy reach of his destination. This can be obtained from the local Social Services Department once he has been registered as disabled.

If a patient with rheumatoid arthritis appears to be eligible for assistance from the Department of Health, an application form (AOF7) is completed by the G.P. or the consultant supervising his treatment and despatched to the nearest Artificial Limb and Appliance Centre (A.L.A.C.). The patient is then called to a Vehicle Clinic at the A.L.A.C., examined by the Appliance Medical Officer, and interviewed and tested by a Ministry Technical Officer. The details of outdoor transport for the disabled are discussed in detail in Chapter 13.

Currently, all disabled drivers suffering from progressive disorders (such as rheumatoid arthritis) and possessing Department vehicles or having Department assistance to convert and maintain their own vehicles are required to report for a yearly medical check-up of their fitness to control their vehicle, followed, if necessary, by a practical demonstration of capability in front of the Department's Technical Officer. This is a wise modification of the old regulations which did not call for regular review and under which it was possible for a patient to deteriorate to a state at which he was unfit to drive without any knowledge of this reaching the supplying Centre.

Hoists

The more severely disabled arthritic patient may need hoisting to enable him to get in and out of bed. The choice lies between a hydraulic portable hoist and an electric hoist.

The hydraulic hoist has the advantage that it can be moved to operate in several places and it is less expensive to buy.

The electric hoist is easier to operate and can be operated by the patient himself. The installation of electric track hoists is expensive and many houses and flats are not sufficiently strongly constructed to bear the combined weight of the equipment and the patient. Free-standing electric hoists which are attached to an overhead gantry supported on four legs are easier and cheaper to provide. Such a hoist usually remains sited over the patient's bed so that he can be transferred from bed to adjacent wheelchair or commode.

The electric hoist is usually chosen for a small helper who is hoisting a tall, heavy, arthritic patient. For such a patient/helper combination the provision of a hydraulic portable hoist is an economy potentially dangerous to both parties. It demands too much physical effort on the part of the small helper who still has to push the heavily loaded hoist from place to place. It may also subject the patient to possible trauma from door frames, walls and furniture as the helper will be unable to push the hoist along and steady the patient at the same time.

DESIGNING AND ADAPTING THE HOME

Many of the day-to-day difficulties of the disabled stem from the structural design of their home, its fittings and furniture. Sensible reorganization and, when necessary, replacement or redesign, can make the life of an arthritic much less difficult and play a large part in maintaining his active life in the community.

Sitting and dining rooms

The sitting and dining rooms used by a rheumatoid arthritic patient must:

(1) Be easy to enter and leave.

(2) Be uncluttered to allow easy circulation within them.

(3) Leave room for the equipment of the patient, e.g. wheelchair or crutches.

(4) Possess at least one easy chair of such a height that the patient can get up and sit down unaided.

(5) Have a table of a suitable height so that a patient with stiff spine and upper limbs may use it in comfort.

(6) Have a carpet rather than a series of rugs on a polished floor, and carpet of such a pile that it does not make it difficult to walk using crutches or other walking aids or to propel a wheelchair.

(7) Have windows and doors which are easily opened and shut.

(8) Have enough space to allow for elevating legrests on a wheelchair or the presence of a long stool of appropriate height so that the patient can sit with his feet up in comfort.

The elderly and disabled tend to spend much of their time sitting down. Selecting a suitable easy chair for them is often difficult. The chair must be of a suitable height so that they can sit down and get up from it without undue effort or discomfort. It must be robust, for such patients tend to 'drop' into the chair and 'lever' themselves out of it, imposing unusual stresses upon it. It must be stable, as the user often tends to slump when sitting and to rock forwards, backwards and sideways in the chair when changing position. The back must be set at a good angle and high enough to give support to the shoulder and head. The seat height is critical and may need to be adjusted by means of 4 wooden blocks attached to the chair legs or by a firm cushion placed in the seat of the chair. It is possible to buy chairs whose legs can be shortened as well as lengthened by means of telescopic 'over legs'. The height of the arms of the chair needs to be such that the patient can push himself up or ease himself down with maximal efficiency and the least possible pain. A patient with stiff, weak hips and perhaps a stiff knee may need a spring-loaded ejector seat for his chair to help him get out of it, or failing that, an ejector seat operated by an air pump or electric motor. Usually, however, precise adjustment of the height of the seat and arms will enable all but the most severely disabled patients to transfer independently.

The shape and contours of a chair contribute more to its overall comfort than the softness of the cushion. There are several chairs marketed for 'geriatric' or hospital use which are likely to be suitable for arthritics, and these are usually available for trial in hospital and residential institutions.

For an arthritic patient with a stiff or fixed hip, sitting can be made more comfortable by using a cushion with a groove cut in the appropriate side. This can be made from plastic foam 3 in (7·5 cm) thick and cut to the shape of the chair seat. A groove is cut 6 in (15·25 cm) wide and 2 in (5 cm) deep on the side corresponding to the patient's affected side and tapered to fit the individual patient. A sheepskin-covered cushion or a sheepskin laid over the standard chair cushion can increase comfort considerably for the patient with very restricted mobility.

Kitchen layout and equipment

A kitchen specially designed or adapted for an ambulant woman with rheumatoid arthritis will differ from that designed for a woman who is chairbound. For the former, the kitchen will be designed to reduce floor space so as to lessen the distance which the patient must walk; for the latter, the floor area will be large enough to permit a wheelchair to be manœuvred easily between cooker, sink, refrigerator and working surfaces. In both kitchens, the heights of the fixtures, the ease with which they can be utilized, and the dimensions and weights of the utensils they contain are equally critical.

In order for the patient to avoid lifting or carrying heavy saucepans, all the working surfaces should be of the same level, so that pans can be slid to and from the stove, working surface and sink. Split-level cookers are helpful and a trolley with one shelf flush with the oven allows oven-cooked food to be slid in and out without lifting. Such a trolley is invaluable, for it can be pushed around the kitchen or even the house, and its many tiers can carry crockery, cutlery and cleaning equipment from place to place. It also acts as a walking aid when equipped with handles and two rubber-tipped legs in addition to its castors or wheels. By doing triple duty as an extra shelf, equipment carrier and walking aid, it saves space in the house which might tend to become cluttered with equipment.

A sink needs to be the exact height at which a woman can stand and work without getting backache, and should, whenever possible, be installed by the plumber with the patient standing beside him to indicate the exact height needed for her comfort. Similarly, the working surfaces should not only be flush with each other, but also of a suitable height for the rheumatoid patient to use them either from her wheelchair or working stool.

Kitchen floors need a surface which is non-slip and easily cleaned, such as plastic tiles or vinyl sheet flooring.

Cupboards and drawers need to be sited at a convenient height calculated to avoid undue stooping and stretching. Doors should open easily and runners should glide smoothly.

Where possible, taps should be fitted with lever handles and sited in whichever position is best for the patient, possibly at the side rather than at the back of the sink. If the kitchen is not purpose built, or structural alterations are not possible, the use of a long-handled tap turner makes the use of standard taps much easier.

Laundry

Washing presents great problems to the rheumatoid arthritic patient, especially when she has a young family. An automatic washing machine, with a tumbler drier, is an expensive but justifiable piece of equipment. If a non-automatic machine and spin drier are used, the use of a rotating clothes-line enables the patient to peg out her clothes while sitting on a stool or in her wheelchair.

Ironing is another chore calculated to cause pain in many affected joints of the woman with rheumatoid disease. If it is done from the sitting position, at a table or board of the right height, using a lightweight iron, much of the effort and consequent pain and stiffness may be avoided. Whenever possible, clothing and household linen should be drip-dry and the total amount of ironing reduced to a minimum.

Heating and electrical supply

Solid fuel heating is contra-indicated for a patient with rheumatoid arthritis unless someone else is responsible for bringing in the coal, making up and cleaning out the fires. Even then, the use of coal fires should be avoided and a more even temperature aimed at by adopting some form of central heating, boosted when necessary by gas or electric fires. It matters not whether the central heating is gas-fired, oil-fired or all electric, provided it is adequate and economical. If cost is an important factor, the use of night-storage heaters, which use electricity at off-peak times, is an economy.

Electric power plug sockets should be installed at waist level and the on/off switches chosen for ease of manipulation.

Bedroom

Bedroom furniture should be stable and strategically placed to provide support and yet permit easy passage around it. A bed which backs on to a wall allows transfers to be made from either side, although it is sometimes preferable to place one side of the bed against a wall so that it is extra stable when it is necessary to push on the bed to stand upright from the seated position. Height is also important when difficulty is experienced in transferring from bed to chair, wheelchair or the standing position, and wooden blocks of the appropriate height, with recesses for the legs of the bed, can be used to raise or lower it to the desired level. A firm mattress, either laid on a hard-based bed or supported by a board beneath it, makes it easier to move within the bed as well as to and from it, and is of prophylactic value in that it discourages spinal and hip deformity. For people with stiff hips, the adjustment of bed height may be critical; but to retain independence for transfers in and out of bed, patients may need more than this adjustment. The use of a bed-ladder facilitates sitting up in bed for those with stiff, weak spines and hips. Such a ladder is made from two lengths of rope or heavy sash cord which are threaded through holes in steps made from short lengths of wooden broom handle and knotted between the steps. One end is attached to the bed rail above the bed-clothes. The patient hauls on the far end, and by climbing the steps with his hands gradually pulls himself to an upright position.

Continental quilts (duvets) or cellular blankets of man-made fibre are lighter than the conventional woollen blankets, and patients may prefer to use them in order to reduce pressure on weak and painful limbs and make turning in bed easier. If traditional heavy bed-clothes are used, a bed cradle may be helpful.

Toilets and bathrooms

Ideally, bathrooms and toilets should have their fixtures specially sited for patients disabled with rheumatoid arthritis. In actual practice, this seldom occurs, and most arthritic patients must manage in rooms of conventional design. There are several relatively minor modifications which can be made to facilitate their use. Often it is only necessary to ensure that the toilet seat is raised to the correct height for the arthritic patient concerned so that he is immediately able to use the toilet without difficulty. In addition, it may be necessary to fit grab rails at appropriate positions on the toilet wall or to fit a standing rail beside the pedestal to make it easier to sit down or rise up from the toilet seat. The toilet door-handle may need alteration, as may the key or bolt, to enable them to be manipulated by the arthritic patient with deformed fingers.

Toilet flush levers are notoriously stiff. and the standard toilet chain may be difficult to reach and painful to pull. The addition of a large knob-like handle whether to the lever or the chain and the extension of the latter to bring the handle to a position which can easily be reached by the patient prevents toilet flushing being an exercise in ingenuity and pain endurance.

The type of toilet seat-raise advocated depends on the needs and wishes of the family, as well as those of the patient. Plastic overseats of several types are available commercially, with special modifications for the person with an arthrodesed hip. These have the advantage that they can accompany the patient when he goes to other houses (suitably transported in a light suitcase). More comfortable, and stable, for the average patient is a fixed wooden, box-like seat reminiscent of Victorian toilets and easily constructed by a local carpenter to fit over the existing pedestal and seat. The top of the overseat is hinged to allow cleaning of the flush pedestal.

Getting in and out of the bath is difficult for the arthritic, and because of the hard, wet surfaces, the activity is potentially dangerous. For the more severely disabled, the elderly and the frail, some assistance from another person for undressing and entering the bath, and for getting out and dressing is more sensible than trying to arrange wall rails or hoists.

The most useful and simple bath aid is a bath seat, and the most useful bath seat is one which fits firmly into the bath at one end and which extends to form a bath-side stool. A second seat, attached and placed in the bath, can be used either as a 'half-way seat' before actually sitting in the bath, or can be used to sit on for the bathing process. Wall rails should be used in conjunction with the bath seat or on their own, but they must have a non-slip surface and must be fitted at the position and angle most useful for the individual patient.

Whenever possible, a practical assessment by an experienced occupational therapist should be carried out in the patient's own home.

It is likely that a combination of bath board, bath seat and wall rail with non-slip surface, together with a non-slip mat in the bath will make bathing an easier and safer activity for the arthritic patient. Whenever there is doubt about the patient's capability, it is wisest to advise that bathing should only be attempted with the assistance of a competent helper.

For the very severely disabled, it is possible to use a hoist, either portable or attached to a ceiling track. If this is not possible, then arrangements can be made for the patient to be given a regular bed bath or to attend the local hospital or day centre where bathing can be carried out by skilled personnel.

MENSTRUATION, CONTRACEPTION AND MARRIAGE

The management of the menstrual cycle and pregnancies of a woman with rheumatoid arthritis occupies an important part of the total management of the disease.

Menstruation

No patient with rheumatoid arthritis who still has persistently heavy periods following treatment of her rheumatoid condition can be considered as fully rehabilitated if rehabilitation is considered as 'return to as full and normal an everyday life as possible'. Anaemia secondary to heavy menstrual loss can be debilitating in any woman but may be particularly so in a woman with rheumatoid arthritis, exacerbating her fatigue and depression and aggravating any anaemia due to the disease itself.

In the treatment of such heavy periods, an investigatory dilation and curretage is an essential preliminary. Preparations of progestogen or combination of progestogen with oestrogen may be used to regulate or suppress menstruation, but this is not without risk. Hysterectomy must be seriously considered as a method of preventing heavy menstrual loss if the administration of regular iron is not able to offset this. If there is some reason why a hysterectomy should not be undertaken, then a radiation menopause—whether by radium insertion or irradiation of the pelvis—should be considered as an alternative, and gynaecological advice should be sought in this matter.

Marriage

When possible, it is desirable that a doctor should discuss the difficulties of a marriage in which one of the partners has rheumatoid arthritis, with both of the partners concerned. The fact that malaise and pain can seriously inhibit both the wish and the ability to make love must not be construed as coldness on the part of the affected partner.

If long continued pain or deformity of the lower limbs makes intercourse in the customary position impractical or impossible, the timely instruction of the husband and wife in alternative postures for intercourse may save the marriage from tension and collapse. Many orthopaedic surgeons now accept that inability to have normal intercourse is a strong indication for corrective surgery, and total hip replacement to permit hip abduction may be undertaken for this reason.

Contraception

In the presence of abnormal periods, pelvic irradiation or hysterectomy may be indicated to prevent both unwanted periods and unwanted pregnancies. When the periods are normal, however, other methods of contraception may be indicated. At the present time there is no evidence that the use of the contraceptive pill is any more risky than for a non-arthritic woman. Indeed, it is probably the contraceptive method of choice, for a cervical cap or diaphragm may be difficult for a woman with painful or deformed fingers to insert, particularly if she also has involvement of the joints of her lower limbs. A tubal ligation is a relatively simple operation, which can be done under local anaesthetic, and provides an effective and permanent method of contraception. The insertion of an intra-uterine device is an alternative method but may cause heavier menstrual loss and may not be feasible in a woman with painful stiff lower limbs and spine.

When the male partner of the marriage has rheumatoid arthritis, it is appropriate that it should be he who adopts contraceptive measures, when no further children are wanted, by procuring a vasectomy. During intervals in which temporary contraception is employed during acute phases of the disease in either partner, the use of a penile sheath by the husband is probably the simplest procedure.

It is a matter for discussion with the family whether contraception is best practised by the wife or the husband. Should it be necessary to use a contraceptive method which could lead to sterility, it has been suggested that there might be good psychological reasons for the affected person, rather than the healthy person, to adopt this. The reasons underlying this view are that disability in one partner often induces resentment in the spouse. Should the spouse be expected to accept sterility as well as a disabled partner, the resentment may well be considerable. However, as with physically able-bodied couples, discussion with a doctor experienced in family planning can help to resolve many of the difficulties. Certainly a woman with rheumatoid arthritis can be saved the risks of the pill and the difficulties attendant upon other forms of contraception if her husband agrees to vasectomy.

Pregnancy

It is impossible to lay down hard and fast rules about the most desirable number of children in a family in which one of the partners has rheumatoid arthritis. The final choice must lie with the affected partner, and the doctor can only help by advising accurately about the factors involved in the choice. It must be made clear to both parents how essential it is to avoid physical and mental strain, and the family should be limited to a size which is unlikely to produce such strain either in the mother who cares for it or in the father who earns for it.

Women with rheumatoid arthritis are often very well during their pregnancy. Symptoms are reduced and disease activity apparently slows down. This often makes them reluctant to accept advice about limiting the size of the family. However, it is necessary to discuss frankly with her and her husband the advisability of having a family, emphasizing that young children can be a considerable physical burden.

In a woman with severe rheumatoid arthritis, when birth must be by Caesarean section because of pelvic abnormalities or severe hip involvement, it may be considered advisable to follow the second Caesarean by bilateral tubal ligation or by hysterectomy.

WORK AND LEISURE

Planning for return to work

In rheumatoid arthritis, as with other disabilities, resettlement in work depends on many factors other than the severity of the disability. The nature of the work, the patient's education and domestic background must all be considered together with social and economic factors. Early planning must be the responsibility of the consultant in charge of the patient, and early decisions can be helped by an efficient rehabilitation and resettlement organization bringing about the necessary integration of the provisions of the Departments of Health, Education and Productivity, and Local Authorities.

The majority of patients with rheumatoid arthritis are able to pursue their usual activities in the early stages of the disease process, and many are able to continue in their chosen employment until normal retiring age. However, most patients are faced with some limitation in their physical activities. This limitation may interfere with employment if it cannot be overcome by some mechanical aid or device and a planned approach to the total management of the disease.

The manual worker and the housewife with a large family will almost certainly have to accept some restrictions. For the housewife, these restrictions in physical activity may usually be offset by the use of appropriate aids and appliances, but the unskilled manual worker may well need to change his employment for something less physically demanding. Office and sedentary workers will usually be able to continue in their previous employment, providing the mode of travel to and from work is well within their physical capabilities. Some skilled workers may have to change their employment if their hands are severely affected or if their work demands awkward positions, prolonged standing at a work-bench, or over-much walking when there is severe involvement of weight-bearing joints.

It is often difficult for the employer to understand the complexity of establishing a realistic prognosis either in terms of persistent handicap or rate of deterioration. It is only by accurate assessment of a man's work potential that a basis for retraining or reallocation of duties can be found. The importance of this assessment cannot be over-emphasized and will depend upon a careful appraisal and recording of:

(1) The patient's symptoms, particularly morning stiffness and joint pain.

(2) His functional capabilities as determined by objective trials wherever possible.

(3) The number of joints involved and the severity of their involvement in terms of pain, reduced range and instability.

(4) Functional expressions of joint range and muscle power in terms of mobility and dexterity.

(5) Clinical tests, e.g. of the sedimentation rate and haemoglobin level, and quantitative tests for rheumatoid factor.

Repeated, careful, quantitative assessments will indicate the rate of progress of the disease and so help the clinician to evaluate the patient's work potential.

Frank discussion between the clinician, patient and employer based upon these assessments will usually bring about a satisfactory readjustment of the patient's working conditions. When it is not possible for the situation to be resolved in this simple fashion, then there may be a need to resort to the official organization designed to resettle and, when necessary, retrain a patient for an occupation more appropriate to his disability.

It is important that the question of return to work should be considered as early as possible during the hospital admission of any patient, since concern about his future may be a potent cause of worry or even depression. In the first instance, return to a patient's last place of work should always be attempted and negotiations for his return to his previous job should be opened by the medical social worker or the patient himself. Failing this, the next best thing is to return to work for his old employers in another capacity. Only when these two possibilities have been adequately explored should re-employment or retraining be considered.

Resettlement in work

In the United Kingdom, there is a Disablement Resettlement Officer at each of the Employment Exchanges, and it is his special responsibility to find suitable work for disabled men and women. A Disabled Persons Register to which any person with a physical impairment can apply for registration, is maintained at every Employment Exchange and certain jobs can be reserved for those who are registered. So far, only passenger-accommodating electric lift attendants and car park attendants are so designated, but many firms employ more than their 'quota' of disabled.

There are 21 Industrial Rehabilitation Units in the United Kingdom providing work assessment facilities. After a period of assessment lasting 6–7 weeks, full training in one of the 40–50 trades at a technical or commercial college or Government Training Centre may be available.

Collaboration between hospital workers, social workers, Disablement Resettlement Officers, Industrial Rehabilitation Units and Government Training Centres must be very close if the disabled person is to be satisfactorily resettled. It is particularly difficult to match the physical capabilities and disabilities of the rheumatoid patient with the available openings in industry, while yet permitting the well-regulated home-based living which is so essential to the successful management of the disease.

For the more severely disabled patients, sheltered workshops provide work under conditions somewhat less stressful than those found in open industry, but the employees in such workshops still have to be capable of a level of productivity not far short of that of open industry.

Occupational Centres provide diversional therapy and are the responsibility of the Local Authority. Patients attending these Centres receive a limited amount of financial recompense ('pocket money', not a wage). Some patients may achieve work at home (e.g. dressmaking, copy-typing or providing a telephone answering service), but this type of work is often poorly paid and unsatisfying.

Hobbies

For those unable to work, hobbies can play a large and important part in their lives, as they may bring about social contacts and creative activities which compensate for the frustrations of disability. Previous training and interests influence the choice of hobby and leisure pursuits, but it is part of rehabilitation to explore the possibilities and to help the patient to develop at least one creative activity over and above his activities of daily living. Even when the disability is severe, with help and appropriate aids, many patients can develop surprising and worthwhile hobbies.

SURGERY IN RHEUMATOID ARTHRITIS

It is becoming increasingly difficult to consider the total care of patients with rheumatoid arthritis without close collaboration between physician and surgeon on both out-patient and in-patient basis. As surgical procedures become a more frequent episode in the management of the disease, it is necessary to consider the part which rehabilitation services play both pre-operatively and post-operatively.

Firstly, a patient's response to simple rehabilitation can be an important measure of his 'motivation' and can indicate whether he is likely to respond well to major surgical procedures. Assessment of the patient as a whole—his personality, social background and attitude to his disease—is one of the important preliminaries to the planning of surgical treatment.

Assessment of clinical condition

A general assessment of the patient's clinical condition is the second prerequisite to surgical intervention. If surgery is proposed for several joints, the surgical programme may be protracted and a long period of hospitalization must be contemplated. The physical stamina of the patient must be carefully evaluated and probable functional gains must be balanced against possible functional losses. Furthermore, any alteration in the functional capacity of one limb may have considerable repercussions on his overall activity. Thus, for example, it is unwise to plan reconstructive surgery of a lower limb if the severity of the involvement of the upper limbs completely precludes the use of walking aids. However, such lower limb surgery may be justified even when walking is not contemplated post-operatively if that surgery can offer either pain relief, a better sitting posture, or an increased mobility of some joint which will facilitate personal care or transfers. For example, the mobilization of extended adducted hips will permit comfortable sitting and easier perineal cleaning and toiletting.

As involvement of the cervical spine in the rheumatoid process is relatively common, pre-operative radiography of this region is essential to exclude atlanto-axial instability. The presence of such instability demands special precautions during anaesthesia. These include the use of an adequate collar throughout the period during which the patient is unconscious and the employment of particular care when the unconscious patient is transferred between bed, stretcher and operating table. Failure to take adequate precautions could be fatal.

Local disease

It is the severity and extent of tissue destruction which the disease causes in each locality that finally determines the choice of joint and type of operation to be selected for its repair. Assessment of the extent of the disease will depend upon:

(1) Pain and stiffness, swelling, loss of active movement, loss of range of passive movement and joint instability.
(2) Radiographic appearance of joints.
(3) Assessment of the amount of joint destruction.

General indications for surgical intervention

Synovectomy is indicated when there is persistent 'boggy' swelling of one or two joints only. In addition to the reliable relief of pain and swelling, the operation may have a dual effect: it may be prophylactic against a more severe involvement of the joint operated upon, while also inducing remission in the general rheumatoid disease.

Reconstructive operations, arthroplasties in various forms or surgical procedures involving tendons are called for when the possibility of functional improvement exists. Finally, in the late stages of the disease when permanent deformity has supervened and the normal anatomical framework of the joints has been destroyed, salvage operations, often involving ablation of certain joints, with arthrodeses and excision arthroplasties of others, may give surprisingly good functional results.

In planning surgery, it is necessary to ask not 'what *is* the functional level' but 'what is the functional level *likely* to be'. The smaller the disability, the better the end result of its surgical treatment. Unfortunately, as patients with rheumatoid arthritis are continually adapting themselves to the slow progress of their disabling disease, they are relunctant to accept reconstructive surgery unless some major disability forces them to do so. In this way the most rewarding procedures are often left unperformed. It is important that patients with rheumatoid arthritis should be educated in the value of simple surgery with known good results and minimal need for rehabilitative treatment (currently the most effective operations in this category are excision of the lower end of the ulna and excision arthroplasty of the metatarsophalangeal joints).

The precise nature of the operation offered for any particular joint must be decided after careful analysis of the patient's functional capabilities and deficits. It aims most commonly at an end result which is a compromise between optimal mobility and optimal stability. Each surgical procedure needs to be followed by early ambulation, early mobilization of the affected joints, and rapid resumption of daily living activities.

The interrelationship between upper limb joints in particular needs careful study before operation is undertaken. A fixed elbow demands good forward flexion of the shoulder and palmar flexion of the wrist if the hand is to be able to reach the mouth during feeding. Loss of pronation and supination can be compensated for by abduction and rotation of the shoulder and, conversely, loss of shoulder range can be partly offset by re-establishing pronation and supination.

In general terms, surgery for a joint should be seriously considered when an intensive trial of conservative measures has been unsuccessful.

Surgery of the upper limb

Shoulder

Primary involvement of the shoulder in the inflammatory polyarthritis of rheumatoid disease, or later secondary involvement following the development of a degenerative arthritis of over-use may both give rise to pain and restriction of movement which are distressing and disabling in their effect.

Nevertheless, provided a regular exercise regime is consistently followed and adequate medication given, in the majority of cases, joint function is comparatively well preserved, even in the presence of considerable structural damage. Local injection of corticosteroids is also helpful but should be used with discretion since evidence is accumulating that bone erosion can follow its repeated use.

Acromionectomy has much to offer in joints in which upward humeral displacement has caused a severe and painful acromial reaction, but surgery on the glenohumeral joint has not provided consistent functional gain or pain relief. Although some centres are assessing total replacement with prosthetic devices, this technique has not yet had the success of total hip replacement.

Protection of the shoulder joint from over-use and misuse may be assisted by:

(1) Prescribing elbow rather than axillary crutches.

(2) Advocating wheelchair use rather than excessive crutch-assisted walking.

(3) Prescribing an electrically propelled chair when self-propulsion becomes painful.

(4) Prescribing a hoist when independent transfers demand excessive shoulder action and induce pain.

The elbow

Synovectomy and debridement with or without removal of the radial head may bring considerable relief from pain. Bilateral elbow involvement is very disabling and is an indication for arthroplasty on one side. Stills Disease is often associated with bilateral ankylosis, and excision arthroplasty of one elbow can restore considerable function. Bilateral excision arthroplasty is seldom performed, as the patient usually requires one stable elbow to push himself up from the chair seat, or to ease his position in a wheelchair. Internal prostheses are being developed which offer stability as well as mobility and are likely to be increasingly used in treatment.

For ambulant patients with elbow involvement, forearm gutter crutches help to distribute the load in a more acceptable pattern.

The wrist

Arthrodesis of one or both wrists has been advocated for many years for patients with painful, unstable joints. However, the wrist cannot be considered in isolation. With restricted shoulder and elbow movement, wrist mobility may be the only movement which provides independence for feeding. Pronation and supination of the forearm can substitute for shoulder rotation and palmar flexion and dorsal extension of the wrist can compensate for loss of elbow movement.

Although popular in the past, arthrodesis of the wrist is seldom necessary. Should it be considered, a light-weight plastic splint will adequately mimic the end result, allowing the functional gains and losses to be assessed by patient and therapists. Excision of the lower end of the ulna often produces good results, but after this operation some patients require a wrist splint while working.

Synovectomy of the wrist joint and excision of the sheaths of tendons where proliferative tenosynovitis is endangering the integrity of the tendons are two prophylactic procedures which may be of great value in preserving hand function.

The hand

Much has been written on the details of surgery of the rheumatoid hand, but the purposes of surgical management can be summed up in two words—prevention and salvage.

Surgical management aims to prevent deformities by early synovectomy and decompression of affected joints and to restore function, particularly punch and pinch grip, by a variety of stabilizing and reconstructive procedures. Synovectomy of the metacarpophalangeal joints is believed to have a valuable prophylactic effect when performed early enough.

Arthrodesis of the unstable, dislocating thumb, arthrodesis in flexion of a hyperextended proximal interphalangeal joint, and arthroplasty of subluxed deviated metacarpophalangeal joints are now routine procedures. Osteotomy may be necessary to convert ankylosed fingers from extension to flexion. Combined with soft-tissue surgery, such procedures can often convert the severely damaged hand into a useful prehensile organ once again, but careful evaluation of the probable functional gain to the patient must be an essential preliminary to the decision to operate.

Surgery of the lower limb

Although the main function of the lower limb is weight-bearing, enough mobility must be maintained to permit comfortable sitting and the performance of everyday activities (particularly toilet). Surgical procedures designed to regain mobility must also give relief from pain and yet retain a reasonable stability for the joints concerned.

Problems often arise later, as the disease progresses, or as degenerative changes supervene or some other disaster occurs. It is paradoxical but often true that in order to achieve walking independence, lower limb operations should aim at joint stability, whereas for a comfortable wheelchair existence, joint mobility is more important. Furthermore, for patients with progressive disease, walking sticks or crutches can be severely destructive for the shoulders.

If the patient is unable to achieve walking and has to remain in his wheelchair, the combination of restricted hip movements and stiff knees can often be disastrous. Inability to flex the knee and thus reduce the overall 'sitting length' make wheelchair existence in a normal house impossible.

Likely surgical procedures for the lower limbs are: excision of the femoral head, total joint replacement for the hip; synovectomy, joint debridement, patellectomy, arthroplasty, proximal tibial osteotomy, and arthrodesis of the knee.

The hip

When rheumatoid disease affects the hip, the resulting arthritis is usually painful and debilitating and leads to flexion and abduction deformity. Walking is voluntarily restricted to prevent the pain which weight-bearing induces, and the tendency to avoid activity by prolonged sitting further encourages the development of these deformities.

Excision arthroplasty of the painful rheumatoid hip should, nowadays, be reserved for the wheelchair-bound patient. For other patients, total hip replacement is the operation of choice.

For both these procedures, and for soft-tissue release operations, certain criteria must be fulfilled. A good range of joint movement pre-operatively, and the ability to perform a rigorous regime of exercises post-operatively are essential if good results are to be obtained. This regime includes continuous balanced traction and prolonged crutch walking and may be a more strenuous programme of activity than a debilitated patient with widespread joint involvement is able to tolerate.

Arthrodesis of the hip is contra-indicated in the rheumatoid patient, both because of the progressive nature of the disease, which leads to increasingly severe involvement of other joints, and also because of the adverse effect which fixation of one hip inevitably has upon the spine and the other hip.

Total hip prosthetic replacement may present technical difficulties in the presence of osteoporosis and may be unjustifiable when many other joints are involved. Nevertheless, total hip replacement, using the prostheses of McKee-Farrer and Charnley, is being increasingly used for the relief of pain and deformity of the rheumatoid hip. Painless movement is produced in 90 per cent of cases, although full range is seldom, if ever, attained, and there is often a residual limp.

Non-weight-bearing exercises are started on the first or second day post-operatively, using either balanced slings or else free movements and an abduction pillow. Although some surgeons permit immediate weight-bearing, many prefer to delay this for a few days. Strong abduction is essential, and abduction exercises must be practised assiduously. Flexion is promoted by use of a slippery board. Although most patients are allowed home 3 weeks post-operatively, there is a definite risk of prosthetic subluxation until adequate fibrous tissue has developed, and patients should be urged to avoid sitting on low chairs or stools which demand a squatting position and the provocative flexion/rotation movements of the hip.

The knee

The achievement and maintenance of full extension of the knee is the constant aim during all stages of rheumatoid arthritis. Without a straight knee, walking becomes increasingly difficult and painful. It is seldom that a rheumatoid patient can be bed-ridden for long without developing a flexion deformity of the knee, particularly if active preventive measures to avoid this are not taken during the period of bed rest, and if he has not subsequently returned to active life.

During the early stages of involvement of the joint, synovectomy is often undertaken to provide relief from pain and swelling. In about 90 per cent of cases, these features are considerably improved, although some loss of movement may result. Early mobilization is encouraged within the support of a firm supporting bandage.

During the later stages, when structural damage has occurred in the articular surfaces of the knee, reconstructive surgery may be indicated. For the moderately damaged joint, partial replacement arthroplasty by means of metal replacements for one or both tibial condyles (MacIntosh, McKeever) or for the femoral condyles (Platt) may achieve realignment, return of joint stability, and 90 per cent of flexion from full extension.

For a more severely damaged knee, similar results may sometimes be attained by one of the total replacement techniques of Walldius, Shiers and Young, in which metal hinges, with or without cement, are substituted for the entire knee joint. There are now several experimental prostheses which attempt to mimic the rolling and gliding movements of the knee and may well eventually replace the metal hinges.

Early active movements are encouraged within the firm bandage which supports the knee post-operatively, and full mobilization follows suture removal.

Total knee replacement should always be considered as an alternative to arthrodesing the joint to relieve pain or restore joint mobility.

Arthrodesis of a knee certainly provides a stable and pain-free joint, but is only suitable for patients with limited involvement of other joints. In addition to causing 3–4 cm of leg shortening, it may exacerbate pain in the hips and spine if active joint disease is present in these regions. Without a good range of hip movement it may cause further disablement, and even when hip movement is adequate a stiff knee is a social handicap. Bilateral arthrodeses should only be undertaken in exceptional circumstances, since two stiff knees make sitting down and getting up independently almost impossible.

Post-operative care

Orthopaedic surgeons vary considerably in the post-operative rehabilitation programme which they advocate. After most surgical procedures, and particularly after synovectomy, early active movement is encouraged within 48 hours of surgery. Indeed, the general principles for physical therapy are not dissimilar from those described for the patient with acute early rheumatoid disease. Activity is gentle, non-resisted and encouraged in short, frequent sessions. The amount and vigour is largely determined by the patient's response to the activity. Passive movements and manipulative procedures are usually unnecessary and often contra-indicated. Total joint replacements are usually followed by early mobilization in the same manner, the surgeon giving clear guidance on the expected rate of recovery and a clear indication of any necessary restrictions on activity.

Many post-operative regimes will depend upon the availability of staff and facilities. Balanced slings and hydrotherapy will often be advised where they are easily accessible to the ward.

General surgical consideration

Arthroplasty by total replacement techniques and arthrodesis are the two forms of lower limb joint surgery which offer immediate post-operative freedom from joint pain.

Many rheumatoid patients have already had long and depressing histories of pain and systemic disease before they come to surgery, and therefore may not tolerate well the relatively long and demanding period of post-operative rehabilitation which some types of reconstructive surgery entail. Convalescence is often further complicated with osteoporosis, muscle wasting and soft-tissue contractures.

Despite the continued advances of surgical techniques, surgery can never be a substitute for suppressive and palliative drug therapy and the general medical care of the rheumatoid patient. It is against a background of well-planned medication that surgery stands its best chance of success. For this reason, the best form of hospital care is provided by special units where medical and surgical care can be shared by physician and surgeon, and surgical treatment and rehabilitation are completely integrated into the patient's total management.

CONCLUSION

Rehabilitation of a patient with rheumatoid arthritis is a complex exercise in general and specific management, requiring close collaboration between general practitioner, rheumatologist and surgeon, together with close understanding of the facilities available for helping the patient to obtain maximal functional independence at home and at work. The balance between rest and activity, the need for aids and appliances, and the timing of prophylactic or reconstructive surgery are all problems which require careful assessment for each patient.

The general clinical care and the physical management of disability cannot be separated, for each is dependent on the other. The problems involved place a considerable onus upon the clinician, but he must not abrogate the responsibility if his patients are to achieve optimal function within the limits imposed by their disease. The rehabilitation of the rheumatoid arthritic must be part of the total patient management and for many patients is the major part of their management.

BIBLIOGRAPHY AND REFERENCES

Conaty, J. P. and Nickel, V. L. (1971). 'Functional incapacitation in rheumatoid arthritis: a rehabilitation challenge. A correlative study of function before and after hospital treatment.' *J. Bone Jt Surg.* **53A**, 624

Duthie, J. J. R. (1967). 'Medical management and prognosis in rheumatoid arthritis.' *Scott. med. J.* **12**, 96

Duthie, J. J. R., Brown, P. E., Truelove, L. H., Baragar, F. D. and Lawrie, A. J. (1964). 'Course and prognosis in rheumatoid arthritis.' *Ann. rheum. Dis.* **23**, 193

Mowat, A. G. (1970). 'Basic medical treatment in rheumatoid arthritis.' *Physiotherapy,* **56**, 450

5—Pain in the Neck and Shoulder

INTRODUCTION

A large number of the patients seeking medical advice complain of pain in the neck and arm, or of a painful stiff shoulder. An even larger number have these symptoms and do not consult a doctor. Of the latter group some consult various unqualified practitioners and others prescribe their own analgesics or palliative treatment. The total number of people involved is enormous.

Of those who consult their general practitioner, many are treated and cured, and it is only those with persistent, severe or frequently recurring symptoms who are referred for consultant advice. Such patients may be referred to medical, orthopaedic, neurological or rheumatological out-patient departments, and they certainly constitute a very large proportion of all patients referred for physiotherapy treatment.

The particular referral depends upon such factors as the frequency of the clinics, waiting list for radiological examination, waiting time for individual clinics, as well as clinical findings. The presence of neurological signs will tend to direct a patient to neurological or neurosurgical consultation, whereas a recurrent wry-neck is more likely to lead to an orthopaedic consultation. A painful stiff shoulder may be considered orthopaedic or rheumatological, often depending upon the waiting time for out-patient appointments.

In all instances there is considerable pressure for the provision of physiotherapy, for there is a general belief that physical treatment is helpful in these conditions.

There is however a wide range of clinical syndromes which present with localized or widespread pain in the neck and arm, with stiffness of the neck or shoulder, with paraesthesia in the arm, or with any combination of these symptoms.

In this chapter we discuss the two main groups of patients: those with a painful stiff shoulder and those in whom the symptoms appear to arise from degenerative changes in the cervical spine.

THE PAINFUL STIFF SHOULDER

General

Pain in the shoulder, with or without restriction of shoulder movements, is a very common symptom. Frequently it is considered to be an accompaniment of cervical spondylosis, although in retrospect the association may be shown to be fortuitous. The condition masquerades under names such as capsulitis, 'frozen shoulder', periarthritis and rotator cuff lesion. Too often authors use these names indiscriminately and as though they were interchangeable; others are precise in defining the different symptoms and signs relating to different and sometimes hypothetical, soft-tissue lesions. Sometimes it is clear that pain in the shoulders is the result of cervical root irritation; limitation of neck movements, the association of paraesthesia with certain positions of the neck, tenderness in the supraclavicular fossa or along the major nerve trunks are all indications of the cervical origin of the symptoms. In all such cases, attention must be directed towards the neck. The majority of patients with shoulder pain appear to be suffering from one of a number of soft-tissue lesions which are self-limiting and rarely associated with prolonged serious disability, but it should be remembered that sometimes pain in the shoulder is a presenting symptom of a serious systemic disease. General limitation of glenohumeral movements, alteration in the scapulohumeral rhythm or limitation of abduction or adduction of the arm and localized pain associated with specific shoulder movements are all signs directing attention to the soft tissues of the shoulder joint. Localized tenderness and pain on 'springing' the acromioclavicular joint can draw attention to a localized and treatable arthritis of that joint.

Shoulder pain can arise from so many causes, the exact pathology of which has not yet been clearly defined, that unless there is definitive radiological or surgical evidence to establish a precise diagnosis, the indication for any particular form of physiotherapy must be correspondingly imprecise.

It is generally accepted that the painful stiff shoulder improves within a period of 9 months whatever the mode of treatment, and sometimes in spite of it. Worthwhile literature on the subject is scanty, the classifications of the cause of painful shoulder are mostly unhelpful and the published trials of treatment frequently unacceptable. Diagnostic factors are debatable; the clinical features, the methods of examination and measurement, and modes of treatment are not amenable to standardization. The symptoms are often associated with an emotional response and influenced by psychological factors.

Rotator cuff lesions

Shoulder pain which is aching in character but which becomes acute when the patient performs certain specific manœuvres is often loosely diagnosed as a rotator cuff lesion, or supraspinatus tendinitis. There are many different causes of this type of shoulder pain. Frequently the nature of the lesion is demonstrable by careful examination.

Supraspinatus lesions are characterized by a painful arc of movement in the mid-range of active abduction and adduction. Sometimes the lesion may be localized by tenderness on palpation along the length of the muscles.

There is some evidence that the critical zone of the rotator cuff, in which tears and calcified deposits tend to occur, coincides with that part of the cuff in which the main anastomoses between osseous and tendinous vessels take place, which is much less vascular than other parts of the musculotendinous cuff.

Bicipital tendinitis can sometimes be diagnosed by elicitation of localized tenderness over the tendon of the long head of the biceps when the upper arm is externally rotated.

Both bicipital tendinitis and supraspinatus tendinitis often respond well to the local injection of hydrocortisone, although there is always a risk that this treatment may precipitate tendon rupture and that repeated injections may cause local necrosis.

Calcific deposits in the tendons of the supraspinatus, long head of biceps or subdeltoid bursa may produce an aching pain and stiffness of the shoulder so severe that surgical intervention becomes necessary. The calcified deposits are removed, adhesions divided, and any tendon ruptures repaired, resulting in considerable symptomatic relief.

Capsulitis

The condition in which pain in the shoulder is associated with a gross reduction in all planes of movement of the shoulder joint is called capsulitis or periarthritis. Sometimes arising for no apparent reason, it may also be associated with a more sinister condition such as:

Angina or coronary insufficiency.
Hemiplegia.
Parkinsonism.
Neoplasm of upper lobe of lung or bronchi.
Neoplasm of breast.

The usual sequence of events in the natural history of capsulitis is one of pain, pain and loss of movement, relief from pain, then slow recovery of movement. The condition usually responds gradually to rest, simple analgesics and physiotherapy directed towards limiting the loss of movement. It may sometimes be accompanied by severe pain and systemic disturbances, and the patient may be found to have a raised erythrocyte sedimentation rate (E.S.R.). Rest and salicylates are usually effective in controlling the condition, but a short course of steroids (7–10 days) has been advocated with a rapid reduction of the steroid dosage as improvement occurs.

Treatment of capsulitis, however severe the initial symptoms may be, must always aim at preventing the development of 'frozen shoulder'.

If conservative measures have not substantially relieved the patient's neck and arm symptoms, and if there is evidence of mechanical obstruction to the rotator cuff as it moves under the acromion, acromionectomy may offer a very successful solution.

Treatment for the painful stiff shoulder

Treatment has two main aims: the relief of pain and the restoration of normal shoulder movement. Treatments recommended include:

Heat.
Ice.
Exercises of various types.
Manipulation under anaesthetic.
Manipulation without anaesthetic.
Local or systemic steroids.
Ultrasonic or x-ray therapy.
Analgesics.

There is no general agreement as to the most effective treatment nor indeed whether any therapy alters the natural history of the condition.

Some patients are much relieved by heat in some form or another, whereas others tend to find that heat worsens their symptoms. Other patients find ice therapy, particularly in the acute early phase of the condition, the most effective form of treatment.

Resting the arm in an elbow-supporting sling is usually followed by relief from pain, but it is important that the patient realizes the need for removing the arm from the sling several times a day to attempt a full range of hand and arm exercises.

The basis of physiotherapy lies in a judicious combination of rest and exercises within the painless range of movement.

Heat, ice, injection of hydrocortisone or of local anaesthetic may offer temporary relief from pain and allow the rest/exercise regime to be instituted. Usually, the symptoms slowly subside, and as the pain goes, so the painless range of motion slowly increases. Attempts to force the shoulder into the painful range, or over-activity of any kind, are usually followed by an exacerbation of pain and loss of joint range.

Not infrequently, and particularly in the elderly, hydrocortisone injections are followed by some symptomatic relief followed by sudden loss of range of movement with or without pain. This is due to complete rupture of the suprasinatus tendon or biceps tendon, depending on the site of the injection.

Manipulation with or without anaesthetic may be needed if the symptoms are improving, but joint movement is not returning. This procedure is probably best avoided unless a full investigation has been undertaken, including electromyography of the appropriate shoulder muscles, to eliminate the possibility of an irritative nerve root lesion.

CERVICAL SPONDYLOSIS AS A CLINICAL SYNDROME

Introduction

There are two main groups of patients presenting with symptoms in the neck and arm:

(1) The young athletic person with an acute intense pain in the arm following sudden trauma, e.g. after a skiing accident, or a whiplash injury in a road accident.

(2) The middle-aged or elderly patient with a recurrent history of neck pain, limitation of neck movement, and brachialgia of root or partial root distribution.

The former is apparently due to a disc lesion and is characteristically made worse by coughing, sneezing and lateral neck movements.

The older patients with degenerative changes in the cervical spine (cervical spondylosis) characteristically complain of pain in the neck and shoulder pain which is worse at night. Women are more often affected than men, and there is frequently a position of the neck which will aggravate the symptoms and another which will relieve them. General body posture also plays a contributory part in the aetiology of this type of neck pain and sitting long over the average-height desk or driving in an incorrect position are aggravating activities. Typical precipitating factors are playing golf, heavy lifting, and carrying.

It is often possible to differentiate between a neck pain which is due to a disease of the joints of the neck and root pains which are associated with irritation of the nerve roots, referred pain or paraesthesia. In either case the pain is usually most severe when the physical signs are least and often diffuse when the lesion is localized. This syndrome has been described repeatedly in the literature and been christened according to the changing theories of its aetiology. 'Acroparaesthesia', 'perineuritis', 'fibrositis', 'thoracic outlet syndrome', 'scalenus anterior syndrome' and 'brachialgia statica paraesthetica' are all terms given to a syndrome characterized by pain in the arm and occurring mainly in women aged 35–55 years. From time to time specific lesions—such as the compression of the brachial plexus at the thoracic outlet, cervical rib, with or without a fibrous band attaching the transverse process of the seventh cervical vertebra to the first rib, and compression of the median nerve in the carpal tunnel—have been shown to account for a small number of patients with these symptoms.

Sir Russell Brain described at length the condition of cervical spondylosis. He described radicular syndromes, acroparaesthesia, shoulder and arm pain of the referred type, 'frozen shoulder', and subacute multiradicular symptoms as all being associated with degenerative changes in the cervical intervertebral discs, and the osteophytic outgrowths on the adjacent vertebral bodies and posterior apophyseal joints.

Precisely what part cervical spondylosis plays in the aetiology of pain in the neck and arm (brachialgia) is unknown. It is generally assumed to be the commonest cause of pain in the neck and arm, and this assumption is based largely on the high frequency with which radiological changes in the cervical spine occur in patients with brachialgia. There is no clear correlation between radiological appearances of the cervical spine and the symptoms and signs which are present in any one patient. For this reason, some authorities have questioned the aetiological significance of cervical spondylosis, pointing out that almost all people over 50 years of age have radiological changes in the cervical spine characteristic of joint and disc degeneration. There is however some evidence to indicate that radiological changes in the posterior intervertebral joints are more likely to be accompanied by such signs and symptoms than are changes in the intervertebral discs.

A discrepancy between severity of symptoms and severity of radiological changes is a characteristic of osteo-arthrosis. It is often the soft-tissue reaction which both precedes and accompanies the joint degeneration which is instrumental in causing a variable degree of associated pain.

In the case of the cervical spine, it is not only bony overgrowth from the perimeter of the intervertebral foramen, but also perineuritic soft-tissue overgrowth within and beyond the foramina which causes the nerve irritation and pain. Of the two, it is probable that the inflammation and later the fibrosis of the meningeal perineuritic sleeve is responsible for the greater part of the pain induced by the radiculitis of cervical spondylosis, since actual mechanical pressure on the mixed nerve produces anaesthesia and weakness, with little pain, whereas irritation of the nerve due to inflammation of the perineuritic tissue is painful.

The persistent irritation of the nerve roots set up by the soft-tissue inflammation, bony outgrowth or joint malalignment of cervical spondylosis may well set up continued stimulation of afferent nerves, providing a background of subliminal sensory stimuli, and thereby increasing the central excitatory state. This would render the threshold for pain lower for other peripheral lesions in the same dermatome and would explain the apparent 'correlation' between 'tennis elbow', carpal tunnel or painful shoulder lesions and cervical spondylosis. It would also explain some of the discrepancies in the response of central and peripheral lesions to local treatment.

The presence of free interneural circulation between nerve roots and the peripheral parts of the nerve may be responsible for the diffuse tenderness of peripheral nerves sometimes found in this condition, as well as for the variability in symptomatology, clinical picture, and response to treatment. It is conceivable that pathological changes in the soft tissues at the site of origin of the nerve roots could influence the vulnerability of the peripheral nerve to mechanical stress. Inflammation and later fibrosis associated with root irritation must diminish nerve sheath elasticity, thus increasing the tension which limb movements put upon it, and in particular predisposing to the sudden pain which patients often associate with certain movements of the neck or arm.

Because in very many people pain in the neck and arm are associated with radiological evidence of degenerative arthritis, cervical spondylosis has tended to become an accepted clinical diagnosis, whereas it is really a radiological diagnosis. Whether the symptoms are mainly pain, or paraesthesia, in the majority of patients, any one attack is likely to settle in 4–6 weeks. Only about one quarter of patients have symptoms persisting beyond 3 months.

With a natural history which is usually self-limiting, the syndrome of pain in the neck and arm is so common and its presentation so variable that it is often dismissed with minimal reference to a few key features. In order to rationalize the many treatments which are at present meted out without any apparent scientific basis for their selection, it is helpful to speculate about the clinical features of brachialgia, and much of this section is unashamedly speculative.

The joints most frequently involved in cervical spondylosis are those between the fifth, sixth and seventh cervical vertebrae, and the clinical features in any one patient vary with the level, type and degree of joint involvement.

Pain and paraesthesia

The common presentation is an attack of pain and paraesthesiae in the neck or arm. Some patients have difficulty in distinguishing between the symptoms, but usually there is a history of some neck pain preceding paraesthesia in the arm. Sometimes the pain is first felt in the muscles of the shoulder girdle, or it may radiate from the point of the shoulder down the lateral side of the arm to the elbow. Coughing, sneezing, active arm movements and active or passive neck movement may all accentuate the pain.

Paraesthesia often takes the form of numbness or tingling in the fingers, hand and forearm, coming on particularly at night. The symptoms are posture-related, and may be eased by deliberate changes in the position of the neck. One or both the limbs may be affected. Occasionally only the hand is involved, becoming cold and blue and feeling numb, although this may be confined to only one or two fingers or the thumb.

A patient, on being wakened in the morning, may complain of inability to use the affected hand, e.g. to turn off the alarm. By careful history-taking it is often possible to distinguish different patterns of presenting symptoms:

Recurrent attacks of shoulder pain These may be induced by disproportionately slight effort and are frequently present on waking. They may be of maximal intensity then or may increase gradually throughout the day. Pain is maximal on rotation and abduction, but in severe attacks pain may increase in severity until all movement is inhibited. Examination may elicit tenderness over the long head of biceps, over the supraspinatus insertion, over either of the spinati bellies or the rhomboids, or at the insertion of the deltoid.

A gradual reduction of range of movement of the neck This may occur over many years and is often accompanied by little pain.

Isolated or recurrent attacks of acute pain in the neck These are sometimes induced by trauma and sometimes come on during unguarded movement, either during the night or during some apparently effortless occupation in the day. The neck is fixed in one position due to intense spasm of the cervical muscles, and voluntary movement is impossible or minimal.

Recurrent stiff neck The patient may complain of recurrent attacks of neck pain and stiffness. Sometimes these attacks are associated with pain or paraesthesia in any of the dermatomes supplied by the nerves C1–7 and the first thoracic nerve T1. Symptoms are therefore located in the upper part of the chest and back, the shoulder, the arm and the hand, and the back of the head. Sometimes such attacks are associated with spastic paresis of the lower limbs caused by cord damage (cervical myelopathy, *see* p. 109).

Attacks of elbow pain Pain in the lateral side of the elbow of the 'tennis elbow' variety and pain in the medial side of the elbow of the 'golfers elbow' variety, especially when recurrent and not attributable to severe unaccustomed activity involving excessive forearm use, may be indicative of cervical spondylosis.

Attacks of pain in the forearm, wrist and hand Pain, paraesthesia, and stiffness of the hand, wrist and forearm may be due to cervical spondylosis. Symptoms referred in the distribution of the ulnar nerve or the median nerve must be distinguished from those arising from 'entrappement' of the ulnar nerve at the elbow or the median nerve in the carpal tunnel. When cervical spondylosis is present, minor trauma can precipitate a full-blown carpal tunnel syndrome.

Pain in the breast and axilla Careful breast examination is necessary to distinguish this type of pain arising from cervical spondylosis from a similar type of pain arising from a neoplastic lesion of the breast with axillary gland involvement.

Pain in the front or back of the chest Localized tender areas in the muscles of the upper limb and pectoral girdle occur frequently in cervical spondylosis and must be carefully distinguished from pain and tenderness in the same group of muscles of neoplastic, traumatic or inflammatory origin. A neoplastic chest lesion involving the upper lobe of the lung can present as shoulder or chest pain; so too can secondary deposits in bones of the thoracic cage. Pain in the upper part of the chest may also result from osteoporosis of the thoracic spine, from a peptic ulcer adherent to the posterior abdominal wall, from pathological conditions of the gall bladder, and from lesions involving the diaphragm.

Headache When due to cervical spondylosis, this is always occipital on one or both sides. It often spreads to, or involves independently, the forehead on the same side. It is associated with arthritic changes in the joints and soft tissues of the upper cervical spine but is not necessarily pure C1–C2 distribution. The headache may occur particularly in the mornings and is often associated with neck stiffness and pain incurred by faulty neck and head posture during the night.

Chin pain radiating to the arms This is rare, but the lower part of the lower jaw and chin are partly supplied by C2–3 (anterior cutaneous nerve of the neck) and such a means of presentation is possible from upper cervical lesions.

Physical signs of cervical spondylosis

As with the symptoms, the signs of cervical spondylosis vary greatly with its phases of activity. Thus, although for the greater part of the time most patients with cervical spondylosis have only minor symptoms and few physical signs, when subjected to trauma, infection, prolonged exposure to cold, sustained posture or over-exertion, their symptoms and signs may rapidly become acute and severe.

During quiescent periods, there may be some limitation of neck movement and mild tenderness on pressure over the spinous processes of affected cervical vertebrae.

During active phases, or 'attacks', or in patients in whom the involvement of nerve roots, nerve cord, or cord vascular supply is permanently severe, the range of neck movement, and often shoulder movement, becomes drastically reduced and may be completely inhibited by pain and muscle spasm. The patient has a tense, apprehensive expression and the head is held in one position of relative ease by muscles whose spasm makes their outlines visible and palpable; the shoulder is held adducted to the body with forearm and hand in neutral position.

If neck movement is possible, the foraminal compression test will frequently be positive, i.e. downward pressure on the head when inclined to the painful side will cause pain in the ipsilateral arm.

Pain and fear of pain are the dominant features of both acute and chronic severe root involvement, but in addition, certain signs identify the source of the radiculitis. Thus, when the sixth cervical root is involved, the patient may complain of pins and needles in the thumb, numbness of the thumb, particularly the tip, and pain shooting down the arm and forearm into the thumb. Examination may demonstrate objective sensory loss in the radial aspect of thumb and forearms, and the tendon reflexes of biceps and brachialis may be weak or absent.

Weakness, when present, is usually confined to the small muscles of the hand, and, less often, to the muscles of the shoulder girdle and upper arm. Weakness may be present irrespective of whether pain is or is not a prominent symptom, and may be the most troublesome feature of the condition. Patients complain of diminishing power of grip or of increasing difficulty with manipulating small tools or implements.

When the seventh cervical root is involved, pins and needles may be felt in the index, middle and ring fingers, and pain may radiate from the shoulder to these fingers. There may be diminished sensation over the back of the hand, the index and middle fingers, and the radial half of the ring finger; the triceps jerk may be weak or absent.

With involvement of the eighth cervical root, pins and needles and pain are located in the little finger, the ulnar side of the ring finger, and the hypothenar eminence, and there may be diminished sensation in the same areas.

Apart from shooting pains to the fingers, patients with severe or active cervical spondylosis complain of tender areas in the muscles innervated by the affected nerve roots. This applies especially to the trapezius, the spinati, the rhomboids, latissimus dorsi and pectoralis major and minor.

Sometimes the symptoms from the neck itself are less distressing than those from the shoulder, elbow, or wrist, and the diagnosis of 'frozen shoulder', 'tennis elbow', 'golfer's elbow' or 'carpal tunnel syndrome' may obscure the underlying lesion in the cervical spine. When a patient presents with symptoms and signs of these 'catch-phrase' diagnoses, cervical spondylosis should always be looked for as an underlying condition.

Differential diagnosis of cervical spondylosis

Because cervical spondylosis can cause referred pain in many distributions, it can be a considerable mimic of visceral disease. Also, because it is a commonly occurring degenerative condition, it may well be an incidental finding in association with other conditions. Thus, the diagnosis of cervical spondylosis is often one of elimination.

Visceral disease Pain referred from pleura, pericardium or diaphragm, including carcinoma of the lung and myocardial infarction.

Upper respiratory infections Infections such as sinusitis or tonsillitis, with secondary adenitis of cervical and paratracheal glands, causing recurrent acute episodes of stiffness and pain in the neck.

Vertebral column lesions Lesions such as rheumatoid arthritis, ankylosing spondylitis, spinal caries, neoplasms or fractures rarely cause difficulty in diagnosis. Congenital abnormalities of the vertebral bodies or the presence of a cervical rib are more common. Localized degenerative arthritis may be associated with injury, deformity or disease.

Central nervous system Lesions of the spinal cord, e.g. syringomyelia, or of the nerve roots, e.g. herpes zoster or poliomyelitis, may give rise to diagnostic difficulties.

Cervical myelopathy and radiculopathy As part of the gradual degenerative changes occurring in the cervical spine associated with aging there is a narrowing of the disc space with a bulging of disc material centrifugally. Osteophyte formation around the bulging disc may lead to significant compression of spinal nerve roots in the intervertebral foramina or lateral part of the spinal canal, or to compression of the spinal cord. This condition is really a late manifestation of cervical spondylosis. Its significance lies in the development of the most important complication—cervical myelopathy.

The symptoms and signs of cord pressure occur far less frequently than those of root pressure, since lateral protrusions from intervertebral discs are more common than posterior protrusions. When cord pressure does occur, it is usually associated with, or preceded by, symptoms of root pressure. Symptoms usually appear gradually, and a patient may complain of weakness in the legs, difficulty in walking in a straight line, and pain and weakness in one or both arms. As in root pressure, the radial position of the prolapsing or bulging part of the disc determines the type of clinical picture which presents. Thus a mid-line posteriorly directed prolapse affects both pyramidal tracts, and possibly both upper and lower limbs.

The onset of cervical myelopathy is insidious, and although the patient may complain of pain and paraesthesia in the arms, these are rarely severe. The important manifestations of this condition are in the lower limbs. The patient may present with some weakness of the legs and difficulty in walking. Enquiry may reveal some paraesthesia of the lower limbs. Examination at this time usually reveals some spasticity and loss of proprioceptive sensation. It has been said that myelopathy does not develop in patients who do not have signs demonstrable at their first hospital attendance.

Treatment of cervical spondylosis

General principles

Many treatments are advocated for patients with pain in the neck and arm:

- Rest of the patient.
- Rest of the neck.
- Palliative physiotherapy, such as heat or ice.
- Collars of felt, rubber, plaster of paris, or plastic.
- Rest of the arm in a sling when brachialgia is severe.
- Traction in extension, flexion, or in neutral position:
    - With weights.
    - By manual traction.

Shoulder-raising exercises.
Manipulation—with or without anaesthetic.
Neck-mobilizing exercises.

There is lack of evidence to show that one treatment of pain in the neck and arm is better than any other. This lack is not a reflection on the efficacy of the forms of treatment, but merely emphasizes the need to make a pathologically based diagnosis of the precise cause of the pain in each patient, so that treatment applied may be appropriate to the underlying cause.

It is unrealistic to consider pain in the neck and arm as an entity, any more than pain in the back or pain in the abdomen can be considered a distinct symptom complex. Future research which defines accurately the source and nature of the pain throughout the course of the condition may well show the need for and the efficacy of specific treatment for each pathological situation.

The several clinical trials which have been carried out have not attempted this and have merely established that both the immediate response and the long-term follow-up are similar, whether patients are treated by the supply of a simple collar, with a time-consuming physiotherapy, or with placebo treatments. Indeed, the only factors which affect prognosis are: (1) the patient's age; (2) the severity of the attack; (3) the number of previous attacks; and (4) the average duration of previous attacks.

Most patients have less pain if their posture is corrected, and the majority are relieved, at least partially, by wearing an adequate collar. The disturbance of sleep can often be reduced by a collar or by instruction in the use of a 'butterfly' pillow. Many patients are greatly relieved by a frank discussion about the nature of the symptoms and, indeed, reassurance may be all that they were seeking, coupled with instruction on how to go about their daily activities in such a way as to avoid future exacerbations of their symptoms.

The basis of treatment of the symptom is rest, followed by graded activity. Rest is achieved for the neck itself by wearing a simple collar; rest for the patient by avoiding strenuous activity, and in severe cases, by rest in bed. Such rest may need to be preceded by or supplemented by traction or manipulation. Dramatic relief can certainly occur with traction or manipulation, but there is no evidence that these procedures influence the natural history of the condition as expressed by recurrences of symptoms, nor is there any guarantee that a repetition of the same procedure will successfully relieve the symptoms in successive attacks.

The clinician and therapist must therefore decide whether the use of any particular procedure is likely to produce relief from the group of symptoms present at the time of examination, and whether the symptoms and the extent of likely relief will justify the expenditure and inconvenience to the patient in attending the out-patient department for its administration.

Although it is apparent that treatment cannot be prescribed collectively but must be selected according to the physical, mental and social state of each individual patient, it is possible to generalize to a limited extent. It seems that the acute lesion with marked limitation of movement and severe pain will respond best to immobilization; the less acute lesion with restricted movement in one direction only will more appropriately be treated by mobilization techniques.

Heat and gentle mobilizing exercises during acute exacerbations of pain and stiffness in the neck usually prove helpful. If possible, heat treatment should be given daily at the physiotherapy department to relax spasm and permit exercises which involve a gradually increasing range of movements. If not, patients should be encouraged to perform their exercises at home in front of an electric fire on the days they do not attend the department.

Daily exercises to maintain the range of neck movement should be continued indefinitely, together with postural exercises and shoulder exercises, and patients should be asked to check their head and neck position in mirrors and shop windows and to correct the tendency to hold the neck protruded and the head bent forward and down.

Manual traction may relieve pain in the acute exacerbations of neck pain and stiffness, particularly if there is an associated radiculitis, with pins and needles in the hand or shooting pains to one or more fingers of that hand. While adequate for people of small and medium stature, manual traction is of little use in the case of a tall, powerfully built patient. For these patients, many physiotherapists feel that mechanical traction may be indicated. This should be applied with extreme care, under expert supervision (*see* Chapter 1).

Such traction may be effective in relieving symptoms, particularly when used in conjunction with a collar worn for the remaining part of the day and during the night as well. If not, when symptoms are severe, bed rest is necessary. A collar should be worn and only one or two soft pillows permitted. If a collar cannot be tolerated then no more than one pillow is allowed. Adequate analgesia and a nightly sedative are essential. Drugs such as diazepam and chlordiazepoxide used in conjunction with analgesics are often helpful in relieving tension and anxiety and in assisting muscular relaxation.

If pain is severe and persists for longer than a few days despite these measures, then admission to hospital and application of sustained cervical traction may be necessary to alleviate pain. However, cervical traction is not without risk, and its use should be carefully considered.

It is seldom necessary to maintain traction for more than a week, and symptoms should then continue to subside with the use of a collar, restricted exertion and daily periods of mobilizing exercises of gradually increasing range and duration.

Collars

As the pathological conditions in both the locomotor and nervous systems cannot be cured, the treatment of cervical spondylosis is a long drawn-out affair which attempts to prevent deterioration of the status quo, and to treat acute episodes of pain and dysfunction as they occur. In the acute stages of mild cases of cervical spondylosis, the symptoms usually respond rapidly to rest in an adequate collar. An 'adequate' collar is effective in preventing neck movement, and effective collars must therefore be rigid. Unfortunately, the more rigid a collar is, the more difficult it is for the therapist to apply and for the patient to tolerate. Most collars are therefore a compromise between ease of application and comfort on the one hand and rigidity and direct therapeutic value on the other. Commonly used materials are sorbo rubber, orthopaedic felt and plastazote. The collar should be worn all day and preferably all night too.

A sorbo rubber collar has one advantage because if taken off and reapplied upside down and back to front it still fits the patient, but it has virtually no mechanical ability to restrict neck movement.

A collar made from orthopaedic felt requires the concavities carved from it to admit the clavicles and to fit round the occipital protuberances and jaw. Thus, a felt collar is more restrictive than a rubber one and produces less pressure on the chin and trachea while the patient is in the horizontal position in bed.

Plastazote collars are made from expanded polystyrene, and their manufacture requires an oven for heating the sheets of material, which the physiotherapist must know how to use. The heated plastazote strip, cut in the estimated length of the collar, is moulded, while still warm, to the patient's neck and allowed to cool into the resulting shape. Its edges are then trimmed, and it is fastened by velcro tapes which may be glued or sewn on to the plastazote. It is important that the collar comes high enough up the back of the neck to cover the occipital condyles, otherwise head movement is not properly controlled nor the neck posture adequately supported. It is equally important that the neck should not be supported in hyperextension.

Once the acute symptoms are improving, the collar should be gradually discarded, the patient being advised to take it off for about an hour in the morning at first and then for an hour longer each day. If there is no discomfort, the period without the collar can be increased steadily. If discomfort is felt, the period should be decreased and then once again increased after a few days. The patient should retain the collar for some months and always wear it for car journeys and heavy work, or if he tends to get a tired, aching neck in the evening while watching television or doing any task which entails neck flexion. Many people wear their collar at night for some weeks after they have stopped wearing it during the day as they find that night posture of the head and neck is a critical factor in determining the pain level of the following day.

If symptoms respond to treatment with a collar, but are severe and likely either to recur or improve, but not completely resolve, it is advisable to try a firmer moulded collar.

Since in the acute episodes of neck pain and stiffness which occur in cervical spondylosis, the position of the neck is frequently abnormal, it is probably better, initially, to provide a collar made from orthopaedic felt as well as a plastazote collar. As pain is relieved, spasm of cervical muscles is reduced, and the head and neck resume their normal relationship with the head held erect and in neutral rotation and the neck in mild and physiological lordosis. At this stage of recovery, a plastazote collar may be worn more continuously. The advantages of the plastazote collar are that it is lighter, less bulky, less obvious, and often better tolerated. There is little difference in its heating effect on the patient. Though it is thinner than felt and may be aerated yet further by punch holes, plastazote is still a very warm material to wear and may be hard to tolerate in the summer. Many patients do not manage to wear a plastic collar at night but can tolerate the softer, felt one, retaining the more restrictive collar for day wear.

Patients with serious disorganization of the cervical spine and, in particular, patients in whom there is danger of a slip of one cervical vertebra upon another, will need immobilization in a collar giving even better support than either felt or plastazote. There are many proprietary types of rigid plastic collar, and one of these may prove particularly suitable for an individual patient.

Rigid plastic collars are of two main types.

(1) All-in-one wrap-over type, with back and side fastening.

(2) Two-piece articulated type, consisting of a front breast-plate reaching as low as the manubrium sterni and in one piece with a moulded neck and chin support, and a back plate extending from scapular level to above the level of the occiput.

Many centres prefer to make their own rigid plastic collars from a cast of the patient's neck. The details of structure vary with the manufacturing centre and the patient concerned—the extent of his disability, his tolerance of a restricting support, and the degree of restriction which it is necessary to impose upon him. Thus, the depth of the collar and its height posteriorly vary considerably. The chin-piece frequently does not cover the chin, but merely provides a shelf for it to rest on. Where maximal control of neck mobility must be maintained, the collar is extended over the lower part of the prominence of the chin, cupping it and controlling its movements.

Rubber collars with parallel horizontal inflatable strips provide an alternative form of collar. Although some patients find them satisfactory, they do tend to leak and may also precipitate skin sensitivity reactions so that their abilities to support and soothe are both uncertain.

If the wearing of an adequate collar is not followed by improvement, the diagnosis should be reconsidered.

Manipulation

Cervical spondylosis may be present without symptoms, but it may so narrow the spinal canal that a sudden hyperextension or acute flexion of the cervical spine can cause a contusion of the cord, with severe neurological consequences. Despite this, millions of patients are manipulated every year by qualified and unqualified practitioners and although occasional tragedies do happen, they are mercifully very rare. There is, however, little evidence that manipulation of the cervical spine has any greater long-term therapeutic effect than the conventional conservative measures used in the management of pain in the neck and arm.

The *indication* for cervical spine manipulation can be defined as pain appearing to originate in the cervical spine which is not associated with signs of cord compression, and in the presence of ligaments and vertebrae which are apparently sound.

Thus, manipulation of the cervical spine is contra-indicated in 'whiplash' injuries where there is any evidence of ligament damage or crush injury of the vertebral body; in rheumatoid arthritis which has a predilection for involving the upper cervical spine; in the presence of hypermobility of the cervical spine, or of congenital malformation or anomalies. The presence of cervical myelopathy is also a contra-indication.

Surgical intervention

Operative treatment of cervical spondylosis is indicated only when there is severe pain which has not responded to an adequate trial of conservative treatment, or when there is progressive neurological involvement. The surgery chosen can be cord decompression or cervical fusion, or a combination of these procedures.

In younger patients, the operative treatment of choice appears to be a fusion of the bodies of the vertebrae on either side of the disc protrusion, through an anterolateral approach. This permits the greater part of the disc and the cartilage plates to be removed and a cancellous bone block to be inserted into the slot cut across the front of the adjacent vertebral bodies. Trauma to the affected nerve roots is reduced or prevented, and the patient is able to get up in a few days, wearing a cervical brace or collar which is discarded when a satisfactory bony union has been achieved. Further disc degeneration and osteophyte increase appear to be prevented by this measure, and it is gradually replacing the older procedure of posterior fusion.

BIBLIOGRAPHY AND REFERENCES

Brain, W. R. (1954). 'Spondylosis: the known and the unknown.' *Lancet* **1**, 687

Brain, W. R., Wright, D., and Wilkinson, M. (1947). 'Spontaneous compression of both median nerves in the carpal tunnel.' *Lancet* **1**, 277

British Association of Physical Medicine (1966). 'Pain in the neck and arm: a multi-centre trial of the effects of physiotherapy.' *Br. med. J.* **1**, 253

Falconer, M. A. and Weddell, G. (1943). 'Costoclavicular compression of the subclavian artery and vein.' *Lancet* **2**, 539

Hazleman, B. L. (1972). 'The painful stiff shoulder.' *Rheum. Rehab.* **2**, 413

Hughes, J. T. (1966). *Pathology of the Spinal Cord.* London; Lloyd-Luke

Irvine, D. H., Forster, J. B., Newell, D. J. and Klukrim, B. N. (1965). 'Prevalence of cervical spondylosis in a general practice.' *Lancet* **1**, 1089

Kellgren, J. H., Jeffrey, M. R. and Ball, J. (Eds) (1963). *Epidemiology of Chronic Rheumatism*, Vol 2. Oxford; Blackwell

Lawrence, J. S. (1963). In *Epidemiology of Chronic Rheumatism*, Vol. 1, p. 100. Ed. by J. H. Kellgren, M. R. Jeffrey and J. Ball. Oxford; Blackwell

Lees, F. and Turner, J. W. A. (1963). 'The natural history and prognosis of cervical spondylosis.' *Br. med. J.* **2**, 1607

Lishman, W. A. and Russell, W. R. (1961). 'The brachial neuropathies.' *Lancet* **2**, 941

Moseley, F. H. and Goldie, I. (1963). 'The arterial pattern of the rotator cuff of the shoulder.' *J. Bone Jt Surg.* **45B**, 780

Russell, W. R. (1956). 'Discussion on cervical spondylosis.' *Proc. R. Soc. Med.* **49**, 198

Steinberg, V. L. and Mason, R. M. (1959). 'Cervical spondylosis: pilot therapeutic trial.' *Ann. phys. Med.* **5**, 37

6—*Backache*

INTRODUCTION

It has often been averred that backache is protean in its origins, that it is not a diagnosis, and should therefore not be dealt with as a separate condition. If this is so, a chapter on backache is superfluous in a book on rehabilitation. But rehabilitation entails the treatment of any patient and his surroundings in such a way as to restore or create for that patient a condition of optimum functional efficiency and maximal comfort, and this, in its turn, demands the relief of pain. Whatever the cause of his backache, the patient attending the Rehabilitation Department asks primarily for the relief of pain and since the measures for relieving this are applicable to the pain from a wide variety of causes, and the long-term management of backache is likewise similar in so many conditions, a chapter on backache has been included.

It is, however, important for those who treat a patient with backache to remember that when they treat the backache, they are treating a symptom; they must therefore take particular care to investigate and treat the cause of the symptom concurrently, lest by relieving the symptom, they permit the underlying pathological condition to progress undetected.

AETIOLOGY

The differential diagnoses of backache of various types are so many that to enumerate them would be to fill the pages with wearying lists. One has only to consider the anatomy of the vertebral column, the structural intricacies of its component parts, its variety of functions, and the plethora of organs to which it is related to understand that this must be so. Small wonder then that dysfunction in any system may present as backache and that the only certain deduction which can be drawn from the complaint of backache is that something is wrong somewhere. Any physiotherapeutic treatment for backache must take place concurrently with, or else follow, accurate definition of the 'something', and equally accurate delineation of the 'somewhere'.

Much has been written about backache as an expression of psychological disturbance. Perusal of the records of patients who have attended orthopaedic clinics over many years illustrates the strong tendency to consider all backache as psychological unless proved otherwise by radiological investigation. While it is undoubtedly comforting for those giving treatment to attribute the backache, which they have not cured, to psychogenic causes, it is less than comforting for the patient. Since the presence of backache is difficult to confirm, or disprove, backache has become the obvious complaint of work-shy, battle-shy or tension-shy patients who require an acceptable reason for opting out of unpleasant circumstances. The popularity of backache among malingerers has discredited its authenticity for those who really suffer from it, and this combined with failure of radiological confirmation of any underlying pathology each year puts a substantial number of patients into the 'psychogenic' category wrongly. It is chastening to recall the number of patients who develop irrefutable radiological evidence of disease some years after a diagnosis of 'psychogenic' has been affixed to their backache.

'NON-RHEUMATIC' BACKACHE

Because many pathological conditions of many systems may present as backache, treatment and rehabilitation cannot be realistic unless the underlying cause is first delineated. A detailed functional enquiry and past history are essential to the accurate diagnosis of this cause, and supplement an enquiry about appetite, bowels, micturition, menstruation and general health.

Information is elicited on:

(1) the duration, time of onset and nature of onset of symptoms;

(2) their relationship to time of day, month or year, to exercise, rest and specific activities and movements;

(3) their present location, and possible variation from their location at time of onset;

(4) their radiation and variation with posture;

(5) sources of exacerbation and relief;

(6) their response to analgesics and anti-inflammatory drugs;

(7) associated presence of pain, swelling or stiffness in any other joints, now or at any time;

(8) the presence or absence of abnormal symptoms and signs in any other system;

(9) the nature of past and present medication—type and duration with particular reference to steroids or to natural or synthetic hormones or pregnancies or abortions;

(10) past operations—with particular reference to hysterectomy and mastectomy in a woman, prostatectomy in a man, or pneumonectomy, thyroidectomy and nephrectomy in both;

(11) past or present reaction to work and leisure activities, particularly to a change or unduly long participation in either.

Such a detailed enquiry is essential in our present social structure, which necessitates a substantial number of people moving from district to district at a speed which exceeds that of their medical records, so that any doctor asked to treat them for backache may well have no information other than that obtainable from the patients themselves.

Disorders of the gastro-intestinal system, such as peptic ulcers or neoplasms situated on the posterior wall of stomach or duodeum and causing inflammatory changes on the posterior abdominal wall, may present as backache in the lower thoracic or upper lumbar region, depending on the location of the lesion. They are usually associated with poor appetite, heartburn and epigastric pain. Dysfunction of the gall bladder, such as cholecystitis, may present with acute pain between the shoulder blades, but will usually be associated with pain in the right upper quadrant of the abdomen and intolerance to fats. Pancreatitis or neoplasms of the pancreas may also be associated with back pain at the thoracolumbar level.

Disease of the genito-urinary system involving the kidney, such as pyelonephritis, may present with backache over the lower ribs and in the costovertebral angle on the affected side, and will usually be associated with frequency of micturition, haematuria and dysuria.

When the prostate is involved, as in prostatitis or in carcinoma of the prostate, backache is usually felt in the sacral region, although secondary deposits from prostatic carcinoma may occur anywhere in the spine, resulting in pain and tenderness in the vertebrae concerned, possibly progressing to greater tenderness and root pain if vertebral collapse ensues.

There is usually, but not always, a history of delay in starting micturition and of haematuria and dysuria. Similar symptoms arise from secondaries due to renal neoplasm, but without delay in starting micturition.

Disorders of the respiratory system involving the pleura on the posterior thoracic wall may also present as backache over the area of the pleura involved. Thus, both neoplastic and infective lesions giving rise to abscess or cavity formation may cause backache which is initially related to breathing and coughing, but may later become constant. Carcinoma of the upper-lobe bronchus frequently gives rise to backache in the subscapular region and sometimes to a painful 'frozen shoulder' as well.

The prodromal period before the eruption of the rash of herpes zoster may be evidenced by severe pain in the back along the cutaneous distribution of the nerve root affected. Persistent pain is limited to one side of the body and the single affected root and may endure for months after the rash disappears. The post-herpetic pain may respond to physical treatments such as ethylchloride spray, ice therapy or the use of a vibrator.

Muscular pain also appears as a symptom of several general diseases. Polymyositis, dermatomyositis and systemic lupus erythematosus may present with pain and muscle tenderness in the sacrospinalis, and certain infections, such as influenza and Bornholm's disease, are frequently accompanied by severe backache. This type of backache usually settles rapidly with rest and disappears as the disease process remits.

Polymyalgia rheumatica usually affects those of late middle age and the elderly and is not infrequently missed as a diagnosis. It is commoner in women than men and is characterized by severe pain and stiffness in the muscles of the shoulder and pelvic girdles. Occasionally there may be an accompanying synovitis of one or more joints, or evidence of vasculitis. Often the patients look unwell and complain of fatigue, lassitude and depression. Because of the age group affected it is usual to find accompanying radiological and clinical evidence of degenerative changes in cervical and lumbar spine. The key to diagnosis is a markedly elevated erythrocyte sedimentation rate (frequently values of 100 mm in the first hour (Westergren) are recorded), coupled with the complaint of incapacitating morning stiffness.

Treatment with corticosteroids is dramatic as far as symptoms are concerned, and probably shortens the course of the disease. Symptoms and the E.S.R. are the best guides to management. This disease runs a course of 3 months to 2 years, and its severity depends upon the vasculitis (if present).

Traumatic myositis may occur after direct or indirect injury, with pain, tenderness and possibly swelling and secondary spasm of the muscles concerned. Treatment of the tenderness with ultrasonic irradiation, the application of ice, or exposure to heat, followed by mobilizing exercises all have their advocates. Occasionally, if the injury is severe, it may be necessary to restrict the mobility of the spine temporarily by the application of a plaster of paris jacket or other form of temporary corset.

Neoplasms

The presence of secondary neoplastic deposits in one or more vertebrae (or even a rib) must always be kept in mind as a possible cause of back pain at any level.

Pain frequently antedates radiological evidence of vertebral involvement, and a scan of patients with symptoms suggestive of secondary deposits in the vertebrae may be necessary to exclude this diagnosis. Local pain and tenderness over an affected vertebra may become intensified and exacerbated by root pain when vertebral collapse and root irritation supervene.

Growths of the thyroid, breast, bronchus, kidney and prostate are particularly likely to give rise to secondary deposits in the vertebrae, and involvement of these organs in any treatment—operative, radiotherapeutic or chemotherapeutic—should always be considered, together with symptoms of possible present dysfunction. Swift referral of patients with secondary deposits for radiotherapeutic or chemotherapeutic treatment is essential, as the relief of pain by appropriate treatment can be dramatic. Where fracture has occurred, or pain persists despite chemotherapy or radiotherapy, the provision of a suitable spinal brace is essential as a pain-relieving measure.

Despite the recognized danger of causing leukemia by excessive radiation, it may be essential to repeat radiographic examination of the spine from time to time if radiological evidence of the presence of a tumour is not obtained, despite clinical evidence to the contrary.

Paget's disease affecting one or more vertebrae may also cause localized pain and tenderness over the vertebrae affected. Considerable relief results from treatments with agents such as calcitonin, mithramycin, and diphosphonates.

Infections of the vertebral column often present with backache, but the more chronic the infection the more insidious the onset. Identification of the infecting organism, administration of an appropriate antibiotic and immobilization of the spine in a plaster of paris cast form the basis of treatment, with or without surgical drainage of any abscesses.

Chronic infection

Tuberculous infection can cause pain and tenderness which may vary considerably with the individual. There may be a large paravertebral abscess without pain; conversely, severe pain may precede abscess formation. Chronic infection of the vertebrae may also occur following typhoid or following a staphylococcal septicaemia when the original infection has been treated with inadequate antibiotic therapy.

Acute infection

Infections such as blastomycosis, brucellosis and tuberculosis, and infections with staphylococcus or other pyogenic organisms cause pain in the back of similar type and distribution, but the onset is swifter and the symptoms of toxicity more pronounced.

Backache may persist after the infection has been healed. Because of mechanical disruption of the normal structure, a plaster of paris jacket or spinal brace should sometimes be worn during the convalescent weight-bearing and discarded later as the vertebral bony structure is reformed.

Metabolic disorders

Demineralization of the vertebrae (osteomalacia) occurs in various metabolic disorders, with resulting vertebral compression, reduction in overall size of the patient, and a variable degree of back pain. Excessive protein withdrawal occurs after prolonged immobilization of the back, and during certain endocrine disturbances, gastro-intestinal disorders, primary or secondary malignant disease or chronic inflammatory states, and prolonged steroid administration. *Osteoporosis* of the vertebrae does not appear to be painful unless vertebral fracture occurs or has occurred from another cause prior to the onset of the osteoporosis. In these instances there is backache at the level of the fractured vertebra, and in the adjacent ligaments and muscles.

Gradually increasing deformity will cause further backache as other parts of the spine attempt to compensate for the collapse of the vertebra, with resulting changes in the tension of muscles, tendons and ligaments.

The aims of treatment of osteoporosis are: to prevent its continuation, to eliminate the cause where possible, to prevent or minimize deformity and to prevent or minimize pain.

The development of deformity may be minimized by a regime of graded, regularly performed exercises, designed to improve posture and reduce strain on the vertebral bodies and their ligaments by strengthening the abdominal and paraspinal musculature. At night, the patient should sleep on a firm mattress underlaid with fracture boards.

Whereas the continued performance of regular exercises is usually regarded as mandatory, there is considerable controversy about the place of a spinal brace or corset in the treatment of the pain and deformity of the osteoporotic spine. However if the pain persists and deformity increases despite strengthening exercises and night postural control, then a spinal corset is needed and should be prescribed. In prescribing a spinal corset, it is sometimes necessary to sacrifice some efficiency to comfort, as most patients will discard a spinal corset if it is too restrictive. Patients wearing spinal supports should be encouraged to perform regular active and static exercises for the abdominal and paraspinal muscles within their pain tolerance.

The relief of pain in osteoporotic fractured vertebrae is attempted by the use of analgesics, combined with strengthening exercises already mentioned for the spinal and abdominal muscles.

Fractured vertebra

A fractured vertebra can often remain undiagnosed as a cause of persistent backache for some considerable time before radiography discloses its presence. Where there is a clear history of trauma, the fracture is rapidly diagnosed and treated. But in certain groups of people, such as those with metabolic disorders such as osteomalacia and osteoporosis, abnormal vertebral configuration such as Scheurmann's disease, or disease such as ankylosing spondylitis, a comparatively minor injury can cause a vertebral fracture, with resulting localized pain, tenderness and loss of function. Immobilization of the spine in a plaster of paris jacket permits the fracture to be rested and supported while ambulation continues. In this way, muscle power and bone protein and mineral content is preserved.

This immobilization should be followed by a regime of graded exercises so that muscles are strengthened to provide physiological splinting for the healed fracture. The patient is traditionally instructed to sleep on a firm mattress with the fracture site well supported, and to maintain at all times a good posture.

Gynaecological conditions

Many gynaecological conditions are associated with low lumbar and sacral backache, which usually occurs or has an exacerbation before and during the first part of the menstrual period. Uterine retroversion and prolapse, endometriosis of the recto-uterine pouch, and uterine fibroids, neoplasm or infection may all give rise to such backache in the lumbar region. Associated symptoms of heavy menstrual loss and intermenstrual bleeding help to indicate a gynaecological cause of the backache.

A large number of women complain of backache during pregnancy, as the lumbar lordosis increases to offset the weight of the protruding abdomen. The performance of regular perineal, spinal and abdominal exercises, the avoidance of lengthy standing sessions, and attention to posture while lying in bed, sitting in a chair, or standing or walking in the upright position, can do much to prevent this.

Many women complain of severe backache after childbirth, or after a gynaecological operation, in which they have remained in the lithotomy position for long periods, often in an unconscious state. There is a very real risk of muscle or ligamentous damage or of joint distraction when the lumbosacral spine is actively or passively held in prolonged flexion, and there is need for a study of the incidence of backache, correlated with the clinical and radiological findings before and after pregnancy, and before and after childbirth. Avoiding the lithotomy position during labour and operation, or else limiting its occurrence to the shortest possible time, would minimize the chance of developing this type of backache. When it has developed, palliative physiotherapy (e.g. heat) followed by gentle extension exercises may ease the pain. Injections of hydrocortisone and lignocaine into tender areas may also be helpful, and the patient should be urged to keep her weight down and to follow the usual programme of prophylactic care for the avoidance of backache.

Acute inflammatory polyarthritis

Severe backache may occur when there is sacro-iliac or intervertebral joint involvement in one of the inflammatory polyarthritides, such as idiopathic ankylosing spondylitis, psoriatic arthritis and Reiter's syndrome, or in association with inflammatory bowel disease.

Treatment of these conditions is designed to control the chronic inflammatory systemic disease with adequate doses of anti-inflammatory drugs, while preserving good spinal posture by bed rest on a firm mattress and a hard-based bed. This bed rest should last as long as the pain is severe and should be followed by gradual mobilization with exercises performed up to just short of the tolerance level of pain and fatigue. Rest in bed in a position of spinal extension is particularly important in ankylosing spondylitis, in which the spine may eventually become quite rigid. Without adequate rest and therapy, the spine may fix in a flexed position. When these are available and used to best advantage, they can at least ensure that the spine stiffens with the patient able to assume an upright posture.

ANKYLOSING SPONDYLITIS

Ankylosing spondylitis is a disease of young men. Of patients with this disease 90 per cent are male, and 80 per cent are between the ages of 15 and 32 years.

The classic description of a patient with a 'poker back', with radiological obliteration of the sacro-iliac joints and 'bambooing' of the lumbar spine, is true only of the late stages of the disease.

In the early stages, there are three diagnostic criteria: stiffness of the lumbar spine; a raised erythrocyte sedimentation rate; radiological changes in the sacro-iliac joints.

Stiffness of the lumbar spine

Stiffness and referred pain in the low back are usually the first indications of the disease and are frequently misdiagnosed as 'growing pains' in the young and 'fibrositis' in the older age groups. A history of trauma can be obtained from most young men, and this, in patients complaining of mild low backache, may be misleading.

A common finding in the earliest stages of ankylosing spondylitis is that the patient wakes up with a slight stiffness in the back which he can 'work off'. In this so-called 'pre-spondylitic stage', the patient finds that he has to steer a careful course between insufficient exercise which makes him stiff, and excessive exercise which gives him pain.

Low backache, the commonest and main presenting symptom of ankylosing spondylitis, has certain characteristics: it is deep seated; it is worse on getting up in the morning and after prolonged periods of sitting; it often shifts from side to side; it is often referred to one or both buttocks; it tends to come and go in attacks lasting for days or weeks, with periods of freedom; it is often accompanied by mild malaise, in contradistinction to backache due to mechanical disorders of the spine, in which malaise is invariably absent.

The most important physical sign in the early stages of ankylosing spondylitis is a stiffness of the lumbar spine. This may be seen as the patient undresses and gets on the examination couch but is frequently not marked enough to be noticed in a fully-dressed patient. This stiffness also shows as limitation of forward and lateral flexion. This restriction of lateral flexion common in ankylosing spondylitis may help to distinguish the disease from chronic disc lesions.

Straight leg raising may be limited due to pain in the sacro-iliac joints, or involvement of the hip joints.

Limitation of chest expansion, which is often given as a criterion of diagnosis in ankylosing spondylitis, does not occur early in the disease process but only when involvement of the thoracic spine leads to arthritis and, later, ankylosis of the costovertebral joints.

Raised E.S.R.

A raised E.S.R. is an almost invariable accompaniment of the active phases of ankylosing spondylitis, but occasionally the E.S.R. may remain within the normal limits for some months after clinical manifestations warrant the diagnosis being made. Conversely, the E.S.R. may remain elevated for some years even though the disease is clinically in abeyance.

Radiology of the sacro-iliac joints

The radiological description of the 'bamboo spine' and the 'tramline' appearance of the lateral radiograph in ankylosing spondylitis characteristic of the established late stages are due to calcification of the intervertebral disc margins and longitudinal ligaments.

The sacro-iliac joints are usually involved early in the disease. A characteristic succession of radiological changes corresponds to progressive joint involvement:

(1) A haziness and indistinctness of outline is associated with marginal decalcification and erosion.

(2) As the erosion proceeds the joint space appears to widen.

(3) Sclerosis appears and is followed by ankylosis until the joint space is obliterated.

The posterior intervertebral joints pass through a similar series of changes, and in some patients the changes are present at a time when the radiographic signs in the sacro-iliac joints are minimal. Thus, in the presence of minimal or dubious changes in the sacro-iliac joints, oblique radiographs of the lumbar spine may confirm the diagnosis.

Difficulty of diagnosis

The greatest problem in making an early diagnosis of ankylosing spondylitis is the difficulty of appreciating the significance of minor symptoms and signs. The natural history of the disease is such that suspicion of its presence is not easily aroused. It is often a slowly progressive condition with minimal symptoms and with a natural tendency to remissions. At the time when many patients first consult a doctor, their complaint is minimal and they are frequently lulled into a sense of false security by a non-specific diagnosis of 'fibrositis' or 'rheumatism', 'disc lesion' or 'postural backache'—terms which the patient knows and is willing to accept. It is only from a detailed history that suspicions may be aroused, by careful examination that the earliest signs may be found, and by full and repeated x-ray examinations that an early diagnosis can be made.

Lack of recognition of other manifestations of the condition may cause delay in diagnosis. Thus involvement of the peripheral joints may lead to a diagnosis of rheumatoid arthritis until spinal deformity supervenes, while iridocyclitis, plantar fasciitis and synovitis of the knee may be treated for a considerable time as separate conditions before the true aetiology becomes apparent.

It is well recognized that some patients are asymptomatic and that ankylosing spondylitis is only discovered as an incidental finding during examination for other reasons. Other patients experience mild symptoms only and consider them too trivial to seek medical advice. Thus the disease is frequently neither manifested nor diagnosed until affected patients reach early middle age, unless regular medical examination reveals it or the exertion of active sport or heavy work provokes further symptoms.

Treatment

The most important aspect of the general management of patients with ankylosing spondylitis is regular physiotherapy in the form of exercises to maintain and restore spinal and costovertebral mobility. Although the later changes involve fusion of the intervertebral joints, the early stages of stiffness and limitation of movement are partially preventable and even reversible. Quite marked increase in joint range and vital capacity can follow a period of intensive physical rehabilitation, and increases of chest expansion of 1–2 in (2·5–5·0 cm) are not unusual. Regular clinical review will enable the clinician to detect deterioration or relapse and will help to maintain the patient's morale and reinforce the clinician's advice to continue regular mobilizing exercises.

The patient's general health must be maintained. Dietetic advice should aim at ensuring an adequate protein intake coupled with avoidance of weight gain.

Regular breathing exercises, postural training and spinal mobility exercises, particularly hydrotherapy (exercising in a warm pool), form the basis of physical treatment. Patients are taught to lift correctly without flexing the spine, for the stiffening back is at greater risk under bending and lifting stress. Periods of intensive rehabilitation of 2 to 3 weeks' duration at about 6-month intervals are an excellent method of maintaining patients in active work. Apart from these periods, patients are encouraged to take regular exercise. Daily breathing and spinal mobilizing exercises are important. All patients are also urged to swim at least once a week. A regular game of tennis, badminton or golf is helpful. Body-contact sports and diving should be avoided as there is a real risk of severe whiplash injury to the cervical spine.

Aspirin affords relief to many patients in doses of 60 gr (4 g) daily, but phenylbutazone or oxphen-butazone have an almost specific effect when given in doses of 100 mg twice or thrice daily. At this dose, toxicity is rarely encountered. Either drug should be taken in divided doses with food or in milk. However, with adequate physiotherapy, many patients do not require analgesics, or else find that doses of these tablets can be reduced. Analgesics should be stopped as soon as the patient can manage without them.

Sleeping on a firm mattress and using a single pillow often reduces not only pain during the night, but also morning stiffness. It also eliminates a factor liable to induce spinal deformity. The use of an electric blanket prior to getting up in the morning may reduce early morning stiffness.

For some patients, a carefully moulded, adjustable spinal brace can reduce severe spinal pain and help to reduce early flexion deformity of the lumbar spine. Other braces have no part in the management of ankylosing spondylitis.

Severe cases and later manifestations

A few patients do not respond to the simple measures described and have considerable unrelenting pain. When this occurs, and the diagnosis is unequivocal, deep x-ray therapy to the painful joints will often reduce the symptoms, but there is undoubtedly an increased risk of developing leukemia as a sequel to this treatment.

Severe stiffness can often be helped considerably by a short course of steroids coupled with back-mobilizing exercises. There is, however, only one absolute indication for corticosteroids in this disease—the development of intractable uveitis. This can rapidly progress to total blindness if these drugs are withheld.

Probably 50 per cent of patients with ankylosing spondylitis have concurrent hip-joint synovitis. In a small proportion, this will lead to ankylosis and be so troublesome as to justify surgery of the hip joints. Cup arthroplasty and total hip replacement have their advocates, but the latter procedure has the advantage of early mobilization post-operatively. Pain relief can usually be provided, but increased joint mobility is not to be guaranteed, as re-ankylosis can occur after arthroplasty.

Occasionally, because of severe spinal deformity, when increasing flexion is markedly diminishing the ability of the patient to see ahead of himself, spinal osteotomy may be considered, but such surgery is acknowledged to be heroic, to carry considerable dangers, and to have rather limited success.

'SPRUNG BACK'

Soft-tissue lesions or tears of ligaments of paraspinal muscles are often diagnosed in the presence of an acute localized pain following an injury, strain or unaccustomed labour. The commonest ligamentous cause of backache is 'sprung back'. This syndrome may be summarized as follows:

(1) Low backache is felt following unaccustomed labour and is worse on slouching, lifting heavy objects with a flexed spine or standing in a poor postural position. The pain may radiate to the buttocks.

(2) Flexion of the spine and straight leg raising may be slightly limited.

(3) Tenderness is found locally over the affected posterior ligaments.

(4) The symptoms and signs are relieved temporarily by infiltration of the affected ligament with a local anaesthetic.

'Sprung back' is commoner in women and may alternatively be called the 'kitchen sink syndrome' as it particularly causes pain when the patient leans forwards over washing-up or other household activities. It may also occur in women or men after athletic activity and in disabled persons with abnormal curvature of the lumbar spine.

Although the acute symptoms of 'sprung back' usually respond dramatically to infiltration of the ligaments with local anaesthetic and/or hydrocortisone, it is wise to institute more long-term measures, particularly to instil into the patient the understanding of the need to prevent unnecessary straining while the spine is flexed.

Back extension exercises, postural re-education, sleeping on a firm mattress and the avoidance of lifting heavy objects with the spine flexed are the usual measures advised.

For the more severe or resistant conditions, a short period spent using a lumbar support or temporary corset may give considerable relief.

'Sprung back' may precede or accompany a prolapsed intervertebral disc. Rupture of the posterior interspinous ligaments can lead to instability and hypermobility between two lumbar vertebrae and this instability predisposes the structures holding the vertebrae together to further damage. The stress on the posterior longitudinal ligament is increased, and rupture of this ligament may occur, leading to prolapse of nucleus pulposus material.

PROLAPSED INTERVERTEBRAL DISC

During the past 40 years, an extensive literature on this subject has grown up, but there is still no universally accepted formula for the diagnosis and treatment of prolapsed intervertebral disc, and unless the patient eventually comes to operation, there is no sure means of confirming the diagnosis. A prolapsed intervertebral disc may present with severe and crippling sciatica of acute onset or as a recurrent, dull, low backache of many years' duration. The signs may vary from minimal limitation of spinal movement to an almost immobile spine accompanied by gross neurological changes in the leg.

Pathological studies indicate that loss of the normal 'turgescence of the nucleus pulposus' (which is associated with age), congenital defects of the cartilaginous end-plates of the bodies of the vertebrae, or of the annulus fibrosus, and a precipitating injury are the main factors concerned in producing a prolapse of the disc. Significant variations in the nucleus pulposus have been recorded in experimental animals in relation to stress.

Radiology of prolapsed intervertebral disc

Radiological evidence of loss of disc space only occurs after prolapse or degeneration of the nucleus pulposus has occurred. A rapid decrease in the affected disc space of some patients has been recorded after removal of the nucleus pulposus at operation, but in other patients the degree of narrowing is variable. The onset of narrowing may be delayed for months or even years after the onset of symptoms.

Radiography can indicate the level of the prolapsed intervertebral disc in approximately half of the patients diagnosed clinically as suffering from a 'prolapsed intervertebral disc' but may be negative in about one quarter of those proven by operation. In general, there is a higher incidence of radiological disc space narrowing and sciatica in the later stages of the condition, but although radiology may demonstrate an established disc lesion, it is of little value (except to exclude other conditions) in the early diagnosis of a disc lesion.

Neurological signs

Neurological signs are due to the physical involvement of the spinal cord or its nerve roots by disc prolapse. Nerve roots can slip away from any lesion which narrows the spinal canal unless that lesion is large enough to encroach significantly on the lumen. Compression, tension or angulation of a nerve root will cause symptoms; and recurrent trauma may well give rise to oedema of the nerve root, an inflammatory response, leading to organization of the oedema fluid, the formation of fibrous tissue and later to adhesions between the nerve root and the prolapse.

The mechanical factors involved are analogous to those met in certain lesions of peripheral nerves (e.g. involvement of nerve in a fracture callus; a neuroma following a peripheral nerve injury; carpal tunnel syndrome). In these conditions, continuous or intermittent mechanical involvement of the peripheral nerve may continue for weeks or months after the onset of symptoms before neurological signs can be detected. It may be assumed that similar conditions are responsible for the development of neurological signs due to prolapsed intervertebral discs, and motor weakness and muscle wasting are usually late signs in disc lesions. The time relationships for sensory changes are less clear.

The early diagnosis of prolapsed intervertebral disc

The syndrome is characterized by chronic or recurrent low backache, followed later by unilateral sciatica which is exacerbated by factors which increase intrathecal pressure. The interval between the onset of backache and sciatica is very variable, and in a few cases acute sciatica may be the first symptom.

The essential physical sign of disc prolapse is a limitation of spinal movement, with a consistent limitation of straight leg raising. Neurological and radiological evidence may confirm or exclude the diagnosis, but are not necessarily present in the early stages.

The severity, location and onset of the backache following the protrusion of the intervertebral disc varies with the size, site and rate of protrusion, and with the precipitating factors. Causing pain which varies from a dull ache to a stabbing pain radiating down the back of one or both legs, disc protrusion usually occurs at the level of L5/S1 or L4/L5 vertebral interspaces. Backache may occur without sciatic radiation, and sometimes sciatic pain without backache, although both are usually present.

Pressure from the disc protrusion may affect cord, cord and nerve roots, or nerve roots, depending on whether the protrusion is directed posteriorly, posterolaterally, or laterally. The exact relationship of the protrusion to the nerve roots crossing its interspace determines the site of the pain radiation and the associated neurological signs and symptoms. Yet due to the fact that the spinal cord ends at the level of the second lumbar vertebra and that disc protrusions may occur simultaneously at more than one intervertebral space, these signs and symptoms do not allow the deduction of the exact site of protrusion of any particular disc. (e.g. Both L5 and S1 roots cross the 4th lumbar disc; S1 root crosses the 5th lumbar disc; therefore a protrusion at the 4th lumbar disc space could press upon the L5 or S1 roots, or both; whereas a protrusion at the 5th lumbar disc space could press upon the S1 root. Thus, an irritation of the S1 root could mean a disc protrusion at *either* the 4th or the 5th lumbar interspace, and an irritation of both L5 and S1 roots could mean *either* a protrusion at the 4th interspace which affected both roots, *or* two protrusions, one at the 4th and one at the 5th interspaces, pressing on L5 and S1 roots respectively.)

Treatment of prolapsed intervertebral disc lesion

Treatment of backache due to an acute protrusion of an intervertebral disc may be considered in three categories—ambulant, bed and operative. Although the initial treatment of choice is bed rest, treatment with the patient ambulant may be tried if the pain is not too severe, and the patient is a non-manual worker.

The choice of treatment of an acute prolapsed intervertebral disc must depend upon the physical and mental condition of each individual patient and upon his work and home conditions.

The choice lies among four basic treatments, which may be used singly or in conjunction with each other: (1) rest in bed; (2) immobilization; (3) manipulation; or (4) traction.

Rest in bed

Most patients with severe backache are best treated in the initial stages by rest in bed and adequate analgesics. Not only the rest, but the position of the spine during that rest is important. To avoid the spinal flexion induced by a sagging mattress, patients are instructed to use a firm mattress laid over fracture boards, planks or a door.

Absolute rest is attempted with the patient in the position of maximal comfort. This he usually finds to be the supine position, with the affected leg flexed at hip and knee, and with only one pillow under his head. Analgesics and/or anti-inflammatory tablets are given for day or night use, and a night sedative supplied.

It is important to control the pain of prolapsed intervertebral disc adequately, since otherwise muscle spasm will continue and a self-perpetuating cycle of pain and spasm will result. When it is necessary to use the more potent analgesics initially, these should be used with caution and tailed off rapidly.

A gentle bulk laxative should be started immediately so as to avoid constipation and straining at stool. Bowel action should be into bedpan, commode or lavatory pedestal, according to the capability and inclination of the patient.

The patient should be encouraged to micturate into a urinal. Male and female urinals made of plastic are now readily available from all large chemists, and their use obviates the need for frequent painful sessions on bedpan, commode or lavatory seat.

Most patients with acute prolapsed intervertebral disc are nursed at home. Severe pain unrelieved by the above measures, or the presence of increasing paraesthesia or of neurological signs in the legs are indications for admission to hospital. Here a patient may be put into a plaster of paris jacket and discharged home if the symptoms and signs are controlled thereby or else treated by bed rest with continuous lumbar traction. Weights of up to 20 lb (9 kg) are gradually suspended from the legs by skin traction, 8–10 lb (3·6–4·5 kg) for each leg. The use of traction for a patient nursed at home is not practical unless continuous care is available.

While traction is applied to the legs, the foot of the bed is raised on blocks and, once again, the patient is nursed on a hard-based bed and firm mattress, using one or no pillows. Traction is maintained for about 3 weeks, depending upon the improvement or otherwise of the back pain. Static exercises are performed frequently and regularly for the muscles of the trunk and lower limbs throughout the period of traction and active exercises for trunk and upper limbs. When pain permits, and the traction is discontinued, graduated active exercises are urged and weight-bearing gradually resumed.

If pain has resolved completely, patients are discharged home without any spinal support and then have a period of regular out-patient physiotherapy, but if there is still unresolved pain, a period in a plaster of paris jacket may be tried, followed in some instances by a surgical corset.

In those few cases when conservative treatment has been tried and has failed, surgical intervention is called for.

Immobilization

Immobilization in a lumbar corset is used particularly for those patients whose financial straits or domestic and work commitments demand that they continue ambulant without repeated attendances for treatment at a physiotherapy department.

For these patients, long-term immobilization in purpose-designed, individually tailored, surgical corsets may provide effective pain relief. When measurements have been taken for these corsets, patients are temporarily immobilized in plaster of paris jackets, in instant corsets made of plaster of paris slabs applied to a tubigrip corset, or else in belts from the store of spinal supports which are stocked in many orthopaedic hospitals. This temporary form of immobilization is worn in each case until it can be exchanged for the finished, made-to-measure corset.

Whichever form of spinal support is worn, it should be kept on at night as well as by day, until the back pain has been relieved. Once this has occurred, and the straight leg raising is almost normal, the spinal support may be left off during the night but worn consistently by day for a further few weeks or even months, depending upon the occupation of the individual patient. Many people discard their supports before they should do because of the discomfort of wearing them. This is reduced considerably if the support is put on while the patient is supine.

As soon as the pain permits, static and then active exercises are introduced for the spinal and abdominal muscles. It is urged upon the patient that a surgical belt is not a substitute for efficient muscular action, and that the strength of the trunk musculature must be maintained throughout the entire period of immobilization. A twice-daily exercise routine before the corset is put on and after it is taken off, together with a further interval of static exercises which can be performed with the corset in situ should prevent the spine from stiffening and the muscles from losing bulk and strength. The exercises should be graduated in intensity and duration, so that by the time the surgical corset is discarded they have increased sufficiently to produce normal or near-normal muscle function.

The corset should be kept available for use when particularly hard physical work, likely to predispose to further disc protrusion, must be undertaken. When it is possible to avoid such work, patients should be urged to do so. Unfortunately, it is not easy to find or pay people to do the manual work attached to the care of the house or the garden, and many people are forced by circumstances to cope with tasks much better avoided.

Manipulation

The following are indications for manipulation.

(1) A thorough clinical examination has excluded the presence of abnormal neurological signs indicative of root pressure or of pressure on the cord.

(2) A radiological examination has excluded the presence of a neoplastic or infective lesion in the vertebrae, or of any indication of vertebral disease or frailty.

(3) A detailed history and thorough clinical examination has excluded lesions in other systems as causes of the backache, and it has been definitely established that the pain arises from the musculoskeletal system.

Even when these conditions have been satisfied, manipulation is by no means universally indicated, or invariably effective. First or recurrent attacks of backache of sudden onset may respond dramatically to a single manipulation. In the management of chronic low back pain, intermittent manipulation may also be useful.

The object of manipulation is to impart involuntary movement to the intervertebral joint from which the disc protrusion has occurred, so to allow the protrusion to be 'reduced' between the momentarily distracted joint surfaces by the tension of the surrounding muscles. When sufficient relaxation cannot be obtained with the patient conscious, manipulation under anaesthesia is sometimes performed. The danger of causing further damage to the patient is greater when he is manipulated in an unconscious state, and special care must be taken to ensure that no greater force is used than that for the conscious patient. Whenever possible, manipulation under anaesthesia should be avoided.

Manipulative treatment must be followed up by a regime of exercises, performed both in the physiotherapy department and at home. These should be initially static or isometric exercises for the erectores spinae and the anterior and lateral abdominal muscles, progressing, as pain permits, to graded active exercises for these muscles.

Contra-indications for manipulation are:

Pregnancy.

Significant root pain in one or both legs.

Marked deviation of the lumbar spine from the vertical when standing as erect as possible, i.e. sciatic scoliosis.

Straight leg raising reduced to 30 degrees on either side.

Continuous paraesthesia in one leg, or paraesthesia induced by standing.

Disturbances of micturition apparently associated with this episode of backache.

Neurological signs associated with the backache and sciatica, e.g. abnormal reflexes.

Sensory loss.

Significant weakness or wasting.

Clinical evidence of sacro-ilitis.

Significant osteoporosis of one or both hips.

Radiological evidence of:

- Osteoporosis.
- Spondylosis.
- Spondylolisthesis.
- Hemivertebra.
- Local bone disease.
- Vertebral anomalies associated with systemic disease.

Intermittent lumbar traction is another active technique which theoretically attempts to reduce the size of the intervertebral protrusion. There are various forms of equipment designed to exert traction on the lumbar spine while patients lie on specially designed traction tables. The efficacy of these is unproven, and a number of patients are in more pain after treatment than before it.

Operative treatment of prolapsed intervertebral disc

The criteria which induce surgeons to undertake operative treatment may be summarized as follows.

(1) Persistent or recurrent low backache.
(2) Limitation of movements of the lumbar spine.
(3) Radiological evidence of loss of disc space.

(4) Persistent sciatica.
(5) Persistent neurological signs.
  (*a*) Limitation of straight leg raising.
  (*b*) Muscle weakness.
  (*c*) Loss of tendon reflexes.

Since the relief of pain following operative treatment of a prolapsed intervertebral disc is not absolutely certain, operation should not be undertaken unless the medical and physical treatment given has been adequate and prolonged. When pain persists and is severe, when neurological signs have developed and are increasing, or when pain recurs in frequent and distressing bouts, operation should be considered. It becomes essential only when paraplegia develops from compression of the cauda equina by a prolapsed intervertebral disc.

Post-operative care depends upon the extent of the surgery. If it has been necessary to remove the lamina then rehabilitation is slower than if the operation was carried out through a laminotomy.

Although post-operative bed rest for up to 2 weeks has been advocated, many surgeons prefer to get their patients out of bed after 2 or 3 days. Static exercises for the trunk are commenced immediately post-operatively, and graduated exercises are increasingly added until there is full recovery of muscle strength.

Post-operative care involves instilling a regimen of 'back care' while encouraging the patient to return to normal activities as soon as possible. Avoidance of prolonged stooping and lifting and carrying of heavy objects with the spine in a position of mechanical disadvantage (i.e. flexed instead of extended), the practice of regular strengthening exercises for the spine, the use of a firm bed and mattress and a well-upholstered easy chair with adequate lumbar support are simple measures which are easily incorporated into the pattern of life for most people.

This attitude of sensible prophylactic care for the back should be encouraged in all patients who have back pain from any cause. Far from preventing them from living active lives, it permits the maximal possible participation in all activities, other than those especially conducive to back pain, by producing and maintaining optimum functional efficiency in the spine and its musculature. The prevention of pain by active conditioning of the affected part rather than by passive abstention from activity constitutes a mode of existence which some patients find hard to understand and harder still to follow. The medical and paramedical staff giving treatment need to emphasize and re-emphasize the necessity of continuing active prophylactic self-care throughout life.

OSTEO-ARTHROSIS OF THE LUMBAR SPINE

A prolapsed intervertebral disc acts as a major aetiological factor in the onset of degenerative changes in the lumbar spine (lumbar spondylosis or lumbar osteo-arthrosis).

It is the gradual transition from acute prolapsed intervertebral disc into general lumbar osteo-arthrosis over a period of years which gives rise to such a broad spectrum of clinical presentation and paradoxical response to therapy. During this process patients with similar symptoms and signs may respond to very different treatments, and one particular patient may respond differently as he gets older.

As prolapse of the intervertebral disc inevitably leads to narrowing of the intervertebral disc space, it also inevitably leads to subluxation of the posterior intervertebral joints. As these joints are synovial, such a mechanical disruption will inevitably lead to osteo-arthrosis. The narrowing of the intervertebral disc will also lead to osteophytosis of the lumbar spine.

Much confusion seems to have arisen from lack of differentiation between true osteo-arthrosis (of the posterior intervertebral joints) and osteophytosis or spondylosis of the vertebral bodies of the lumbar spine.

The diagnosis of osteo-arthrosis of the lumbar spine will depend on the radiological demonstration of generalized changes in the posterior intervertebral joints of the lumbar spine, usually in the middle-aged or elderly patient.

CONGENITAL ABNORMALITIES OF THE LUMBAR SPINE

Congenital deformities of the lumbar spine depend on radiography for their diagnosis. Those which can be associated with low back pain are:

- Spondylolisthesis.
- Spondylolysis.
- Abnormalities in the number of mobile lumbar vertebrae.
- Transitional vertebrae.
- Spinous process impingement.
- Spina bifida.
- Abnormalities of the posterior articular facets.

The incidence of congenital defects has been estimated variously as 0·5–27 per cent in patients with backache and 2–7 per cent in controls. The clinical significance of the defects is thus far from clear.

It is likely that congenital deformities of the lumbar spine are significant mainly because they represent a mechanical defect and, as such, are a contributory factor to the development of degenerative changes in the intervertebral joints.

'POSTURAL DEFECTS'

'Postural defects' have been variously recorded as being present in from 5 to 50 per cent of patients with backache, the incidence depending upon the patient group surveyed and the reporter's interests. These variations are partly due to selection of cases, and partly to the diagnostic criteria applied (which are seldom defined). All 'postural defects' are variations from the accepted 'normal' posture which can be corrected by the active effort of the patient. It is seldom that one part of the body alone is involved, and usually the entire posture is at fault. The main source of difference of opinion is the definition of 'normal posture'.

The 'postural defects' commonly met may be classified into three types, depending on the primary defect:

(1) Anterior-posterior curves of the spine.
(2) Lateral curves of the spine.
(3) Foot defects.

A few patients with 'postural defects' present with backache; many others present with foot defects; others are asymptomatic. As far as treatment is concerned, general postural re-education is more important than treatment of the feet alone.

'SHORT LEG' SYNDROME

The incidence of differences in leg lengths will depend upon the method of length assessment and upon the criteria by which patients are selected for leg measurement. The smaller the unit of measurement, the greater will be the incidence of length difference, and the larger the unit of measurement, the greater will be the agreement between observers.

The amount of leg difference which is clinically significant has been assessed at figures varying from $\frac{1}{4}$ in (0·625 cm) to $\frac{5}{6}$ in (2·10 cm). Differences of this magnitude demand considerable accuracy in measurement, which is difficult to ensure when it is generally accepted that it is impossible for one person to measure leg length more accurately than to within $\frac{1}{2}$ in (1·25 cm), and when there is considerable variation among individual observers. Until the technique of measurement can be standardized and its degree of accuracy improved, it is not possible to estimate the magnitude of the clinical problem attributable to difference in leg length.

Significant differences in leg length have been recorded in association with chronic infection of one joint (e.g. T.B. hip); local hypertrophy (e.g. angiectatic hypertrophy); haemangioma or lymphangioma; neurofibromatosis; injury; muscle disease (e.g. poliomyelitis) and congenital malformities; but the commonest form of leg length difference appears to be idiopathic.

Differences in leg lengths of less than $\frac{1}{2}$ in (1·25 cm) have little clinical significance, and there is an incidence of asymptomatic leg length difference of $\frac{1}{2}$ in (1·25 cm) or more in 7 per cent of the general population. The association between leg length differences and low back pain is emphasized by the fact that among patients with this type of pain such a difference in leg lengths occurs 3 times more commonly than it does among members of the population as a whole.

The clinical diagnosis of 'short leg' has been defined as depending on the presence of $\frac{1}{2}$ in (1·25 cm) leg length differences or more. The clinical diagnosis of 'short leg' syndrome assumes the presence of 'short leg' with associated symptoms.

'Short leg' syndrome is a condition commonly presenting as low backache of gradual onset, but occasionally as low backache of sudden onset, or pains in the legs, in which the only physical findings are those directly related to a leg length difference of $\frac{1}{2}$ in or more.

Although the symptoms are usually of gradual onset, they may sometimes by precipitated by minor trauma. In either case they are made worse by standing and activity, and relieved both by rest and by correction of the deformity (providing structural changes do not prevent the correction).

When associated with postural or congenital defects of the lumbar spine, however, the symptoms are not relieved by correction of the difference in leg length. 'Short leg' syndrome may prelude the development of a prolapsed intervertebral disc and may contribute to the aetiology of this condition. 'Short leg' may also be associated with idiopathic structural scoliosis.

Post-traumatic 'short leg' may interfere with functional recovery from the causative injury; this is a short-term effect of leg length discrepancy. The more serious effect is the long-term resulting degenerative disease which may develop in the weight-bearing joints of both shortened and normal limb, when excessive changes occur in the mechanical stresses to which they are subjected.

This relationship between 'short leg' and low backache resembles that between congenital defects of the lumbar spine and backache. Both defects may or may not cause symptoms in their own right. Both probably predispose to the development of ligamentous strains and consequent discomfort.

Although it has been estimated that 'short leg' occurs in approximately 7 per cent of the population without giving rise to symptoms, it would seem desirable to correct any inequality in leg lengths of more than half an inch, whether or not it is currently asymptomatic. Long-standing deformities need to be corrected in stages, but length discrepancies of short duration (e.g. post-traumatic 'short leg') may be corrected by a single procedure. In all instances, correction may be made simply by raising one heel and/or lowering the other to produce an adjustment of up to 1 in (2·5 cm). Raises of more than $\frac{1}{2}$ in (1·25 cm) in one heel should be accompanied by some thickening of the sole of the shoe.

CORSETS AND SPINAL SUPPORTS

The advisability of prescribing corsets or spinal supports is a matter about which there is a considerable difference of opinion. Some doctors prescribe a corset, or a support, almost routinely for any patients with recurrent backache; others refuse to prescribe either. It is interesting that such an 'all or none' attitude is adopted by many advocates of either policy, when the analogous prescription of a collar for pain in the neck is more laissez-faire. It has been adequately shown that consistent external support is beneficial for attacks of acute neckache, but as symptoms decrease, most doctors introduce a period of 'weaning off', allowing the collar to be removed for an increasing number of short intervals, and then for increasingly longer intervals.

A spinal support of some kind is appropriate for the patient with acute backache:

(1) Who needs or wants to remain ambulant but for whom manipulation is not indicated and physical measures such as heat or lumbar traction are insufficient to effect prolonged pain relief.

(2) Who has tried bed rest at home and has found it ineffective in controlling symptoms, but is not sufficiently inconvenienced to need hospitalization for continuous lumbar traction or for surgical intervention.

(3) Who has recurrent attacks of backache, despite an adequate programme of prophylactic exercises and strict attention to back care in all activities of daily living.

When back pain is acute the need for back support is equally acute and can be fulfilled by the provision of:

(*a*) A plaster of paris spinal jacket.

(*b*) A spinal jacket made of thermoplastic material (e.g. expanded polystyrene—plastazote).

(*c*) A standard surgical corset, ready-made in a range of different sizes and available 'off the shelf'.

(*d*) An 'instant corset' made from tubular elastic bandage strengthened in the back with slabs of plaster of paris bandage or of thermoplastic or of orthopaedic felt.

The disadvantages of the plaster of paris jacket are that it is heavy, does not allow for adjustment, and often produces a condition of unbearable claustrophobia. Its main advantage is that it does provide a very real restriction of all spinal movements. Less effective in producing such restrictions are the 'ready-made' surgical corset, the 'thermoplastic' corset and the 'instant corset'. All these forms of support, however, act as deterrents from attempts at flexion, lateral flexion and rotation of the spine, as well as reminders that patients must keep within their range of pain-free movements.

Application of a temporary back support during an acute episode of back pain should be preceded by the measurement of the patient for a more permanent form of corset. Both made-to-measure corsets of cotton material reinforced with steel strips, and the more complex spinal supports take several weeks, with one or more fittings to be made satisfactory. The temporary, or 'instant', corset attempts to keep the patient's back relatively immobile until the definitive brace or corset is completed. Often the patient becomes symptom-free before the permanent corset arrives. In this case the corset is retained and kept for use during long car journeys, heavy work (when unavoidable), prolonged activities which tend to cause backache, recurrences of back pain, and periods of malaise or fatigue. Prophylactic use of a corset can be very helpful in preventing the occurrence of severe back and sciatic pain. If the patient is *not* pain free when the definitive corset or support is ready, it should be worn until freedom from pain has lasted for several weeks, and then should be very gradually discarded.

The more rigid surgical braces are usually reserved for conditions more serious than prolapsed intervertebral disc or idiopathic low back pain. Whichever type of spinal corset, brace, belt or support is worn, it is important that static exercises should be carried out for the spinal extensor and abdominal muscles as a part of the regime involved with its use.

GENERAL MANAGEMENT OF PATIENTS WITH BACKACHE

Although the treatment of backache in its acute stages must necessarily vary with the causative lesion, the management of a patient who has backache or recurrent backache, or who is likely to have backache, has many constant features. Such management attempts to achieve a balance between the demands of family, work and environment upon the patient's back, and his functional capacity to fulfil those demands. It seeks to enable him to enjoy the fullest possible life without precipitating further attacks of pain.

The clinician and physiotherapist combine in advising regular exercises for spinal and abdominal muscles, weight control and the correct position of the spine during daily living activities. The occupational therapist advises how such activities may themselves be modified in order to avoid the fatigue or strain which may lead to further backache.

Prolonged standing, standing with the weight mainly on one leg and standing in a slumped or stooping posture should be avoided. A standing patient should never attempt to pick up heavy objects while his knees are extended but should squat down to grasp them and should lift by straightening his legs.

Prolonged sitting without adequate lumbar support should also be avoided. Drivers may need a small firm cushion, a backrest or one of the specially designed seats for drivers with painful backs. Patients who work in the sitting position for most of the day should avoid using stools or unsuitable chairs. The use of an upright chair is best, with a seat of such a height that the patient can sit comfortably with thighs horizontal, both feet flat on the ground and the lumbar spine well supported. Such a chair is appropriate also for the housewife with backache, so that she may sit to iron, wash up and do as much of her kitchen work as possible. In an easy chair, patients are advised to avoid sitting with knees crossed or with their feet tucked under them and to place a firm cushion behind their backs. Prolonged stooping almost invariably precipitates backache. To avoid this patients are asked to sit or kneel whenever possible for tasks which otherwise require a stooping posture. Alternatively, the heights of working surfaces, sink, ironing board etc. can be lowered to enable patients to sit at them comfortably.

Lifting or carrying heavy objects should be left to others, but if it is unavoidable, the patient can protect her back by balancing the load on her hip or abdomen.

Prophylactic organization of housework, shopping and gardening for the patient with backache is based on similar principles to those established for the patient with cervical spondylosis. This is particularly important when the two conditions occur in the same patient, as they frequently do.

Leisure activities should not include sporting activities which involve heavy lifting and pulling. During sedentary activities such as reading, writing, painting, sewing, knitting and crocheting, the patient with backache needs to sit in the type of chair already described.

Insufficient care is at present given to the design of chairs for children at school, young people working in lecture rooms, classrooms and libraries, and adults who follow sedentary occupations. Backache is not as infrequent among the young as it should be, which is not surprising when 2 hours at a stretch are often spent sitting on a high stool during double science periods and when there is no choice of seat heights available. It seems ludicrous that a tall and a short child must sit on chairs of the same height and lean over horizontal tables of constant height. A return to the sloping working surfaces of earlier school desks and a realistic approach to the need to relate the seat height to the height of the working surface for each child could do much to improve matters. The spines of the young are resilient, but when children are subjected to unnatural conditions and prolonged sitting they need the assistance of a well-positioned chairback constructed to provide lumbar support; equally they need to have their feet firmly on the ground—to assist a good spinal posture, to enable them to change position easily in the chair and to provide some weight relief to their buttocks.

BACKACHE AND THE DISABLED

Here it is appropriate to consider, in particular, the parent, spouse or child who cares for a disabled relative. The incidence of prolapsed intervertebral disc and consequent back pain among such patients is high, and as both patient and helper become older and less resilient, and the disabled person becomes heavier, the strain on the helper's back increases. The provision of adequate aids in the home to prevent the onset of back pain of such intensity as to necessitate bed rest for the helper, with consequent breakdown of the home situation, becomes a matter of urgency. Unfortunately, many people are reluctant to accept help until such a crisis has been precipitated. Once it has occurred and its consequences become apparent, the affected helper can usually be persuaded to wear a supporting corset, to follow a definite regime of prophylactic self-care, and to pay proper attention to the maintenance of the strength of spinal and abdominal musculature, while avoiding further provocation of disc prolapse by using a hoist for transfers and encouraging the patient to lose weight.

The general practitioners who treat disabled patients have particular need to anticipate the onset of serious back trouble in those giving the most care. They can ensure the early provision of a hoist through the local social services and a visit by an experienced domiciliary occupational therapist to advise both patient and helper on possible problems associated with activities of daily living.

If difficulty is experienced in providing a hoist suitable for patient, helper and the home in which they live, referral of patient and helper to a disabled living centre or rehabilitation unit is indicated, where accurate assessment and prescription of the most suitable type of hoist can be made.

The cost of installing an electric hoist with an overhead track or of rehousing a family in a house where a portable hoist can be effectively used is insignificant compared with the cost of accommodating a disabled person permanently in an institution, simply because the relative giving care has also become disabled with back pain.

AGE GROUPS AT PARTICULAR RISK

When examining patients who present with backache, it is important to recall that backache from certain causes is particularly likely to occur in different age groups, and to be vigilant in excluding these causes.

Young people

In young people complaining of backache, symptoms may arise from:

Scoliosis (1) idiopathic or primary; (2) secondary to (*a*) vertebral anomaly; (*b*) paraspinal neuromuscular dysfunction.

Kyphosis secondary to bony abnormalities such as Scheuermann's disease.

Infection such as vertebral abscess or osteomyelitis from TB, staphylococcal or typhoid infection.

Injury such as crush fracture following accidents at sport and work or on the road.

Involvement of the posterior vertebral joints in one of the acute arthritides (including ankylosing spondylitis).

Young women

In young women complaining of backache, in addition to the causes listed above:

Structural or functional abnormality in the genital system must be excluded.

Backache of locomotor origin is especially likely to occur during pregnancy, after labour and after gynaecological operations.

Middle-aged patients

In such patients more frequent causes of backache presenting for the first time are:

Degenerative joint disease.
Vertebral metastatic involvement.

Older people

In older people likely causes are:

Osteoporosis.
Degenerative joint disease.

SUMMARY

The structure of the lumbosacral spine predisposes to mechanical problems, and it is not in the least surprising that low back pain is so common. Indeed, mechanical causes are responsible for most cases.

Identification of cause entails a detailed examination of the patient and careful attention to his history. Appropriate treatment demands not only the elimination of serious and removable causes of pain, but also the reassurance of the patient, an adequate explanation of his symptoms and advice on future care relative to work, leisure and daily living activities.

Certainly, if the patient has an acute disc lesion, with persistent neurological signs, there is good reason to consider surgical removal of the offending disc. If bony inadequacy is present (e.g. spondylolisthesis) or persistent pain associated with other congenital deformities, there is a good case for considering spinal fusion. Polymyalgia rheumatica, osteoporosis, neoplasm, myelomatosis, tuberculosis, ankylosing spondylitis or fracture call for special care and treatment.

The majority of cases of backache are associated with minor strains with or without associated degenerative changes. The patients are often reassured by old-fashioned non-specific terms—'lumbago' is often more acceptable and sounds less disabling than a slipped disc or 'arthritis', which are emotive terms with serious connotations.

At some stage, most of these cases of low back pain respond to:

Palliative heat.
Rest on a firm bed.
Restriction of movement by a corset.
Active mobilization by exercises, preferably in warm water (hydrotherapy).

In the majority of cases, the natural history is one of progressive radiological changes of osteo-arthrosis and osteophytosis (spondylosis) and progressive loss of joint range, associated with intermittent symptoms of backache with or without referred pain in the buttocks or legs. The more acute the symptoms, the more restrictive and intensive should be the treatment prescribed.

Acute, severe, disabling pain warrants immediate radiological examination, whether or not there is a history of trauma, and in the absence of serious causes, the best treatment is rest in bed with a firm mattress. Chronic recurrent low backache responds well to palliative physiotherapy.

In both types, the immediate acute phase, the exacerbation and the recurrence will respond to total rest. The period of immobility should be followed by a period of back-strengthening (extension) exercises and then mobilizing exercises.

Pain is the guide. Exercises and other activities that cause pain should be avoided. Static exercises of the extensors are rarely painful and more active mobilizing exercises including extension, flexion, rotation etc. can be introduced when they can be performed without pain.

The indication for rest in bed or rest in a spinal support will be determined by the severity of the backache experienced by the particular patient and by his physical, psychological and social state.

When loss of movement is a significant feature, stretching and manipulative techniques may achieve dramatic results.

At all times, postural re-education and strengthening exercises are essential except when they themselves precipitate severe pain, when treatment by further rest is indicated.

There are a number of serious conditions which may present as low back pain, with or without sciatica, and these must always be excluded. Haemoglobin estimation, E.S.R. and appropriate radiographs are mandatory investigations supplementing full clinical examination.

Backache tends to be a recurring symptom, for the sufferers are notoriously reluctant to abide by the advice given them. They will not exercise to strengthen their spinal musculature, lose weight, limit their activity to a level below the threshold of pain onset, abstain from precipitating activities, limit the duration of their activities, limit the time for which they take up any particular spinal posture or organize their leisure/work/household activities to avoid exacerbations of their pain. They persist in 'finishing the job' instead of changing from task to task to avoid becoming fatigued. They refuse to cut down their arduous physical activities and supplement them with mechanical aids or to acknowledge the passage of time. They will not accept that the older a man is the shorter the time for which he can hold any particular trunk posture without causing muscular pain. Above all they refuse to recognize the particular precipitating cause of their backache and are therefore unable to effect its removal, or else, recognizing it, do not, or cannot, choose to remove it.

BIBLIOGRAPHY AND REFERENCES

Barnes, C. G. (1971). 'The differential diagnosis of backache.' *Br. J. Hosp. Med.* **5**, 219

Brain, W. R. (1954). 'Spondylosis: the known and the unknown.' *Lancet* **1**, 687

Brav, E. A. (1942). 'Diagnosis of low back pain of orthopaedic origin: analysis of 62 cases.' *Am. J. Surg.* **55**, 57

Charnley, J. (1951). 'Orthopaedic signs in the diagnosis of disc protrusion.' *Lancet* **1**, 186

Clymer, G., Mixter, W. J. and Mella, H. (1921). 'Experience with spinal cord tumours during the past 10 years.' *J. nerv. ment. Dis.* **53**, 229

Falconer, M. A., McGeorge, M. and Begg, A. C. (1948). 'Observations on the cause and mechanism of symptom-production in sciatica and low back pain.' *J. Neurol. Neurosurg. Psychiat.* **11**, 13

Floyd, W. F. and Silver, P. H. S. (1951). 'Function of erectores spinae in flexion of the trunk.' *Lancet* **1**, 133

Hart, F. D., Robinson, K. C., Allchin, F. M. and MacLagen, N. F. (1949). 'Ankylosing spondylitis.' *Q. Jl Med.* **18**, 217

Hurst, A. (1943). 'Treatment of sciatica: essay in debunking.' *Br. med. J.* **2**, 773

Jayson, M. I. V. (1970). 'The problem of backache.' *Practitioner* **205**, 615–21

Kellgren, J. H. (1939). 'On distribution of pain arising from deep somatic structures with charts of segmental pain area.' *Clin. Sci.* **4**, 35

Kellgren, J. H. (1941). 'Sciatica.' *Lancet* **240**, 561

Mixter, W. J. and Barr, J. S. (1934). 'Rupture of intervertebral disc with involvement of spinal cord.' *New Engl. J. Med.* **211**, 210

Mowat, A. G. and Camp, A. V. (1971). 'Polymyalgia rheumatica.' *J. Bone Jt Surg.* **53B**, 701

Newman, P. H. (1952). 'Sprung back.' *J. Bone Jt. Surg.* **34B**, 30

Nichols, P. J. R. (1960). 'Short leg syndrome.' *Br. med. J.* **1**, 1863

Pearce, J. and Moll, J. H. M. (1967). 'Conservative treatment and natural history of acute lumbar disc lesions.' *J. Neurol. Neurosurg. Psychiat.* **30**, 13

Rush, W. A. and Steiner, H. A. (1946). 'Study of lower extremity length inequality.' *Am. J. Roentg. Rad. Ther.* **56**, 616

Tegner, W. S. (1954). 'Physical medicine.' *Proc. R. Soc. Med.* **47**, 389

Van Leuven, R. M. and Troup, J. D. G. (1969). 'The "instant" lumbar corset.' *Physiotherapy* **55**, 499

Wright, V. and Moll, J. M. H. (1973). 'Ankylosing spondylitis.' *Br. J. Hosp. Med.* **9**, 331

Wyke, B. D. (1967). 'The neurology of joints.' *Ann. R. Coll. Surg.* **41**, 25

Wyke, B. D. (1970). 'The neurological basis of thoracic spinal pain.' *Rheum. phys. Med.* **10**, 356

7—*Osteo-arthrosis*

INTRODUCTION

Osteo-arthrosis is a pathological condition of a synovial joint, which though occurring spontaneously in the middle-aged and elderly, may also be precipitated by injury, disease or deformity. It is a progressive condition involving the destruction of hyaline cartilage and ultimately involving all the structures of the joint in changes which are mainly degenerative. Clinically, there may be crepitus on movement, restriction of the range of motion and effusion into the joint cavity with enlargement or alteration of the joint contours. The diagnosis is established by the occurrence of the characteristic radiological changes of narrowing of joint space, subchondral sclerosis and cyst formation, and osteophytosis. Such a joint has become worn and mechanically defective, and is more prone to mechanical strains. Clinically the condition may be symptomless, and the severity of the symptoms is rarely related to the severity of the radiographic changes. Symptoms are more frequently associated with trauma and are thus often more significant in the weight-bearing joints of lower limb and spine than in the upper limb joints.

As the condition progresses, joint range becomes increasingly restricted, often reducing the severity of the symptoms. However, osteo-arthrosis in a weight-bearing joint, such as a hip or knee, associated with a mechanical abnormality due to old injury or disease, can progress with considerable speed and rapidly lead to painful joint destruction.

SYMPTOMS

It is helpful to review the symptoms associated with osteo-arthrosis, as they are usually a guide to treatment. Patients with osteo-arthrosis commonly complain of pain, stiffness and reduced range of movement. In addition, they may complain of intermittent swelling, due to effusion, or to permanent increase and change in size, due to bony enlargement. Joint laxity, locking or grating may also be presenting symptoms.

Pain

The pain is often worst after prolonged exercise, though it may be relieved by exercise once the initial stiffness on commencing movement has worn off. Depending upon the nature, severity and location of joint involvement, bed rest may relieve or exacerbate it: frequently, osteo-arthritic pain will light up as the muscles relax after the patient has been in bed a short time and will disturb sleep. Persistent maintenance of any one body posture also tends to bring on pain.

Most patients assert that as long as they can 'keep going', 'chop and change' and 'take their own time' about their various tasks they can also reduce their pain. For every arthritic joint there will usually be one 'position of ease' in which maximal relief of pain for long periods is experienced. The pain from osteo-arthrosis is not constant but varies with position, activity and weather. Although it is not accompanied by the systemic upsets of rheumatoid arthritis, it is nevertheless distressing, and has a 'wearing' quality remarked upon by the majority of those who suffer from it; and under certain circumstances it can be intensely painful.

Stiffness

Unlike that of rheumatoid arthritis, the stiffness of osteo-arthrosis is not necessarily worst in the mornings. It may be evident at any time of the day in which a posture is held constantly for a long time. A patient with osteo-arthrosis of the knees and spine may complain of the need to assist himself out of an easy chair either by pushing on the arms of the chair or else by rocking himself in increasing arcs until he manages to stand at the end of the forward rock.

Some stiffness is muscular in origin, and some of it may be due to a permanently diminished range of movement due to alteration in joint structure. Stiffness of the former variety wears off with exercise and is minimized by frequent changes of posture. Conversely, it is exacerbated by prolonged exercise. As with the pain of osteo-arthritic joints, this muscular stiffness is less when patients are able to change often from task to task, so varying their patterns of movement.

Diminished range of movement

In the early stages of osteo-arthrosis, restriction of joint movement may be partly due to a voluntary decision to avoid pain, and partly to the involuntary spasm of the muscles to which pain is referred from the inflamed joint structures. In the later stages, in which cartilage destruction and bony overgrowth have occurred, this restriction follows the actual mechanical block to joint movement which such overgrowth can produce. Pain may be felt while some movement remains in the joint.

Swelling

The swelling complained of may be due to bony overgrowth or to an effusion or it may be due to inflammation in the periarticular tissues, as in the Heberden's nodes of the interphalangeal joints. Occasionally swelling may be apparently extra-articular and yet derive from the joint itself, as in the case of cystic swelling, particularly of the knee and elbow.

'Locking' or 'giving way'

'Locking' or 'giving way' of weight-bearing joints are occasional symptoms usually associated with an effusion in the joint. The knee joint is particularly prone to these symptoms which are probably due to detached fragments of osteophytes, cartilage or menisci lodging momentarily between opposing joint surfaces.

MEDICATION

Either simple analgesics or preparations with analgesic and anti-inflammatory action are given in sufficient doses to eliminate pain or reduce it to a reasonable level. Soluble aspirin, enteric-coated aspirin, aloxiprin, phenylbutazone, indomethacin and paracetamol alone or combined in the same tablet with salicylate may be found effective. There is a great deal of individual variation in the responses of different patients to these various drugs.

Side-effects are frequent, and are most commonly upsets of the digestive tract. Care is needed when salicylates, phenylbutazone or indomethacin are given to patients with past history of indigestion or peptic ulceration. Whenever possible soluble or enteric-coated tablets should be used, and administered during meals. Persistent indigestion is an indication for stopping any particular type of tablet, as haematemsis or melaena may result if this symptom is ignored.

Sometimes a reduction in dosage level, the use of the same medicament in an enteric-coated capsule, or the addition of an antacid permits medication to be continued.

More recently, ibuprofen, aclofenac and benorylate have been added to the armamentarium of drugs for the treatment of osteo-arthritis. Their long-term effects have not yet been fully evaluated and therefore they should be reserved for patients who are intolerant of, or unhelped by, the longer established preparations.

The establishment of a satisfactory drug regime presents a very real difficulty in a large number of patients. In effective doses, many of the drugs commonly used have untoward side-effects which outweigh their usefulness as analgesics. Apart from the tendency of the salicylates, phenylbutazone and indomethacin to cause gastro-intestinal pain and bleeding, phenylbutazone and indomethacin may both cause fluid retention and indomethacin may produce insomnia and depress normal intellectual function. Many patients need to strike a balance between an effective and a tolerable level of medication.

When sleep is regularly disturbed by a serious joint pain, and operative corrective treatment for the joint concerned is not feasible, a stronger analgesic may need to be given at night in addition to the sedative.

It is important that patients with osteo-arthrosis who are on a regular drug regime should be instructed how to prevent constipation, both by dietary means and by taking regular doses of bulk laxatives such as bran or methylcellulose preparations.

PHYSIOTHERAPY

Physiotherapy can be a great help in osteo-arthrosis. The procedures employed must naturally depend upon the particular joint or joints involved and also on the amount of articular and periarticular damage which is present. The patient's pain threshold, his degree of functional disability and his commitments both at home and at work must be taken into consideration.

Physiotherapeutic treatment is usually combined with medication, and with advice by the medical adviser and the occupational therapist on the day-to-day management of the patient as a whole.

The aims of physiotherapeutic treatment of osteo-arthrosis are:

Pain relief.
Restoration of function.
Prevention of further deformity.
Stabilization of unstable joints.
Enforced rest by splintage or bracing.

When, despite adequate medication and physiotherapy, it is not possible to prevent progressive joint destruction, or to achieve adequate pain relief, surgical treatment must be considered.

Symptomatic treatment

Osteo-arthrosis manifests itself clinically as a painful, swollen joint with some restriction in joint range and with associated muscle wasting and weakness.

Passive palliative physiotherapy in the form of heat (wet or dry) can be very soothing and pleasant for the patient. Such treatment forms an excellent way for the therapist to establish rapport with the patient, and to pave the way for the acceptance of other treatment, whether this be advice or active strenuous exercise.

Radiant heat, infra-red heat, short-wave diathermy, ultrasonics, hot packs, hot-water sprays, hydrotherapy or wax are all methods of applying heat, and there is no convincing evidence that there is any physiological reason for selecting one rather than another. The choice should be left to the physiotherapist and will depend on the availability of the apparatus, the time available for treatment and the personal predilections of the therapist and the patient.

Muscle power and joint effusion

It is universally accepted that the quadriceps muscle is the guardian of the knee joint. When an acute effusion of the knee joint occurs, whether due to minor trauma, surgery or an exacerbation of arthritis, the quadriceps muscle shows a tendency to waste. This wasting appears to be a prelude to an exacerbation of arthritis, and thus a vicious circle of events is initiated to perpetuate a progressive disorganization of the joint.

There is some evidence that the quadriceps wasting is associated with an inhibition of its normal contraction; increasing the tension within the knee joints by intra-articular injection has been shown to induce temporary inhibition of voluntary contraction of the quadriceps. Certainly from the clinical standpoint, acute effusion of any aetiology is often associated with difficulty in obtaining active quadriceps contraction and leads to marked wasting. The condition can be helped by active stimulation of the quadriceps muscle with electrical impulses. Usually 3 or 4 treatment sessions over 2–3 days is enough to re-establish voluntary contractions.

This vicious cycle can be broken by a combination of intensive non-weight-bearing quadriceps exercises and passive splinting and support of the knee during essential weight-bearing. A simple back-splint of plaster of paris, plastic, or other available materials may be adequate.

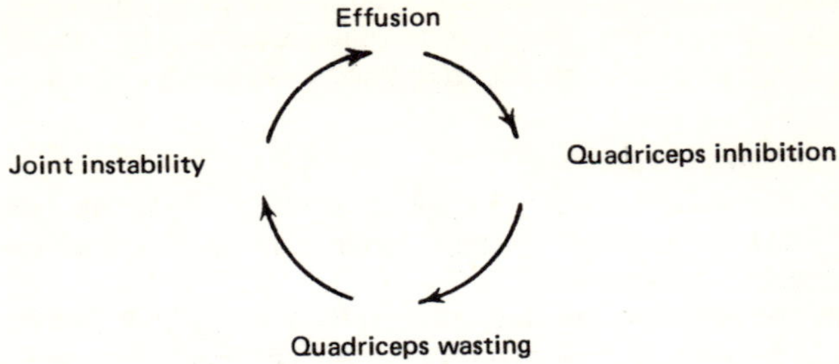

A plaster of paris cylinder is sometimes necessary. For more chronic and severe conditions, weight-relieving calipers are useful.

It may be that other muscles or muscle groups are the 'key' muscles for various other joints and of the same importance to their stability as the quadriceps is to the knee. Certainly abduction of the hip is often weak and painful during an exacerbation of symptoms due to osteo-arthrosis of the hip, and intensive non-weight-bearing abduction exercises of the hip are often followed by a reduction in pain. Perhaps the gluteus medius is inhibited by effusion in the hip joint. Similarly, the calf muscles are often slow to respond to strengthening exercises in the presence of ankle injuries.

Obesity

The part that obesity has to play in the aetiology of osteo-arthrosis may be subject to discussion, but the reduction of obesity in the presence of symptomatic osteo-arthrosis of weight-bearing joints is universally recommended. Indeed, the loss of surplus weight in the presence of osteo-arthrosis of hips, knees, ankles and spine should be a primary aim. There are many who will refuse to introduce other forms of treatment until weight has been reduced to 'normal'. The process is often difficult for patients in active employment or in the lower income groups, and for some a short period of hospitalization and the administration of a low (800 calories per day) diet may be the only way of initiating weight reduction. For most patients a sympathetic dietician, and membership of a group of 'weight-watchers' are successful once they understand the real need for reducing their weight.

GENERAL ADVICE

Living with osteo-arthrosis is an exercise in invention, substitution, compromise and, above all, organization. When a doctor says to a patient 'You have wear-and-tear arthritis. We can help you a great deal, but we cannot actually undo the damage which has been done—you will have to learn to live with it', this should not be seen as a negative attitude, and it does not call for passive acceptance on the part of the patient.

Where osteo-arthrosis follows direct trauma or infection, one joint only may be involved, but in the older patients, osteo-arthrosis seldom strikes at a single joint. Several joints are usually affected, albeit to varying degrees. The patient who could cope well with the vicissitudes of one abnormal joint is faced with the knowledge that to do so would be to precipitate pain in several others. He lives therefore in a state of perpetual compromise, where the joint or joints giving most discomfort at any one time are managed with concessions consistent with the optimal good of the body as a whole.

The essence of living fully and successfully with osteo-arthrosis is the mutual acknowledgement by doctor and patient that osteo-arthrosis may have repercussions affecting every aspect of life, and the recognition of the importance of managing the life of the patient in such a way that these repercussions are minimized. This can only be achieved by a broad outlook on the work and leisure activities of the patient.

Probably the most important contribution that can be made to the management of osteo-arthrosis in a rehabilitation department is the dispensation of reassurance and good general advice. The confident reassurance that the symptoms do not herald a serious, progressive, crippling disorder is based upon accurate diagnosis. The patient should be given a clear and simple explanation of the pathology, the likely prognosis, the alternatives of long-term and short-term treatment available and a rational explanation of the reasons for choosing or changing a particular treatment regimen. The importance of preventing obesity and other forms of excessive strain and of maintaining general physical fitness and local muscular strength must be stressed.

Emphasis must be placed on the need to rest during a period of acute joint pain while yet avoiding prolonged inactivity during quiescent phases. The difference between non-weight-bearing exercises and free activity must also be clearly demonstrated and the necessity of avoiding undue stress and trauma to the affected joints explained. Such advice may range from discussion concerning the patient's work (particularly for those in heavy industry) to the problems of inadequate or unsuitable housing. It may also include instruction on the use of a simple appliance such as knee bandage or wrist support whilst undertaking certain tasks.

The dispensation of useful advice is a time-consuming activity if it is to be relevant and meaningful. Unfortunately, it is not always possible for the doctor to spend as much time as is really necessary in explanation. In these circumstances, it is incumbent upon the clinician to ensure that someone else is given the time to accomplish this most important part of the patient's care. Much of this important work properly falls to the physiotherapists and occupational therapists. For many patients, the doctor's reassurance is the most important part of the treatment, but the majority will benefit from more general advice and direction from the therapists.

DETAILED ADVICE

Detailed advice may with advantage be the combined responsibility of the physiotherapist and occupational therapist attending the clinic or concerned in treatment. It is well recognized that patients do not remember clearly the instructions and advice given by doctors. Repeated enforcement of this advice during treatment sessions or follow-up clinics is often better remembered and therefore of greater use. Thus, the more relaxed interview with the therapist following that at which the doctor has made his enquiry, examination and prescription for investigation and treatment, is often the more important for the patient's rehabilitation.

The therapist translates the doctor's advice into domestic terms. She enquires further into difficulties with activities of daily living and gives detailed advice on how to minimize pain and exertion. In addition, she suggests alternative methods of arranging domestic routines and ways of rearranging furniture and household fixtures, and she will also supply essential aids, or arrange for them to be supplied. Although it is traditionally the occupational therapist who does this, ideally this aspect of management should be the combined responsibility of physiotherapist and occupational therapist working together. The physiotherapist supplements the necessary knowledge of the home situation from further information which she gathers during treatment sessions. Under the warmth of the heat lamp, relaxed and confident, because the fear of being left with pain has been removed, a patient will often reveal details which have been concealed from the doctor. Some aggravating factor at work or home is described which has precipitated or contributed to the present state. This may be a financial difficulty, a marital problem or a work situation, a clinical fear or some domestic or social stress.

When a patient has pain and dysfunction from osteo-arthrosis, the discovery of predisposing factors in the history is of considerable importance. Since the condition cannot be cured, it must be managed, and the more detailed the knowledge of a patient's pain, the more likely it is that the pain can be reduced to a minimum. As in so many other fields of rehabilitation, the wiser the therapist, the less therapy she will need to dispense. Counselling pays better dividends than empirical physical therapy.

Many of the key factors in a particular patient's pain pattern can be quickly elicited. Others can only be discovered by detailed questioning. One of the greatest values of a period of palliative physiotherapy is that it provides time for the patient to relax and establish a rapport with the therapist. During these periods much essential and therapeutic discussion can take place.

If the patient is not clearly and authoritatively informed about his symptoms and their prevention, he will acquire a great deal of uninformed folklore or invent concepts for himself. Thus, an adequate explanation to the patient of the natural history of the disease, so that he understands the part which he can play in influencing its progress, is the corner-stone of his management.

Work

The elimination or reduction of predisposing factors which cause exacerbations of the patient's symptoms necessitates a frequent reassessment of their relationship to his work, transport, home, leisure activities and personal care. Some of the most important advice to be sought and given relates to a man's work. To give sensible and relevant advice, considerable information is needed. Careful enquiry is needed about his postures and movement during work, and their duration, repetition and capacity to cause pain or stiffness. It is helpful to the doctor and therapists if the patient is able to describe in mime the sequence of movements which make up the basic pattern of his day's work so that the causes of the pain can be made apparent.

Gratuitous advice to 'take it easy' or to 'find a light job' may precipitate a sequence of events leading to permanent unnecessary unemployment. Detailed advice regarding work activities should only be given when an accurate prognosis can be matched with a detailed knowledge of the type of employment. Preferably such advice should be constructive, indicating capability and not negatively restricting activity. Many patients have lost their jobs through ill-considered advice. Many others have kept them in relative comfort following suitable alterations to equipment, working surfaces, seating heights, or the method in which they use these.

Transport

Here, too, pertinent questioning often reveals a host of precipitating factors leading to pain and dysfunction in affected joints. Such questions include:

Does the patient drive a car—what make is it?
Does it cause any discomfort?
Does the seat cause backache?
Do the controls cause wrist, elbow or shoulder discomfort?
Are the door handles stiff and do they cause pain in the wrists or hands?
Is there an awkward stretch to reach the handle or lock on the back door?
Does he get pain when he looks around to reverse?
Does he get pain when he brakes suddenly?
Does he do minor car maintenance and repair jobs himself?
Does he wear a seat belt?
Has he a well-designed headrest.
Does he ride a bicycle?
Can he dismount easily?
Can he mount it easily or must this be done from a kerb?
Can he pedal it easily?
Does he travel by bus or train?
If so, does he fall asleep while travelling?
Does he strap-hang for long intervals, and must he stand frequently?

Home

Enquiries about a patient's home establish:

Does he have a warm house?
What is his usual chair like and does sitting cause pain?
Does he fall asleep often in his chair?
Has he difficulty in getting up and down from the toilet?
Or climbing up and down stairs?
What is his bed like, and does he get pain at night?
What is the layout of his house, and does any of the work in the house cause particular pain?

Housework and leisure activities

Everyday activities at home are often a potent source of pain. A patient should therefore be questioned about his home, hobbies or other household commitments.

Leisure activities are particularly important and become increasingly so in the older age groups. Relevant questions to a patient include:

In general.
What are his hobbies?
Does he do a lot of gardening?

Does he do a lot of decorating and do-it-yourself work, or participate in a competitive or exacting sport?

If a housewife:

Does the patient clean, cook or polish excessively?
Has she a part-time job? If so, what?

Family commitments:

Are there children? How many and how dependent?
Are there lodgers? How many and how dependent?
Is there family or outside help for domestic work?
Is there difficulty or pain with personal care—washing, dressing, grooming and toiletting?

For patients in hospital, such assessment is the province of the occupational therapist and indirectly of the physiotherapist, but for patients seen in the G.P.'s surgery, out-patient departments or their own homes, it is the G.P. or consultant who needs to initiate the assessment. Though time-consuming, it is an essential preliminary to the correct management of osteo-arthrosis and indicates in which of the many aspects of daily activity help is required.

With the wide range of assistance from the Department of Health and Social Security now available, it is usually possible to provide considerable help for patients in need, but the provision of the right help at the right time, and in an acceptable form, is difficult; without accurate functional assessment it is impossible.

SUMMARY OF POSSIBLE TREATMENT IN OSTEO-ARTHROSIS

These are the essential parts of the *management* of all patients with osteo-arthrosis:

(1) An adequate explanation of the natural history of the disease and of the part which the patient can play in influencing its progress.

(2) Instruction in activities of daily living so that he avoids fatigue and pain whenever possible.

(3) Initial instruction and advice by the doctor caring for him, confirmed and re-enforced by the therapists who treat him.

(4) Instruction in the importance of maintaining optimal general physical fitness and correct body weight.

(5) Organization of house and garden to minimize effort, fatigue and pain during their maintenance.

(6) Organization of working conditions to ease or avoid discomfort—if necessary by changing occupation.

(7) Assessment of transport, hobbies and leisure activities. Reorganization to avoid pain and effort.

Some, or all of these forms of *treatment* need to be incorporated in the overall management of the condition:

(8) Medication by means of analgesic drugs, night sedatives and laxatives.

(9) Injection of hydrocortisone with or without local anaesthetic, into and around joints, bursae, tendons and muscles.

(10) Support or stabilization in the form of splints and calipers to prevent the exacerbation of pain caused by movement of painful joints and by excessive mobility in unstable joints. This includes collars, spinal braces and corsets.

(11) Intermittent attendance at the rehabilitation department for appropriate palliative treatment, general assessment and advice.

(12) Surgical intervention to alter the stresses on a joint by means of an osteotomy, to fix a joint in one position by means of an arthrodesis, or to change its internal structure by means of excision, interposition or replacement arthroplasty.

(13) The issue or aids and appliances to enable a patient to compensate for the grossly restricted or absent function of lower limb joints, whether this stems from pain, stiffness, weakness or a combination of all of these symptoms. Such aids are those offering weight-relief or stabilization to joints of the lower limbs:

Weight relieving calipers.
Sticks, quadruped sticks, crutches or walking frames.
Wheelchairs.
Outdoor transport.

(14) The issue of aids and devices to improve function and reduce stress for upper limbs. Such devices:

(*a*) Increase the range of upper limb movement, e.g. lazy tongs, helping-hand aids, curtain-pulling stick, stocking aids.

(*b*) Decrease the effort needed to manipulate household fixtures or equipment, e.g. tap turner, padded glove.

BIBLIOGRAPHY AND REFERENCES

Dixon, A. St. J. (Ed.) (1965). *Progress in Clinical Rheumatology*. London; J. & A. Churchill

Golding, D. N. (1969). 'General management of osteoarthrosis.' *Br. med. J.* **3**, 575

Law, W. A. (1967). 'Surgery in the treatment of osteoarthrosis.' *Hosp. Med.* **1**, 612–616

Licht, S. (Ed.) (1969). *Arthritis and Physical Medicine*. U.S.A.; E. Licht

8—Fractures, Dislocations and Other Injuries

INTRODUCTION

The rehabilitation of a patient with a fracture should start as soon as the fracture is reduced and the reduction has been firmly held. Indeed, the most important factor in determining the end result and therefore in determining the need for rehabilitation is the quality of the treatment of the fracture and the associated soft-tissue injury.

For each fracture, there is an ideal rehabilitative routine which falls into several sections:

(1) The routine followed during the period the fracture is consolidating:

(*a*) In hospital, whether as an in-patient or out-patient.
(*b*) At home.

(2) The routine followed when the fractured bone ends have joined in a well-consolidated union.

(*a*) In hospital, whether as an in-patient or out-patient.
(*b*) At home.

(3) The issue of appropriate aids to assist the function of the fractured part and the patient as a whole.

(4) Training and advice on personal care and daily living activities during the period of fracture consolidation and the ensuing one of patient mobilization.

Throughout the entire period of rehabilitation it is essential that five separate aspects of the healing of the injured part should be considered concurrently: bone healing; soft-tissue conservation; joint mobility; maintenance of muscle strength and co-ordination; total patient health.

Bone healing

The prime object of the treatment of a fractured bone is to cause the two ends to unite in a firmly consolidated union in the optimal functional position.

Soft-tissue conservation

Soft-tissue conservation encourages the repair and resumption of the normal functional interrelationship of the various soft-tissue components—muscle, nerve, blood vessels, lymphatics, connective tissue and skin.

Maintenance of joint mobility and muscle strength

The maintenance of joint mobility seeks to retain a full range of motion for the unimpeded joints of the whole body and to regain the maximal possible amount of movement for any joints immobilized during the period of fracture consolidation. The regular performance of active exercises throughout the period of fracture consolidation is the key-stone to the total rehabilitative treatment of the patient. Such activity:

(1) Assists the preservation of the mobility of the joints of the fractured limb.

(2) Promotes the circulation of blood, lymph and tissue fluid.

(3) Prevents disuse osteoporosis in the bones of the fractured limb.

(4) Minimizes adhesion formation.

(5) Preserves muscle power, tone and co-ordination.

Total patient health

Total patient health may well be inadvertently allowed to deteriorate while the fracture site is receiving maximal attention during the early stages of fracture healing, particularly if the patient is confined to bed or chair during a prolonged period of non-weight-bearing. The rehabilitative treatment for the whole patient should be started when the fracture has been reduced and continued throughout the period of immobilization required for bone healing. A programme of planned, graduated activity should be supplemented by mobility and independence training when the healing of the fracture permits, and is completed only when optimal functional efficiency has been restored to the injured part and the patient as a whole.

The rehabilitation of a patient with a fracture varies so much with the type of fracture that it may conveniently be considered in four sections:

Rehabilitation of
- Upper limb fractures
- Lower limb fractures
- Spine and pelvic fractures
- Fractures associated with multiple injuries

The differences in the problems presented by the rehabilitation of fractures of these various types relate to:

The relative independence of people with upper limb fractures from the time the fracture is reduced.

The need to avoid weight-bearing and to protect lower limb fractures during the healing phase.

The difficulties of combining the needs of adequate nursing with adequate measures to ensure the achievement of maximal power and mobility in spinal and multiple injuries.

In each case rehabilitation presents problems of specific and general management. The specific problems relate to the maintenance of muscle power in the injured part during the period of fracture healing and to the re-establishment of maximal mobility and power when movement of the part is introduced.

The general management is concerned with the maintenance of general physical fitness, morale and motivation during prolonged immobilization of the injured part which may possibly involve immobilization and hospitalization of the patient. It is concerned also with the assessment of the probable outcome of injury and the preparation for work resettlement. This may entail return to the patient's original work, initiation into a different but more suitable type of employment, or preparation for prolonged or permanent disability of a minor or major degree.

As far as the rehabilitation of adults is concerned, the primary responsibility of rehabilitation personnel is to:

Minimize or prevent residual disability.

Utilize normal daily and work activities to maintain or regain physical function and to re-establish a patient's confidence in his physical capability.

Frequently patients remain away from work or fail to return to full normal activities. This is commonly due to lack of authoritative guidance on the therapeutic advantages of a rapid return to those everyday activities within their capabilities. Some patients who have severe multiple injuries or special injuries such as crush injuries of the hand, or who are engaged in particularly heavy physical labour or competitive sport may need special intensive rehabilitation.

The rehabilitation of children with limb fractures rarely presents problems. Most children need to be restrained from over-exertion rather than encouraged to exercise. Indeed, adequate immobilization is usually the only post-reduction therapy which is required. Some instruction in the importance of preventing plaster becoming immersed in water, together with some instruction in the use of crutches or similar appliances is often all that the physiotherapist is called upon to do.

LINES OF COMMUNICATION

Communication with the patient

When patients are treated as out-patients following fractures or dislocations, it is often difficult to ensure that they supplement exercise sessions at the physiotherapy department by regular sessions in their own homes. This is partly because they do not understand that they are expected to do so. It is also partly because they do not appreciate the benefits which can accrue from muscular exercise nor the damage that may result from inactivity.

Reiteration of the need and reason for frequent exercise sessions should be started by the doctor supervising rehabilitation, and followed by the physiotherapists, nurses and occupational therapists who combine to give their care. Even with such repeated explanation, it is advisable to present patients with a small information card, detailing the type and timing of exercises which they should perform, what signs of improvement can be looked for, what to do if their condition deteriorates and whom to consult when they are worried. These cards should also carry the telephone numbers of the hospital and the G.P. and the time of the next appointment.

Communication with the general practitioner

A brief notification should be despatched to the general practitioner from the consultant at the Fracture Clinic or Accident Service, before or at the time of departure of the patient for home. Ideally, this should be backed by a telephone call to the surgery or health centre attended by the patient. Such liaison enables the general practitioner and his team of ancillary staff to take over smoothly their task of supporting the patient in the immediate post-fracture period. This may involve the supply of analgesics or hypnotics, nursing care or domestic help. It will also consist of checking the circulation in a plastered limb, and, if local facilities are available, initiating physiotherapy so that long ambulance journeys are not needed.

Communication with social services

Patients with fractures or dislocations who are not independent personally, domestically and socially, should not be sent home from hospital until the presence of adequate family or social service backing has been confirmed. This is often best done by direct contact between the medical social worker or ward sister and the family or area social service concerned. It is not enough to ask the patient about this. Many old people are confused and often imply that their home situations are as they would like them to be rather than as they are. Others are simply too proud to accept what they consider as 'charity'.

Those living alone, particularly when elderly, may find themselves unable to manage at home without assistance during the period of rehabilitation following a fracture or dislocation. The ideal solution will often be transfer to a local community hospital. They will be near friends, and the G.P. and his staff will be able to carry on with their care. If this is not possible, the local health visitor, social worker or domiciliary occupational therapist may be able to visit and give care at home. However, many old or solitary people strongly resent what they consider to be an intrusion on their privacy by unasked visitors, and refuse the help which they need. It is wise therefore to make a routine referral via the hospital social work department to the social services so that a direct check can be made on the real needs at home. Through such a referral the following help can be provided:

The district nurse may make a regular visit to help with personal care activities and any dressings or slings, and to assist with the weekly bath.

The domiciliary occupational therapist will check on the need for help in all activities of daily living (washing, dressing, toilet, cooking, housework), and supply necessary aids.

The home help may be particularly concerned in managing some of the heavier housework (cleaning the grate, laying the fire, shopping, collecting the pension, and doing the washing). Once it is safe to attempt them, the domestic activities provide an excellent form of rehabilitative exercise for fractured limbs, and patients should be encouraged to reassume them at the earliest opportunity.

FRACTURES AND DISLOCATIONS IN THE UPPER LIMB

Fractures and dislocations in the shoulder region

Since the immobilized, traumatized shoulder joint readily stiffens, treatment of injuries in the shoulder region aims at the minimal period of immobilization for the glenohumeral joint. This must be consistent with the stable union or reduction of the fracture or dislocation concerned, and must aim to produce optimal conditions for the maintenance of joint function during this period and throughout the period of remobilization.

Four principles of rehabilitative treatment of shoulder injuries therefore emerge as being applicable for fractures of the upper end of the humerus, or of the scapula and for dislocations of the glenohumeral joint.

(1) If reduction is unnecessary or impossible, treatment is concentrated on regaining shoulder movement, and the fracture or dislocation is largely disregarded.

(2) If the reduction is necessary and possible, it may need to be held, and shoulder movements must then be regained by active exercises as soon as possible.

(3) Whether or not reduction is effected and whatever treatment is given, in all shoulder injuries the elbow, wrist, thumb and fingers must be kept freely mobile from the start.

(4) Active use of the hand for personal and domestic tasks is encouraged even while the shoulder is supported by a sling or plaster.

In the later stages of rehabilitation progressive active exercises for the shoulder are introduced early and practiced assiduously to re-establish the range and power of shoulder movement. But the timing and degree of such exercises must vary with the type of fracture or dislocation under treatment, the age and general condition of the patient, and the nature and severity of any associated lesions in the shoulder region.

Diagnosis of these associated lesions at time of injury may be difficult or impossible and the anticipation of their occurrence and recognition of their presence during rehabilitative treatment is therefore vital. Thus, whereas shoulder stiffness may well be due to neglect, fear or prolonged immobilization, it may also be due to:

Damage to the rotator cuff, which may be clearly localized (e.g. supraspinatus rupture) or less well defined (e.g. capsulitis or 'frozen shoulder').

Nerve damage. The circumflex nerve is particularly at risk and more severe injuries may damage the brachial plexus.

Damage to the articular surfaces of the glenohumeral joint.

Unrecognized associated fracture.

Detachment of the greater tuberosity or fracture of the humeral neck. These may accompany other injuries around the shoulder and may not be apparent until delayed recovery of function suggests the need for further investigation.

Some shoulder stiffness is likely to follow the period of immobilization of the arm in the sling, which forms an essential part of the treatment of so many shoulder injuries. Necessarily, the glenohumeral joint is internally rotated and adducted while held in the sling position, and in this position damaged muscle and capsule soon lose the ability to stretch. Loss of external rotation and limitation of abduction ensue. For this reason the period of immobilization of the glenohumeral joint following shoulder injuries is the minimal one consistent with stable reduction and is always followed by early active movements. Active exercises may prevent stiffness and can usually cure it. Passive exercises are usually contra-indicated, but the shoulder is the one joint which may respond to passive movements or mobilization techniques when recovery of joint movement ceases to improve with active exercises. Such techniques are contra-indicated when the joint shows evidence of active synovitis and should be used with the utmost care in elderly people.

The painful stiff shoulder can be a very disabling complication. It may respond to ice packs or to applications of heat. Active exercises for the shoulder and entire arm in a warm pool are often beneficial and this form of therapy can be introduced early even before consolidation has occurred, while the arm is still supported in a sling between hydrotherapy treatments.

Purposeful occupational therapy provides active exercises to overcome shoulder stiffness in the early stages of active mobilization. It is important that the activities should be chosen and adapted for each patient so that elevation of the shoulder should be required in doing them. In the early stages, traditional craft activities have their value. Later, heavier activities such as carpentry and gardening can be introduced, progressing to log-splitting, cement-mixing and heavy digging, to build up muscle bulk and strength. The harder tasks of housework such as window cleaning, furniture and floor polishing, and eventually interior decorating, provide the same power-building exercise for women.

Fracture of the humerus

Whether the fracture is of the neck of the humerus or of the shaft, transverse or spiral, union is usually rapid and rehabilitation relatively straightforward. Immobilization may be accomplished by a simple sling or 'U'-shaped plaster. In all instances, finger and hand movements are essential from the outset. 'Pendulum' exercises (practised with the patient leaning forward while the arm hangs supported by plaster or sling) for the shoulder joint can usually be introduced early, but abduction exercises are avoided until there is evidence of consolidation.

Radial-nerve damage requires special treatment with the early use of a simple lively 'radial-nerve' splint. Such a splint should not impede the active use of the finger and hand during the recovery phase.

Fracture of the elbow

Fractures in the region of the elbow are notorious for producing some loss of range in all planes of movement—flexion, extension, pronation and supination. The combination of these movements is of paramount importance in placing the hand at the appropriate distance from the trunk and face. Thus, in the majority of daily living activities and in all those movements involved in personal care, elbow movement plays an essential part, and marked restriction of elbow range may lead to a significant loss of independence.

Because of its tendency to become stiff after injury, the elbow joint should only be immobilized for the *minimal* time consistent with a stable reduction of the fracture or dislocation concerned.

Except in a supracondylar fracture with forward displacement of the lower fragment in children, the elbow is immobilized in flexion rather than extension. Should elbow stiffness follow immobilization, whatever range of movement is recoverable is of far more use from a position of 90 degrees of flexion than from a position of full extension.

Closed reduction of fractures and dislocations in the elbow region is preferred, and open reduction and internal fixation are only employed when it is necessary to hold the fractured fragments in the reduced position.

Whenever possible, reduction of an elbow fracture is maintained by gravity traction, and the forearm is held in a collar and cuff sling with or without a supporting backslab. Simple sling immobilization is usually needed for 3 weeks only, but when a backslab is used the sling is usually retained for up to 3 weeks after the slab has been removed.

Active finger movements are practised immediately following reduction and are maintained assiduously throughout the period of elbow immobilization. Active shoulder and wrist movements are added when fracture healing permits. Their early institution is particularly important in adults in whom a 'frozen shoulder' may easily follow sling treatment of elbow injury.

Elbow movement is regained when the period of elbow immobilization has been completed by means of active non-resisted exercises, but some limitation of extension is almost inevitable following severe elbow fractures. Formal physiotherapeutic treatment seldom needs to be prolonged since normal use of the injured arm at home or at work will encourage recovery of movement over a period of at least 6 months.

Passive elbow movement must be avoided at all times, and elbow manipulation by physiotherapists, relatives and patient is *absolutely* contra-indicated. So is 'therapeutic stretching' by carrying heavy shopping bags and suitcases.

Apart from complications which may accompany fractures or dislocations in the elbow region, further injury to the upper limb may occur during the actual treatment of these conditions. Volkmann's ischaemia and myositis ossificans are the two most serious sequelae which may occur, and these must be diagnosed early and treated promptly unless serious functional loss is to result.

Forearm fractures

In the treatment of fractures of the radius and ulna, perfect apposition of the fractured bones is necessary to avoid a rotation deficit. Thus, although closed reduction of such fractures is usually initially attempted, unless this reduction can be held by an above-elbow plaster, open reduction and plating of the bones is indicated.

In all cases, shoulder and finger exercises are practised regularly and frequently from the start, and elbow flexion/extension and forearm pronation/supination are regained by progressive active exercises when the plaster is removed. As with fractures around the elbow, elbow and forearm movement must never be forced or assisted, and the elbow must not be passively manipulated.

Non-union, mal-union, joint stiffness and ischaemia of the hand are possible complications to be avoided by careful reduction and immobilization.

The commonest fracture of the wrist, a Colles' fracture of the lower end of the radius, is treated by closed reduction and a below-elbow plaster slab which extends to the metacarpal heads. Swelling of the hand and fingers frequently occurs shortly after reduction and any medical or paramedical personnel treating a patient who has developed blue, swollen or painful fingers needs to split the bandage holding the slab immediately. The development of oedema is discouraged by the elevation of the arm at night and its support by day in a sling for the first few days after fracture. Active shoulder and finger exercises are prescribed, and the use of the hand for light tasks is encouraged. The sling should be withdrawn within a few days so that secondary capsulitis of the shoulder due to immobilization may not develop.

Shoulder stiffness should be preventable and is certainly treatable either by ice and active exercises, or heat and active exercises. Finger stiffness may arise from disuse. Repeated explanation and demonstration of finger exercises may be needed to convince elderly patients that they are not doing irreparable damage by moving their fingers. Rarely, stiffness of the fingers is persistent and arises from Sudeck's atrophy, in which pain and stiffness of the fingers with puffiness, patchy discoloration and moist hyperaesthetic skin come on a few weeks after injury. Regular, persevering physiotherapy assists recovery over many months and with heat, elevation and progressive exercises, the fingers gradually approach normality.

Severe and persistent stiffness of the wrist seldom follows a simple Colles' but is more likely to occur when the fracture line involves the joint or when there has been associated dislocation of one or more carpal bones. Mobilization of such stiff, weak wrists by progressively active exercises preceded by heat or ice is greatly assisted by appropriate occupational therapy.

Rehabilitative treatment of other fractures of the lower end of the radius is similar to that following a Colles' fracture. Out-patients are able to follow recommended occupational therapy in their own homes in household and do-it-yourself activities.

Fractures and dislocations of the carpal bones

Following reduction of fractured or dislocated carpal bones, the forearm and hand are immobilized in plaster. Finger movement is encouraged by directing the patient to undertake as many normal activities as possible, consistent with preserving the plaster's integrity. Only when this advice is not followed, or cannot be followed, should it be necessary to institute regular sessions of formal physiotherapy and to instruct the patient in active exercises for the fingers in the hospital rehabilitation department.

Scaphoid fractures are usually treated by 8 weeks in plaster. If union has occurred and the fingers have been actively exercised throughout the period of immobilization, rapid recovery of wrist movement and power follow plaster removal. Non-union of the fracture and possible avascular necrosis of the proximal fragment may occur, and a weak and painful wrist results. Should this be so the wrist is immobilized for a further 3 weeks after the customary 2 months in plaster. If this fails to relieve the pain and weakness, excision of the radial styloid and the removal of the necrotic segment of the scaphoid may be considered. Wrist function is regained by active exercises post-operatively, and by an early return to normal activities.

When osteo-arthritis results from non-union of the scaphoid fragments, provision of a plastic wrist-splint and possible intra-articular steroid injections at weekly intervals for 3 weeks may be sufficient to ensure comfort, but arthrodesis may become necessary to produce a pain-free stable wrist.

Lunate dislocations may occur separately or in association with a fracture of the scaphoid. Simple dislocations are treated by closed reduction and held by a plaster of paris slab, while active exercises for shoulder, elbow and fingers are started at once. Damage to the arterial supply of the lunate may follow dislocation, and avascular necrosis may develop. Operative removal of the bone becomes necessary, and permanent stiffness of the wrist is likely to result. This is treated, as is the wrist stiffness following injury to the scaphoid bone.

Fractures and dislocations in the hand

Fractures in the hand almost always unite, and immobilized fingers almost invariably stiffen. The treatment of fractures and dislocations in the hand therefore aims at the minimal period of finger immobilization and at the restoration of maximal functional efficiency rather than exact anatomical outline.

Constant factors of management therefore involve:

Control of swelling By elevation of the hand and early active exercises for the fingers.

Minimal splintage Only the finger which is injured should be splinted, either individually, or else by a narrow garter attachment to an adjacent finger. The functional position of partial flexion is adopted for fractures of any digit other than the thumb under certain conditions. When external splintage would immobilize several fingers unnecessarily, internal wire fixation is used instead.

Skin care When skin damage accompanies bone injury, treatment of the skin takes precedence over treatment of fracture.

Maintenance of finger movement During the period of immobilization of the fractured bones, use of the remaining fingers is encouraged and the arm as a whole is used and exercised regularly. Following the removal of the splintage, finger movement is regained by active exercises. Playing a musical instrument is excellent occupational therapy, and craftwork and housework are also helpful in restoring co-ordinated finger movement.

During the period of remobilization after removal of the supporting splintage, home physiotherapy in which both hands are exercised several times daily, supplements, or follows, the more sophisticated treatment offered in the physiotherapy department. Specific regimes involving, for example, the immersion of the hand in warm water, help to impress the habit of regular exercise upon the patient.

Patients with severe hand injuries in which, in addition to bone fracture, there has been much soft-tissue damage and subsequent fibrous contracture, need admission to hospital for specialized intensive care. To correct the contractures, warm-oil massage and gentle, gradual stretching are repeated for short intervals several times daily, and the correction is maintained by application of a light plaster splint, renewed daily in the early stages and at longer intervals later, according to response to treatment. Manipulation and sudden stretching are absolutely contra-indicated. Specially programmed occupational therapy assists in the structural and functional recovery of the fingers and hand and their reintegration into the body image.

Crush injuries of the hand are relatively common in heavy industry and frequently lead to considerable time off work and loss of earning power. Intensive rehabilitation in the purposive atmosphere of an active rehabilitation unit can reduce morbidity and improve the end results of treatment. When nerves are involved in the injury, careful, detailed supervision of the rehabilitation is even more important, and close collaboration between the orthopaedic surgeon or plastic surgeon and the rehabilitation team is of the highest importance.

INJURIES OF THE SPINE

General

The immediate and rehabilitative treatment of fractures of the spine vary according to the stability or instability of the fracture and the actual or potential cord damage involved. This book is not concerned with the management of paraplegia and tetraplegia associated with spinal injury but only with the rehabilitation of patients without cord injury.

Cervical spine

The reduction of fractures of the cervical spine is followed by a period of immobilization in which the fracture is held reduced by traction, plaster or internal fixation.

After the period of continuous immobilization, a polythene collar is usually prescribed and worn for some weeks. The patient should be instructed to take this off for gradually lengthening periods each day, and the physiotherapist teaches him to perform gentle strengthening exercises for practice during the unsupported intervals. Manipulation and passive movements are contra-indicated. Prolonged attendance for out-patient physiotherapy is common but usually unrewarding. Movements return with natural usage when the immobilization is discarded.

Fractures of the thoracic and lumbar spine

The treatment of spinal fractures uncomplicated by neurological deficit may be divided into two distinct groups: (1) Patients with potentially unstable fractures, who are treated by strict immobilization. They progress through a sequence of bed rest, with or without traction, plaster of paris immobilization, spinal brace and then spinal corset. (2) Patients with more stable fractures, who may progress directly from a period of bed rest to a spinal brace or corset. A few of these patients may return immediately to full activity.

In all cases the rehabilitation programme is concerned with:

(1) Maintaining the power and volume of the paraspinal musculature and the function of all other muscle groups.

(2) Instilling into the patient the concept of maintaining the optimal position of the spinal column while undertaking many activities.

(3) Teaching the patient to lift by using the power of his legs while his back is held straight.

(4) Graduating and increasing the general activity and physical fitness of the patient and strengthening his trunk musculature proportionally.

(5) Preventing unnecessary fear and inactivity by active demonstration of the progressive increase in functional capability.

In such a programme, the rehabilitative activity is always in parallel with the progress of the clinical and radiological stabilization and eventual consolidation of the fractured vertebrae.

In the past, many injuries of the spine from industrial accidents have been associated with unnecessarily prolonged immobilization. In recent years, it has been clearly demonstrated by the routine treatment of personnel injured in the armed services, and with careful and understanding rehabilitation, such injuries need cause no more than a few months relative inconvenience preceding a return to full activity.

Fractures of the pelvis

Following simple, isolated fractures of the pelvic ring, bed rest without reduction is advised until the patient is comfortable. He is then gradually mobilized, first standing and then walking with whichever walking aid gives him greatest confidence and stability.

Following pelvic-ring disruption in which the ring is fractured in two places and displacement and complications are common, immediate and rehabilitative treatment varies with the type of disruption produced. As a general principle, however, non-weight-bearing exercise in bed will maintain muscle power, and when the fractures are united, increasing weight-bearing activities can be introduced. Exercise in the swimming pool is particularly valuable in this type of injury as it enables the physiotherapist to introduce a wide range of activity before weight-bearing is allowed.

FRACTURES AND DISLOCATIONS OF THE LOWER LIMB

General

The management of all fractures falls into four phases which follow the natural history of bone healing:

Fracture reduction and holding.
Union.
Consolidation.
Remodelling.

But the treatment of fractures of the lower limb differs from that of those of the upper limb in the longer periods which must elapse before full function may be restored. This is directly related to the need for a healed fracture of a lower limb to be able to bear weight.

To reduce the long period of immobilization in bed which adequate fracture healing might otherwise necessitate, whenever possible, a lower limb fracture is protected from abnormal lateral and rotation stress by internal or external fixation, weight relief is provided by a caliper or crutches, and preconsolidation ambulation is encouraged. Despite this technique of fracture treatment which permits early protected walking, most lower limb fractures entail some period of bed rest since during the immediate post-reduction stage the swelling consequent on soft-tissue damage necessitates elevation.

During the intervals between the different stages of healing, physiotherapeutic treatment consisting of bed rest, assisted ambulation and protected and unprotected activity is essential. The overall rehabilitative programme following a lower limb fracture involves:

(1) Exercise in bed following reduction and immobilization, usually restricted to static exercises only for muscles acting over the fracture line and immobilized joints. Active exercises for all movable joints of all four limbs and trunk.

(2) Early mobilization during the interval from reduction to union, with supervision of non-weight-bearing activities and introduction of partial weight-bearing on the injured limb; continuance of progressive exercises to maintain strength and mobility of all four limbs and trunk.

(3) Later mobilization during the interval from union to consolidation, with supervision of the gradual resumption of full weight-bearing and the maintenance of regular exercise sessions while fracture protection is being maintained.

(4) Final rehabilitation following fracture consolidation and removal of external plaster protection when muscle power and co-ordination and joint range are developed; retraining for work, sport and full activity may now occur.

Early phases of treatment

Patients with upper limb injuries can get up, walk about and become independent using one hand, and thus, almost inadvertently, accomplish their own rehabilitation and resettlement as the injury recovers. They usually only require instruction and encouragement. Patients with lower limb injuries, however, present a very different problem. Both during the initial period of bed rest and during the ensuing period of active rehabilitation to achieve walking, they may need considerable support, training and active encouragement from experienced staff. Elderly and fragile people are at severe risk while recumbent in bed, and the secondary effects of immobilization—pressure sores, chest infection, and sheer inanition—may often be more disabling than the original injury. Thus, the early part of the period of mobilization is often critical and is a period in which not only physical improvement in muscle power, joint mobility and stamina are to be achieved, but considerable psychological barriers may have to be overcome, such as fear of further injury, fear of the future, anxiety about family, compensation and loss of work. Much of the routine suggested is directed towards the patient's general rehabilitation as well as to specific recovery from lower limb injury.

During the initial stage of physiotherapeutic management of the lower limb fracture, reduction has been effected, union is awaited, and it is essential to ensure that fracture immobilization is not synonymous with patient immobilization. Whether internal fixation, traction or plaster of paris is being used to hold reduction while the patient is at bed rest with his leg elevated, his exercise regime is designed to promote rapid removal of oedema fluid from the fractured limb. The patient must safeguard muscle action and joint mobility by static contractions of the muscles spanning the fracture and the joints immobilized in its treatment, and by active exercises for all the mobile joints in all four limbs and trunk.

A specific exercise programme is devised, taught and rehearsed with each patient at least twice daily by the therapist giving treatment. In addition, a group or class session can be held for the ward each day in which static exercises for gluteal, quadriceps and calf muscles can be taught and practised together with breathing exercises and exercises for upper limbs and trunk. More active exercises can be introduced on an individual basis and graded by the use of springs and slings attached to an overhead beam or to the foot of the bed.

Bed rest may be of short duration, merely until the swelling disperses in fractures which involve the distal part of the limb and are simple in nature and uncomplicated in mode of reduction. It may be prolonged for weeks or months following fractures which involve the proximal part of the lower limb, or which form part of a multiple injury complex with associated damage to the brain or cord. However severe the total clinical picture may be, regular physiotherapeutic treatment should be started as soon as it is medically allowed and pursued energetically throughout the period of recumbence.

Nursing and physiotherapeutic care overlap each other considerably during this initial post-reduction phase. Seriously injured, frail, elderly or relatively immobile patients need to be nursed on firm-based beds in which the heights of both ends are adjustable and on mattresses which both support the spine and protect the skin. Often a firm sponge-rubber mattress is adequate, but when skin ulceration is a possibility, the use of a sheepskin, a ripple mattress, or a 'cubex' mattress may be indicated. (The 'cubex' mattress consists of aerated polystyrene granules compartmentalized into various patterns to make a firm whole.) Alternatively, large foam blocks may be used to make a composite surface from which removal of appropriate blocks allows toiletting, washing or the easier performance of exercises. When skin health is severely threatened, a water mattress or 'flotation bed' is occasionally indicated.

For a female patient especially, the early days following reduction and fixation of a fractured femur can be fraught with unnecessary additional pain. Use of a bedpan for micturition, particularly when only one nurse is available to assist the patient on and off, is intensely painful. The alternative use of one of the many plastic female urinals which are now obtainable could minimize the discomfort for the patient and the work for the nursing staff. A bedpan should be reserved for defaecation only and it should be mandatory that two nurses should be present to administer and remove it. The use of a bedside commode should be introduced as soon as it is possible.

Physiotherapists attend each patient only twice or thrice daily, while nurses are in the ward throughout the day and night. With collaboration between the physiotherapist and the nursing staff, an extended supervision of the patient's exercise regime becomes possible. Particularly when backed by a written exercise chart, explanation by the physiotherapist to the nurse of her requirements can ensure that the requisite exercises are performed more regularly because they are monitored and encouraged by the nurses giving care.

Routine use of a physiotherapy chart, kept at the foot of the patient's bed with other charts and medical notes, not only facilitates closer supervision by the nursing staff, but also enables all staff to make detailed enquiries and observations of a patient's rehabilitative progress.

Early mobilization

In the absence of associated injuries, unless maintenance of fracture reduction demands external traction, once swelling has been reduced patients with lower limb fractures are allowed up. Periods of dependence of the limb, during which exercises are performed within the plaster cast, are then alternated with periods of elevation, when the limb is elevated on chair, stool or the elevating legrest of a wheelchair.

Sitting with the foot dependent and inactive should be forbidden as this quickly leads to hypostatic oedema, swollen toes and all the discomforts of an overtight plaster. A dependent foot must be an active foot. Toe-wriggling and static contractions of muscles controlling immobilized joints should be regularly and frequently practised.

Non-weight-bearing is taught at this stage, using elbow crutches initially, and progressing to sticks if and when fracture stability permits. Accurate adjustment of the height of the handrests of the crutches and sticks is essential so that this corresponds with the level of the tip of the greater trochanter when the patient is standing in a shoe.

Occasional walking is not enough in itself to ensure the steady functional gain required of the patient as a whole and the injured limb in particular. It is still necessary to continue with regular exercise sessions for all four limbs and trunk several times daily.

There are many theoretical and practical advantages and disadvantages of allowing early weight-bearing, and each fracture must be considered individually. Decision will depend upon the position and stage of healing of the fracture itself, the amount of soft-tissue injury, whether internal fixation has been used, and the general state of the patient. The after-care of fractures of the lower limb calls for the utilization of much of the art and skill of clinical practice, and critical decisions taken by the orthopaedic surgeon will often depend upon the calibre of the rehabilitation services available to him.

During the first few days after removal of plaster or caliper, walking is supervised closely. Initially the patient reverts to the use of crutches and partial weight-bearing, gradually increasing the weight taken by the fractured limb until full weight-bearing has been achieved.

Control of weight-bearing

Unless some disability prevents their use, standard elbow crutches are used to teach crutch walking. The length of the crutch upright from handgrip to tip is adjusted for each patient, the presence of an adequately grooved ferrule is checked, and handgrips and forearm grips are tested for comfort. In many cases this entails winding plastic foam round the rigid plastic from which the grips are made and then covering the padding with chamois leather or rexine.

Once weight-bearing begins, the patient is encouraged to take steps of equal length and to swing the injured leg in the natural rhythm of walking. Walking sticks are later substituted for the crutches and are retained until normal balance and a limp-free walk have been re-established. Regular class work in the gymnasium at this stage is designed particularly to improve the power and co-ordination of the calf muscles and so to promote a springy step, preparing the way to running, jumping and sporting activities as rehabilitation proceeds. For this reason also it is important to use two sticks and not one, when crutches are eventually discarded, since two sticks permit a more symmetrical walking pattern. They should be retained until rehabilitative treatment is completed and weight relief is no longer needed.

Assisted walking with crutches gives considerable weight relief to the fractured limb, but involves extra work for the other lower and both upper limbs. The performance of regular exercises for all four limbs and trunk throughout the period of patient immobilization and the gradual introduction of longer intervals of crutch walking interspersed with intervals of rest and elevation of both lower limbs is esential if discomfort and oedema are to be avoided.

Plaster walking

Efficient walking with a limb encased in plaster of paris involves the provision of a walking plaster which not only protects the fracture from stress, but also permits as normal a gait as possible. While the strength of the plaster protects the fracture, its shape and size influence gait. For ease of walking and to prevent unnecessary strain on other joints, the foot of the plastered limb needs to be in the plantigrade position (i.e. the neutral position) and not in the 10 degrees of flexion which is commonly advocated.

A rocker may be incorporated into the plaster sole and the patient is taught to walk by rocking himself vertically over the rocker which he uses as a fulcrum, assisting the following swing-through of the plastered limb by a pelvic ‘hitch’ from the quadratus lumborum, and using gluteal action to level the pelvis during the action of the rocking. The spring of the uninjured leg and the upward thrust from the crutch handles provide additional propulsion and lift for the plastered leg and help to prevent external rotation while pivoting on the rocker, and also circumduction during the swing-through phase.

An alternative to a rocker incorporated in the plaster sole is the use of an overboot with a rocker-type sole, which is worn over walking plaster. This has many advantages, not the least being the greater ease with which a normal heel–toe gait may be acquired during its use. It protects the toes from trauma and cold and the plaster from rain. It facilitates the active participation of the long toe muscles during walking and the performance of exercises for the intrinsic muscles of the feet while at rest.

In patients who are frail or elderly or have a disability of the uninjured leg, a raise fitted to the shoe of the non-plastered leg may be needed to facilitate a more normal swing-through action of the plastered one.

Walking in calipers

The reduction of certain lower limb fractures is held by means of traction. This is maintained until the fracture has united, and the patient is then mobilized in a weight-bearing caliper. A simple half-ring caliper, ischial-bearing and of adjustable length, permits partial weight-bearing with fracture protection until consolidation has occurred. Use of such a caliper reduces the long period of bed rest otherwise necessitated by the treatment of some inherently unstable fractures and allows muscle strength and joint range to be built up by the greater range of exercises which ambulation makes possible. The caliper is removed for non-weight-bearing mobilizing exercises during the regular sessions of physiotherapy in the gymnasium and warm pool which are incorporated into the daily routine of the ambulant patient. Repeated instruction and possible adjustment of the caliper is essential to ensure that it is fully weight-relieving and is providing adequate protection against stress for the fracture concerned.

Walking without protection

When fracture consolidation has been confirmed by radiological and clinical examination, full weight-bearing without fracture protection becomes permissible, and caliper and plaster alike are discarded.

The success and comfort of the ensuing period of rehabilitation depend upon the extent to which the patient has carried out his earlier exercise programme of muscle exercise and joint movement, the efficiency with which hypostatic oedema of his fractured leg can be controlled, and his total motivation to regain normal function.

The time at which protection is removed varies with the type of fracture, the blood supply to the fractured limb, and the age, constitution and associated injuries of each patient. Allowing for these variable factors, it is nevertheless possible to make an approximate forecast of the probable times at which union and consolidation are likely to occur in any particular type of fracture.

BIBLIOGRAPHY AND REFERENCES

Apley, G. A. (1968). *A System of Orthopaedics and Fractures* (3rd edn). London; Butterworths

Gardner, D. C., Goodwill, C. J. and Bridges, P. K. (1968a). 'Absence from work after fracture of the wrist and hand.' *J. occup. Med.* **10**, 114

Gardner, D. C., Goodwill, C. J. and Bridges, P. K. (1968b). 'Cost of incapacity due to fractures of the wrist and hand.' *J. occup. Med.* **10**, 118

Nichols, P. J. R. (1963). 'Rehabilitation after fracture of the shaft of the femur.' *J. Bone Jt Surg.* **45B**, 1, 96–102

Nichols, P. J. R. and Parish, J. G. (1959a). 'Rehabilitation after fractures of the tibia and fibula.' *Ann. phys. Med.* **5**, 3, 73–87

Nichols, P. J. R. and Parish, J. G. (1959b). 'Rehabilitation of malleolar fractures of the tibia and fibula.' *Ann. phys. Med.* **5**, 128–40

Nichols, P. J. R. and Wynn Parry, C. B. (1958). 'Rehabilitation after reconstruction of the shoulder for recurrent forward dislocation.' *Ann. phys. Med.* **4**, 8, 281–7

Watson-Jones, Sir R. (1955). *Fracture and Joint Injuries* (4th edn). London; Livingstone

Wynn Parry, C. B. and Nichols, P. J. R. (1966). 'Rehabilitation.' *Clin. Surg.* **12**, 236–64

Wynn Parry, C. B., Nichols, P. J. R. and Lewis, R. N. (1958). 'Menisectomy, a review of 1723 cases.' *Ann. phys. Med.*, **4**, 6, 201–15

Wynn Parry, C. B. (1973). *Rehabilitation of the Hand* (3rd edn). London; Butterworths

9—Strokes

THE NATURE AND SIZE OF THE PROBLEM

There are probably at present about half a million patients in the United Kingdom suffering from hemiplegia following a cardiovascular accident. Hemiplegia is therefore one of the most commonly occurring physical disabilities. The severity of the disability in any one hemiplegic patient depends on the density of the initial ischaemia, the adequacy of collateral circulation and the severity of the residual brain damage; these in turn vary with the type of acute lesion with which circulatory dysfunction presents.

Cerebral thrombosis associated with hypertension and arteriosclerosis, intracerebral haemorrhage, subarachnoid haemorrhage and cerebral embolism are the four main cerebrovascular lesions which may result in hemiplegia. Prognosis and the delineation of a programme of rehabilitation depend on a knowledge of the natural history of each condition. Unfortunately, it is often only possible to establish the diagnosis accurately at autopsy, since the presentation of all four lesions during life may be remarkably similar. Despite the difficulty of making an early differential diagnosis of the causative lesion, various general characteristics of the patient assist in prognostication of life expectancy and rehabilitation potential.

Mortality

Life expectancy varies inversely with age, severity of preceding hypertension, severity of accompanying cardiac dysfunction, and duration and depth of initial unconsciousness. As far as *cerebral embolism* is concerned, about 1 in 3 patients dies within 3 months of the initial episode and a further one third die within 3 years. Thus two thirds die within 3 years, and the average survival period is 2 years. *Cerebral infarction* carries a slightly better prognosis, since only 1 in 4 patients with this condition dies within 3 months and another quarter die within 3 years. Only half are therefore dead in 3 years and the average survival time is 3 or 4 years.

Morbidity

The delineation of a realistic rehabilitation programme following stroke entails accurate and repeated assessments of the residual disability and functional capacity of any one patient. An early single assessment is often of little value, since the patterns of recovery from stroke are so variable, and the earlier the assessment is made the less likely it is to give an accurate prognosis. Yet some initial tentative prognosis is urgently needed, so that the type of long-term care required may be given the earliest possible consideration, and an approximate plan of management formulated. Patient, relatives and remedial staff need information on the rate and extent of probable recovery, the ability to return home, and the care which will be needed either in the home itself or, alternatively, in a residential institution should return home prove impossible.

Such information requires not only an assessment of the patient's physical and mental condition both before and after the stroke, but also a knowledge of his premorbid education, training and skill, and an assessment of his home and social conditions.

Assessment of the clinical condition after a stroke embraces that selection of particular signs and symptoms, variable in number, association and degree, which follow stroke in any one patient. These signs and symptoms are:

Loss of motor power.
Loss of sensation.
Hemianopia.
Aphasia.
Apraxia.
Dementia.
Incontinence of urine.

In addition to the characteristics of the stroke itself, assessment of the clinical condition of a patient must take into account any associated disabilities which may be present.

Seventy-five per cent of the patients with stroke are over 60 years of age, and of those referred for rehabilitation to a hospital or a rehabilitation unit, 70 per cent are over 50 years and 25 per cent are over 60 years. Commonly associated disabilities in stroke patients are, therefore, arteriosclerosis, hypertension, diabetes mellitus, cardiac insufficiency, osteo-arthrosis, visual defects, hearing defects and the general frailties of the elderly.

The onset and the pattern of recovery from stroke is itself of prognostic value. The onset may be sudden or insidious; a gradually extending paralysis and prolonged, deepening unconsciousness indicate a bad prognosis. Usually the initial paralysis which develops is flaccid with absent tendon reflexes, becoming gradually hypertonic with exaggerated reflexes during the course of the first few days; persistence of flaccidity seems to carry a poor prognosis, and so, too, does intense hypertonicity. Spontaneous recovery starts soon after the initial episode and continues for many months, but usually the greatest degree of recovery is seen in the first few months and often in the first 6 to 8 weeks. Subsequent recovery is slower and correspondingly less likely to affect ultimate functional capacity; thus a patient who has not regained much of his personal independence and some ability to walk within 3 months of the onset of the stroke is unlikely to do so at a later date.

The rehabilitation potential of young hemiplegic patients naturally differs from that of patients in the older age group. Their functional recovery is likely to be swifter, and the prognosis is often less gloomy. Management is correspondingly different in detail, and rehabilitation should be planned on a more energetic basis.

REHABILITATION IN THE EARLY STAGES

General care

The immediate care of the patient with stroke depends on the severity of the cardiovascular accident and its effect on his condition, and is initially concerned with the maintenance of the life processes, the diagnosis of the causative lesion and its treatment, and the prevention of deterioration in the locomotor system while its control is no longer properly co-ordinated.

During the acute phase, physiotherapy is directed towards:

(1) Passive movements of all limb joints of the affected side to prevent contractures.

(2) Prevention of deformity by the use of a bed cage, foot-boards, axillary pillow, palmar wrist-splint.

While the patient is in bed, whether during the period of unconsciousness or during the early recovery stage, a foot-board to discourage foot drop and a bed cradle to remove the weight of the bed-clothes from the legs should always be used. During the early comatose phases, a pillow in the axilla may help to prevent a fixed adduction of the shoulder. These passive preventative measures are used to supplement more active measures to maintain joint range and prevent contracture. These will consist of putting all affected joints through the full range of movement several times each day. If the patient is unconscious, then the movement of the shoulders in particular, and all joints of both arms and legs should be carried out at regular nursing sessions. During these sessions the patient is turned, washed and cleaned, pressure areas are attended to, oral hygiene is carried out, and catheterization is undertaken when necessary.

During the initial phase of the acute post-stroke stage, the hemiplegia is usually flaccid and passive movements are relatively easily elicited. Great care and gentleness are required to prevent over-stretching of muscles and ligaments and consequent soft-tissue damage. As spasticity supervenes, there is a continuing need for skill and experience if soft-tissue injury is to be avoided. The risks of a musculotendinous tear which later becomes calcified cannot be over-emphasized. If the patient is dying, then unwarranted disturbance should be avoided, but if there is a reasonable chance of recovery, it is essential to avoid delay in active prevention of unnecessary stiffness and deformity.

The length of time the patient needs to be kept strictly bedridden will vary with the cause and severity of the lesion but should be minimal. As soon as possible, sitting and bed-edge activity are introduced (sitting, leaning and balancing exercises). At this stage, physical treatment is directed towards:

Prevention of chest complications—breathing exercises, postural drainage (particularly for patients with a history of bronchitis).

Continued mobilization of joints (particularly shoulder).

Prevention of contractures of hip, knee and foot.

Retraining in balance and postural control.

A stiff, painful shoulder may well permanently complicate the weakness and spasticity of the upper limb of the hemiplegic patient, unless the physiotherapist has been gentle in her handling of the arm and the nursing staff have refrained from pulling on the paralysed arm during nursing, toiletting and bed-making. A hemiplegic patient should *never* be moved by *one* member of the nursing staff unaided during the acute stage of stroke, but always by *two* nurses using a grip which obviates the need for traction on the paralysed arm.

Between sessions of exercises with the physiotherapist, the patient should lie on alternate sides when unconscious and should alternate between side and back when consciousness returns. When side-lying, the pelvis should be positioned so that the underlying half is displaced backwards, the legs should be partly flexed, and the hemiplegic arm supported on one pillow and held in partial abduction by another. If the paralysed hand tends to become swollen, the arm may be elevated and supported by a forearm cuff-sling from an upright stand beside or attached to the bed.

Early mobilization

As recovery begins, active rehabilitation is introduced. Standing, walking and arm mobilizing exercises, supplemented by passive movements of those joints which the patient cannot move himself, form the basis of early active treatment. The importance of regular exercise sessions on the bed cannot be over-emphasized and should be started as soon as the patient can be mobilized. Achieving the sitting or standing position is often complicated by defective balance and an apparent increase of spasticity when changing from the horizontal to the vertical position. However difficult they may be, voluntary movements of trunk and limb muscles and active attempts to sit and stand several times daily should be encouraged. Standing up and sitting down independently may be practised in the ward (or bedroom) if a stable 'geriatric' chair is placed facing the foot of the bed. The patient then grasps the bed-end and assists himself out of bed and into this chair. It is usually necessary to fix a foot-stop between the legs of the bed to prevent the patient's feet from sliding away from him while he practises these movements.

As soon as the patient is able to sit up and stand, his paralysed arm should be supported in a suitable sling. There are various designs which are suitable, their common features being that they give some support to the arm at or under the elbow to prevent glenohumeral subluxation and that they support the hand at such a level over the opposite breast that they prevent oedema of the hand and fingers. The common slings are the 'double loop' sling (with a loop over the hand and a loop over the upper forearm) and the 'trough sling'. Although the use of one of these slings prevents swelling of the hand and distraction of the shoulder, it may also predispose to stiffness of the shoulder and elbow unless the arm is removed from it frequently. Regular exercise sessions for the arm are particularly important for the patient who wears a sling.

The early walking training of a patient with a stroke is a time-consuming activity. At first it is necessary for the physiotherapist to have a colleague or a helper so that the first stages of standing and walking are controlled by two people, one on either side of the patient. While the leg is flaccid, a temporary back-splint made from plastic or plaster of paris may be helpful to prevent the leg 'giving way'. As spasticity supervenes, temporary drop-foot springs, slings, or even simple bandages may be used to help the patient through the swing phase of movement of the hemiplegic leg. Progression to walking bars, walking frames, quadruped sticks and walking sticks depends upon the patient's general rate of recovery.

After the first few weeks, rehabilitation can be directed towards functional activity, and it is at this stage that the complications and associated disorders which may accompany strokes play a dominant part in determining the rate of progress in the pattern of achievement.

Incontinence

While the patient is unconscious, catheterization may become necessary. Unless a highly efficient team is present to ensure regular aseptic, intermittent catheterization at frequent intervals, it is better to use an indwelling catheter, changing it weekly or fortnightly.

When consciousness returns, the patient may recover his ability to control micturition. The return of this ability may be indicated when the spigotted catheter is released at 2-hourly intervals and the patient attempts to micturate. The catheter is then removed, the patient is given a bottle or bedpan at frequent intervals, and, if co-operative, instructed how to assist micturition by tapping, pressing, squeezing or rubbing the abdominal wall overlying the bladder. Particular care is needed during this period with aphasic, demented, hemiplegic patients, as well as patients with sensory loss, since incontinence may be suspected merely because of urine spilt from receptacles which cannot be properly supported or utilized.

Most patients affected by incontinence regain some degree of control. If a normal micturition pattern does not return, it is possible to build up in many patients the ability to stay dry by frequent visits to the lavatory, regulated drinking of moderate quantities of fluid, and timed stimulation of the bladder to contract by manual stimulation of the abdominal wall, assisted by forward flexion of the abdomen and contraction of the abdominal muscles.

Some patients will remain incontinent, and no recovery of control of micturition of any sort can be taught them. The use of an indwelling catheter then becomes necessary as a permanent measure to keep female patients comfortable and socially acceptable. With the plastic disposable bag now available for catheter attachment, it is possible to fasten this around the thigh and so to retain some personal dignity. Women patients need to be persuaded into wearing longer skirts or else trouser suits if they are to wear the urinals inconspicuously. Small taps are fitted to the lower end of the plastic bags to enable them to be emptied. Male patients can more easily be fitted with satisfactory drainage appliances, and they have their trousers to conceal these urinals.

Particular care should be taken by all those giving care to a hemiplegic patient to ensure that these urinals are emptied regularly and remain concealed as much as possible. A burst, detached or leaking urinal may cause great distress to the fastidious patient for whom the idea of catheterization is often extremely distasteful.

Relationship of clinical findings and rehabilitation

Early assessment of the long-term prognosis is very difficult, but is all-important if realistic decisions and plans are to be made. The characteristics of strokes which bear most relevance in the long-term rehabilitation are: loss of motor power; disturbances of sensation, including perception of body image and visual field defects; spasticity; impairment of speech; impairment of mental status.

Motor problems

Loss of muscle power, muscle control and muscle tone all contribute to the disability, but motor defect alone is seldom a real bar to functional recovery. A patient with hemiparesis from polio may have complete independence, and a patient with an arm and a leg amputated on one side, although clearly handicapped, can achieve considerable functional skill. It is the disturbance of muscular tone inherent in stroke which has such a profoundly disabling effect. Not only must the patient who is hemiplegic from stroke compensate for the weakness due to loss of motor power, but he must also overcome the spasm of the affected muscles when he attempts voluntary movement of the hemiplegic side. This spasm is often cumulative in effect—a man who can walk 2 steps easily, may be forced to a halt after 20 because of inability to move his spastic limbs.

Sensory defects

A variable amount of sensory defect may accompany the unilateral loss of power and occurs in about 10–15 per cent of strokes. These are most frequently defects of superficial sensation, but in a few patients there is a disturbance of proprioceptive sensation or of two-point discrimination (astereognosis). Sensory disturbances have a profound bearing upon rehabilitation. A patient with defects of position-sense or astereognosis, or disturbance of spatial orientation and perception, is unable to respond to a training programme requiring the redevelopment of many functional activities. Thus, the failure of a patient to perform and improve as well as might be expected may well derive from sensory disturbance. Among those who care for hemiplegics, there is therefore a need for greater awareness of the possibility that such sensory disturbances may co-exist with the spastic hemiparesis. In their presence, the conventional rehabilitation programme and the expected standard of achievement may need considerable modification.

Anoscognosia is the denial of the true self-image and occurs when a patient is either completely unaware of the hemiplegic side or refuses to admit that it is an integral part of himself. It is associated with right (non-dominant) hemisphere lesions, and although the clinical picture may improve slowly over many months, recovery is seldom significant. The condition indicates a poor prognosis for functional recovery. Such a patient may initially be thought unco-operative until anoscognosia is recognized. He is not, however, failing to co-operate, but is failing to achieve what is required of him because he is not properly aware of the presence and activity of affected parts of his body.

Any disturbance of body image leads to a sensation of instability associated with a fear of falling, which is quite distinct from the disturbances of balance which may occur through involvement of the vestibulocerebellar system or through impairment of visuospacial perception.

Impairment of perception of the body image interferes with even simple activities such as dressing and walking. Persistent attempts to achieve these activities may be doomed to failure unless the patient can be taught to recognize, understand and compensate for his disturbed body image. A simple test is to ask the patient to draw himself. A characteristically distorted drawing is a clear indication that the patient is likely to have difficulty in activities requiring an awareness of the paralysed side.

Apraxia is the inability to perform previously learned, skilled tasks and can be demonstrated by the patient's inability to copy simple drawings of various designs. It should be distinguished from *ataxia* which is muscular inco-ordination. *Agnosia* means loss of ability to recognize the impact of sensory stimuli, and results in an inability to understand the function of the articles although the patient can clearly describe them. *Perseveration* is a response which is more appropriate to previous instructions than current ones and can be applied to speech and thought as well as action.

The disturbances of co-ordination of muscular action which result from such disturbances of sensation provide early indications that physical therapy and rehabilitation regimes are likely to be unavailing. At best, their achievements will be minimal and will be accomplished only with great effort by the therapists concerned over long periods.

Spasticity

The intensity of spasticity demonstrable in a hemiplegic patient is variable, and depends upon both cerebral and non-cerebral factors.

It is the extent and location of the cerebral damage which primarily determines the degree of spasticity or flaccidity of the affected muscles. Many non-cerebral factors exert a secondary affect upon the muscle tone, and it is important that those giving care should recognize these factors and enhance or counteract them to increase the patient's mobility.

Particularly important is the influence which body posture has on spasticity. A patient whose arm is semi-fixed in the typical hemiplegic position when the body is erect will often be able to move the arm through a wide range of movements when his body is supine. It is therefore incumbent on the physiotherapist to instruct the patient to exercise his hemiplegic limbs night and morning while lying on the bed, so that joint movement may be better maintained.

Intense or noxious stimuli of many kinds may provoke increased spasticity, particularly when due to infection, injury or increased mechanical tension. Thus, pressure sores, bladder distension, bladder infection or paronychia of the toes may be provocative. Cold also increases spasm, and spastic limbs need to be warmly clad in cold weather. Stretching of affected muscles likewise effects spasm, and for this reason the provision of a toe-raising spring to combat foot-drop in a hemiplegic patient tends only to increase the flexion which it attempts to counteract.

Mental factors as well as physical ones influence the degree of spasticity which a patient exhibits at any one time. Conditions of stress and strange surroundings exert an unnaturally potent effect upon the labile emotions of the stroke patient and are likely to increase spasm.

Many of the techniques of physiotherapy introduced in recent years attempt to employ spasticity on the one hand and to inhibit it on the other. It is sometimes necessary to teach the patient to use, for example, an extensor spasm to achieve standing or walking. More frequently, the physiotherapist attempts to reduce spasticity in order to achieve some more functional movement, or to increase the muscle power of those muscles which can oppose the effect of the spastic ones. The use of ice, the use of relaxation techniques, and many of the 'proprioceptive neuromuscular facilitation' techniques are directed towards this end. The use of drugs, such as diazepam during the day, will often enable the physiotherapist to achieve more active function and will also reduce uncomfortable nocturnal spasm. This drug's value must, however, be balanced against its soporific effect, and its tendency to inhibit intellectual activity and produce intractable lethargy. Its withdrawal frequently produces several days of malaise and depression. Nevertheless sustained stretching of a spastic muscle during 8–9 hours' sleep appears to be of more value than a few minutes' stretching 2 or 3 times a day. Thus adequate night doses of diazepam and the use of a lightweight plaster splint with some dorsiflexion of the ankle (vide infra) is more likely to prevent contractures of the calf muscles than intermittent treatment in a physiotherapy department. During the day, ice will often relax spasticity enough to allow the physiotherapist to assist active exercise for the antagonists of the spastic muscles.

Injections of alcohol (40–45 per cent) into the muscle belly near motor points often gives some temporary relief. More accurate injection of the motor nerves with small quantities of 2 per cent aqueous phenol will usually have a more prolonged effect. Intrathecal phenol will destroy large motor and sensory nerve fibres with consequent reduction of voluntary power as well as interruption of the stretch reflex arc.

The presence of continuing pain or discomfort, or persistent interference with active function in an otherwise well-rehabilitated patient, should be an indication for considering surgical procedures to produce a more permanent reduction in the spasticity or its effects.

Speaking and writing

Right-sided hemiplegia is frequently accompanied by aphasia or dysphasia. The effects vary from complete inability to understand the spoken or written word, with failure to express thoughts and needs in speech and writing (global aphasia) to a mild difficulty in finding the right word or a slowing in the formulation of sentences, slight spelling difficulties or slowness in reading. Some speech defect is present in about 50 per cent of strokes.

Persistent aphasia (or dysphasia)—particularly global or receptive aphasia—has an adverse effect on rehabilitation. This accompanies about 15 per cent of strokes, and for these patients formal speech therapy appears to be useless.

In the treatment of aphasia other than the global variety, the precise contribution of the speech therapist in re-establishing a patient's ability to speak has not been clearly established. There are some indications that it may be a supraliminal barrage of afferent visual and auditory stimuli which recalls speech in some cases; in others, the painstaking teaching of speech and reading from first principles may be needed as well.

Aphasia presents considerable problems as it is often accompanied by intellectual impairment shown even in a non-verbal test of intelligence. Repetition of words, with persistent use of wrong words, is common. Occasionally, there may be true anarthria or dysarthria when the muscles of speech are neurologically affected.

In all circumstances of difficulty after a stroke, it is important to establish a sympathetic, encouraging and stimulating environment; this means that all the personnel working with the patient, including nurses, physiotherapists and relatives, should collaborate with the speech therapist in working towards re-establishing normal speech.

For each patient, it is necessary to assess the level of understanding of speech and the written word and to establish a simple method of communication (sign-board writing, pad and picture). Difficulties in comprehension (receptive dysarthria) can be helped by training with visual clues accompanying spoken or written instructions. Executive dysarthria (difficulties in formulating words in the presence of normal understanding) can be helped by formal speech training using oral exercises (e.g. reading, word games and general social activity with friends, relatives, staff and other patients). Defects in reading (*alexia* or *dyslexia*) are difficult to treat but can sometimes be helped by simple practice in reading. The more severely affected patients require special techniques.

Agraphia or *dysgraphia* is in part due to the muscular paralysis of the right arm and in part due to central defects. Some dysphasic patients without paralysis have dysgraphia which may improve with practice. Writing practice is however very boring, and it is necessary to devise ways of maintaining interest, e.g. writing letters and compiling records of activities. There is a general belief that speech and writing ability will either recover, or not recover, whatever treatment is given, and there is little objective evidence of the benefits to be derived from speech therapy. However, most rehabilitation units treating hemiplegics find that speech and writing therapy are an important part of the patient's programme. These activities are often a reflection of the general active and encouraging approach of such a unit. Co-operation and collaboration between physiotherapist, occupational therapist and speech therapist is essential if optimal results are to be obtained. Patterns of activity are so interdependent that each therapist must have an understanding of the skills and contributions of the other.

Mental status

Successful rehabilitation depends upon the patient's ability to comprehend, accept and adjust himself to the level of physical disability and inconvenience inherent in any particular stage of recovery, as well as upon his ability to co-operate with procedures designed to improve function, e.g. exercises and use of aids and appliances. It therefore follows that the final functional efficiency of any particular patient is as much a product of his mental state as his physical condition. The patient who has sustained severe intellectual damage from his stroke, with little residual paralysis, may indeed be the more difficult to restore to his premorbid status. The various types of mental impairment which may accompany stroke differ widely in the effects which they have both on the retraining potential of the patient and on the actual retraining programme which is planned for him. Recognition of the particular type of impairment in any particular patient is therefore essential for the therapists and for the doctors who care for him, so that realistic goals of achievement may be set and presented to patient, relatives and employers alike.

The classification of the psychological effects of brain damage into (1) impairment of perception, (2) impairment of intellectual function, and (3) changes in personality, is within most therapists' capability to apply in the evaluation of their patients. With the assistance of clinical and educational psychologists, specialized objective techniques may be used to further evalute and analyse the important variables of motivation, frustration, co-operation and adaptability. Such an evaluation can provide a useful assessment of a patient's residual mental ability.

Personality impairment loss of drive and vitality, irritability, easily provoked anxiety, dependence and emotional liability.

Psychiatric symptoms depression or anxiety symptoms, separately or together, are those most frequently occurring.

Intellectual impairment loss of memory, inability to appreciate and co-ordinate new and previously learned facts, inability to calculate.

From such an assessment it is possible to classify patients as:

Minimally disabled those with minor memory impairment or transient anxiety/depressive states.

Mildly disabled those with intellectual impairment permitting adequate functioning in non-intellectual occupations; those with personality change insufficient to prejudice maintenance of family and other relationships; those with depression or anxiety states responding to treatment.

Moderately disabled those with intellectual deficiency sufficient to impair work status, and/or produce deterioration in personal relationships and subjective well-being, and/or promote severe or prolonged depressions not responding fully to in-patient treatment.

Severely disabled those with impairment of personality and intellect severe enough to lead to unemployment or marked fall in employment status, and/or to marked deterioration in family relationships and subjective well-being; and those with severe prolonged depression not responding fully to in-patient treatment.

Such a classification is essentially a practical one, grouping patients according to the effect that their mental status may have upon their rehabilitation potential, but there is a very real need for further research into the mental disturbances following strokes.

One further indication of cerebral damage which has a poor prognosis is the persistence of emotional lability. This may be manifested by rapidly changing emotions, temper outbursts or attacks of inappropriate crying or laughing. Although the premorbid personality will determine the emotional reaction of the patient with a major illness, in strokes, the physical and mental effects of the illness must be carefully assessed. It is the patient's ability to change which is important, and much more clinical and psychological data is needed to establish clear guidelines for the clinician and therapist.

Ability of the patient to respond to rehabilitation

Strokes usually occur in older patients who not only have diseased cardiovascular systems, but degenerative disease in other systems as well. The presence of such disease must influence the effort which a patient can put into practising his exercises and may indeed be the limiting factor which decides the final level of functional competence which he attains. Thus, a patient with chronic bronchitis or coronary insufficiency finds that his exercise tolerance is lowered by the early onset of dyspnoea.

The locomotor assistance which the parts of the body unaffected by the stroke are able to give to the affected parts may likewise be limited by their own dysfunction. Thus, a patient with arthritis in the contralateral leg may find that he cannot stand mainly on that leg as hemiplegics tend to do, because of the pain which weight-bearing induces. Similarly, a patient with arthritis in the hand or arm cannot use bars or walking aids effectively to assist the weight-bearing of the paralysed limb. The compensation which one limb can supply for the deficiencies of the other is therefore diminished and the patient's ability to participate in an active rehabilitation programme is diminished accordingly.

A patient with defective special senses such as blindness or deafness is less able to comprehend and is therefore more likely to experience difficulty during rehabilitation. In particular, a blind patient with hemiplegia has almost insuperable difficulties in recovering functional independence. If he needs a stick to enable him to walk, he holds it in his unaffected hand. This leaves him without a hand to feel before him for obstacles and for steadying himself. He cannot use visual feedback information to supplement defective cortical sensory appreciation and he is unable to instigate muscular contraction so as to assist his balance and bolster his confidence.

LONG-TERM REHABILITATION PROGRAMME

From the very early stages of recovery, it is helpful to impose upon the patient (and the hospital staff) a detailed, regularly performed, programme of activity.

The programme should involve:

(1) Daily exercise by the patient on the bed, with and without the slings: lying down, sitting up, leaning back on both hands, sitting on the side of the bed, sitting in the chair, getting on and off the chair, wheeling himself in his wheelchair.

(2) A daily visit to the gym for mat work in the lying, sitting, kneeling and crawling positions; bar work to promote arm and hand movement; and parallel bar walking.

(3) A daily sleep on the bed after lunch, followed by a short session of bed exercises.

(4) Alternating periods of elevation of the affected leg on a stool, and periods of dependence with the sole of the foot resting flat and comfortably on the ground.

Such a programme requires that the patient has outdoor shoes to wear for most of the day and certainly for exercise and walking sessions. A tendency to hypostatic oedema in the affected foot and leg may be checked by wearing tubigrip or an elastic stocking, elevating the leg at frequent intervals and performing regular and frequent exercises for ankle and foot. The establishment of such a programme demands liaison between the occupational therapist and nursing staff to teach the patient independent dressing, toilet, grooming, washing and feeding activities, so that independence training is interdigitated with the daily regime of exercises from the earliest possible moment.

Although it may be necessary during the early days of recovery to issue a hemiplegic patient with various simple aids to encourage his independence, the aim of treatment is to dispense with such aids at the earliest possible moment. There are some who would even deny the value of supplying a patient with a reaching aid, such as a 'helping hand' or 'pick-up stick', or feeding aids such as a non-slip table mat, a detachable vertical lip for a plate, a spork, or a drinking beaker with a wide handle and pliable straw. But issue of such equipment may lead to independence for reaching, feeding and drinking, and this will produce an immense boost to the patient's morale.

It is, however, important to stress to the patient recovering from hemiplegia that he should consider aids and equipment as a young child learning to swim does his water wings. They are a necessary part of learning and should be dispensed with once it is possible to manage without them.

Dressing

Minor alterations in the clothes of a hemiplegic patient will often make independent dressing possible relatively early in recovery. The substitution of velcro fastenings for buttons and the strategic resiting of zips, with the addition of a curtain ring to the zip opening, when necessary, are useful for the clothes of both men and women alike. Men find shirts and coats difficult to manage and need to be shown how to lay them on the bed and how to get into them and out of them again. They also usually need to be shown how to put socks on. The use of elastic shoelaces instead of cotton ones eliminates the difficulty of tying and untying laces one-handed. Women have special difficulties with brassieres, corsets, pants, and stockings or tights. If possible, it is far better to accept that these difficulties exist, and to select a form of apparel which will avoid incurring them. The fashionable long trousers in non-iron man-made fibre with tunic tops now available for women are ideal for the hemiplegic patient. Worn with knee-length socks, panti-girdle and front-fastening brassiere, they provide a form of apparel which is easy to manipulate, easy to wash and needs no ironing, besides looking well on the older woman. Low-heeled shoes are essential, and if a caliper is to be worn, the shoe to which it is fixed must be strong and well made.

If a woman will not accept an alteration to her mode of dress, she will usually have to accept some assistance with getting in and out of her clothes, since the average corset of an elderly lady is beyond the ability of a hemiplegic patient to manage, and the use of conventional stockings held up by back and front suspenders necessitates twice-daily feats of agility which try the able, let alone the disabled. A stocking aid is helpful to get the stockings on and up, but nothing except sheer manual dexterity will cope with a suspender.

Even when possible to achieve, dressing may be very tiring to the more disabled hemiplegic patient, and it may be expedient to accept some help in order to avoid unnecessary fatigue and exasperation. When independent dressing is a practical proposition, the occupational therapist will show the patient how to lay his clothes down in the reverse order to that in which he will require them next day to dress. He will be shown how to place them by the side of the bed or chair opposite to the hemiplegic side, to prevent him from falling over when he reaches for them.

Washing and grooming present fewer difficulties to the hemiplegic patient and can usually be performed one-handed with little special equipment other than that designed to stabilize the soap.

Visiting and using the lavatory demands far more co-ordination than is generally appreciated. Hemiplegic patients may have difficulty in getting their pants up while standing after defaecation or micturition. The use of braces for men prevents the trousers falling down too far for the patient to be able to retrieve them one-handed. Velcro-fastening or zip-fastening flies help those with urgency of micturition and will give a patient a small but valuable addition to personal dignity by preventing the need for assistance with refastening fly buttons.

Returning home

Once it is apparent that sufficient recovery of physical and mental power is likely to make living at home a realistic possibility, the home circumstances of a hemiplegic patient must be discussed and assessed. This may be done by the occupational therapists and medical social workers liaising direct with the domiciliary occupational therapist, or with the health visitor attached to the practice of the patient's general practitioner. A trained person *must* actually see the patient's home to determine whether any equipment or minor structural alterations are needed. Both patient and relatives are apt to prove biased and uninformed, and the information they proffer needs confirmation by a dispassionate third party.

Often neither equipment nor structural alteration is necessary apart from the removal of slippery rugs and the advice to avoid over-polishing the floors. Heights of bed, chairs and water closet pedestal may however be critical, and the supply of sets of blocks of the requisite height for bed and chair, and a raised toilet seat attachment may be indicated. The *lavatory* itself needs careful checking. A grab rail and an outward opening door may need to be installed. If the lavatory is indoors and easily accessible, only the supply of a night commode beside the patient's bed may be necessary. When access to the lavatory is difficult, as for example when it is upstairs, and the patient is unable to climb stairs, then arrangements will have to be made to convert a downstairs room for the patient's bedroom and for him to use a commode both by day and by night.

Kitchens

Sometimes the question at issue is not merely whether a patient can live at home, but whether she can manage to cope with the running of the home. Active participation in domestic tasks obviously demands a higher degree of functional competence than merely living there as part of the furniture, and the *kitchen* is likely to prove the stumbling block in attaining this competence. Appropriate alteration of heights of sink, stove and working surfaces, so that pots and pans may be slid rather than lifted, does much to facilitate the preparation and cooking of meals, and here a split-level cooker is particularly helpful. For the younger hemiplegic patient, alterations of structure and equipment in the kitchen and other parts of the home are amply justified. But for the older hemiplegic, a drastic refashioning of the kitchen is usually an unrealistic solution to the problem.

Whenever possible, the patient should be assessed in a well-equipped occupational therapy department kitchen, or in the assessment flat of a Disabled Living Unit, so that the requisite alterations may be determined and effected before she leaves hospital for home.

When alterations to the kitchen are not contemplated in the case of the elderly hemiplegic man or woman living alone, or that of the elderly hemiplegic spouse, whose marital partner is incapable of increasing assistance, then outside care such as home help, family help and meals-on-wheels may be the only alternative.

Care in the home

When there exists adequate and willing family backing or outside help, a hemiplegic patient may remain happily in the home. When the available assistance is inadequate for the patient's needs, this ceases to be possible.

If the hemiplegic patient is attempting to run the house, removal to a purpose-built downstairs flat or bungalow may make this a feasible proposition. If not, then a warden-assisted flat or Part III accommodation are the only other alternatives. If the patient is not attempting to run the home, but is living as a guest in the home of a relation or with an able-bodied spouse, the ratio of patient's needs to help available is equally critical. With the best will in the world, a busy young mother or the elderly spouse or sibling of the patient can only integrate a certain amount of extra work into the existing daily routine. If the hemiplegic makes too much extra work, he can no longer be cared for at home and must be transferred to Part III accommodation.

If all this information is available for a discussion in case conferences between all the medical and paramedical members of staff looking after the hemiplegic patient, a realistic decision can be made before discharge from hospital is arranged and the possible distress of a failed attempt at independent living may be averted.

When the hemiplegic patient *does* return to live at home, both patient and those giving care will need considerable support from the social and health services. This takes the form of regular visits by the district nurse for bathing and catheter changing; regular visits by the health visitor to detect need for further assistance whether monetary or in kind; regular visits to the nearest day hospital to give relief to those giving care; monthly chiropody, when needed, at the day hospital—this can substitute for the traditional follow-up at the out-patients' department of the unit which was responsible for his in-patient care. Frequent follow-up attendances at a hospital physiotherapy department are essential for the maintenance of the continuing well-being of the stroke patient *only* when adequate care is not provided in community-based services.

Regular visits to a local day centre give relief to those giving care. Such visits will enable the patient to be reviewed by the visiting staff, doctor, physiotherapist, occupational therapist and chiropodist. Under ideal conditions, these would be the general practitioner and paramedical workers. They would be responsible for providing the continuing care that is so essential to the well-being of the stroke patient.

Stroke is not a notifiable disorder and its true incidence has never been determined. Certainly it is very common and its incidence is probably around 2 per 1000 head of population per annum.

Undoubtedly many strokes are treated at home by the patient's general practitioner. Factors making home treatment difficult even in the presence of adequate nursing facilities are incontinence, delirium and prolonged unconsciousness. All survivors of the actual stroke who exhibit these features will usually be admitted to hospital. Others will also be best treated in hospital because of concurrent illness (e.g. diabetes mellitus) or so as to avoid stressing unduly other members of the family.

The vast majority of these patients are elderly and require predominantly nursing care. This can often be provided in a community hospital near to the patient's home and staffed by people known to him. (Of course, this can only be second best to his own home where, surrounded by familiar objects and familiar faces, he has maximal incentive towards recovery.)

Ideally, each community hospital and each general practice should have the part-time services of remedial therapists seconded from the district general hospital. Their activities should be co-ordinated by the general practitioner and dovetailed into the patient's management. Provided that the therapists work in both community and district hospitals, and provided that there is good liaison between general practitioner and rehabilitation consultant, it should be possible to rehabilitate a large number of strokes in the community. Those patients creating difficult problems could be moved to the district hospital rehabilitation centre under the care of the same remedial therapists.

Following discharge from either the community or the district hospital, the patient would continue his rehabilitation at home under the guidance of the general practitioner and the remedial therapists. Regular domiciliary visits by one of the members of the team, coupled with the patient's regular attendance at the day centre will ensure the essential continued care, repeated assessment, and support for the family as a whole.

TREATMENT OF THE RESIDUAL PARALYSIS OF THE LOWER LIMB

Most hemiplegics will require a walking aid for some weeks or months, and the elderly hemiplegic will often be unable to give up such an aid. Initially, the best aids are 'quadrupeds' or 'tripod' sticks with a wide spread (some 'tripods' tend to be unstable in some circumstances) or walking frames. Later, some patients will graduate to the use of a walking stick. It often appears to be a false move to encourage over-rapid progression from walking frame to quadruped, for the use of the frame encourages the use of the hemiplegic hand, and encourages a better balance.

The patient should continue for many months to have periods of prone-lying each day in order to prevent the development of hip flexion contractures. Similarly, the bed foot-board should be retained for some months to prevent foot drop.

Braces, calipers and splints

Occasionally, the leg remains flaccid and a full-length caliper appears to be necessary, but the weight and complexity of the conventional device usually outweighs its usefulness. In early stages, a back-splint to brace the knee is a useful aid for walking training.

About 50 per cent of hemiplegics need some immobilization and support for the ankle because of instability. A boot with a T-strap may suffice, but the more unstable will need a double iron and a drop-foot stop.

As far as below-knee splints are concerned, the problem is usually that of controlling an equinovarus spastic foot. The type of short leg-brace used is determined by the severity of the spasticity. If it is mild, with no clonus, and gives easily, simple piano-wire splints are suitable. But usually the spasticity is too great and any stretching of the spastic muscles tends to increase their spasticity. In these circumstances, ankle dorsiflexion (toe-raising) springs have little value. The spring accentuates the spasticity and only serves to distort the shoe. Thus the lower-leg braces usually need to be 'holding' braces, maintaining the foot and ankle in a functionally optimal position. However, if the foot is not dorsiflexed, there will be a tendency for the knee to hyperextend during the stance phase (if weight-bearing occurs) because of the tight Achilles tendon.

The solution is to get the ankle correctly positioned and 'stop' the caliper. If dorsiflexion can be achieved without increasing spasm then this is an advantage. If, however, Achilles-tendon shortening is present and the patient cannot stand on the hemiplegic leg because of weakness around the knee, a wedged heel-raise will prevent hyper-extension of the knee.

The varus deformity can be corrected by an outside iron which is cranked into valgus at or above the ankle, or by an inside iron with an outside T-strap.

In all instances, it is essential that the shoes fit properly. The heel of a suitable shoe is firm and well shaped so that it holds the heel of the foot firmly and prevents it lifting out of the shoe. An instep strap is sometimes necessary to assist in this, yet the shoes need to open widely to admit the foot easily and thus avoid stimulating a full Babinski response when pulling the shoe on. Furthermore, the shoe needs a firm sole-plate which cannot be deformed by the caliper or toe-raising device. Finally, the brace must be firmly attached to the shoe.

Hemiplegics, it must be remembered, are usually elderly and are one-handed. It is very unusual for a hemiplegic patient to manage to put on a below-knee caliper, and it is virtually impossible for him to manage a full-length caliper. This means that calipers and braces must be very simple or must be accepted as therapeutic training devices to be put on for walking exercise by the physiotherapist.

For all these reasons, it is strongly recommended that, whenever possible, simple lightweight plastic splints are made. New rigid plastics (e.g. polypropylene) have made it possible to produce aesthetically acceptable lightweight drop-foot splints. Their manufacture entails very careful casting, for a plastic moulded splint is only as good as the cast allows it to be. For below-knee walking appliances, it is essential to cast the foot and the lower leg with the distortion created by weight-bearing. Technicians skilled in plaster work can reproduce this by the use of a board placed on the sole of the foot and held in longitudinal compression while casting; others may use an impression-taking machine. Providing the splint is accurately shaped and the foot-piece is correctly positioned, the ankle can be held in a position of slight dorsiflexion to suit the patient's requirements. Plantar flexion is completely stopped, but some increase in dorsiflexion should be possible.

Walking training

Much time is wasted in walking training. The spastic gait is always ugly and awkward looking, but if it allows the patient to cover the ground well, and walking is stable, it matters little if the leg is circumducted and there is some degree of foot drop. Even if a patient does achieve a relatively normal gait under supervision, he usually relapses into the typical spastic gait when he returns home. Thus, it is more important to teach the patient to use extensor spasm than to overcome it, e.g. step up stairs off the affected leg and step down on to the affected leg, taking one step at a time.

Evaluation of walking potential is less important than evaluation of potential for total mobility and this must include not only those factors which are obviously directly related to the motor aspects of walking, but also such features as sitting and standing balance, visuospatial perception, weakness or spasticity in the appropriate muscle groups, competence in walking under different conditions (levels, slopes, rough ground, steps), and contractures of hips, knees and ankles.

Furthermore, the evaluation should include a reappraisal of the general clinical status and exercise tolerance, since it may be that correction of some other pathological conditions unrelated to the stroke may be of the utmost value in improving the total capability of the patient.

TREATMENT OF THE RESIDUAL PARALYSIS OF THE ARM

The spastic arm is more difficult to manage than the spastic leg, and its chance of recovery is slim.

Inability to abduct the shoulder is a serious and often painful handicap, interfering considerably with almost all activities of daily living. The spastic adducted shoulder can be mobilized by a combination of passive and active movements, particularly while in the warm treatment pool or after injections of local anaesthetic and hydrocortisone if pain is a predominant feature. Ice packs are often useful in relieving spasm and may be followed by several hours of reduced spasticity, during which time active and passive movements can be achieved. Pulley exercises combining active and passive movements can be carried out as part of the regular daily routine at home.

At all stages, it is important to prevent, and if present to treat, oedema of the hand and fingers. Gravitational drainage, the use of the high sling and passive movements will all have this object in the early stages. Unless oedema is prevented, stiffness will inevitably develop.

Hand splints to assist extension of wrist and fingers, e.g. banjo splints, are ungainly devices. They have to be complex and large, both to overcome the powerful flexion spasticity and to pull the fingers in the correct direction. Most lively splints seem only to hyperextend and sublux the metacarpophalangeal joints, and stabilizing splints are usually more helpful.

There are few procedures which will improve the upper limb. Relaxation of the entire flexor muscle mass with phenol or alcohol will often improve the appearance of the hand and facilitate the use of splints, since splintage of a flail hand is easier than splintage of a spastic one. Similarly, injection of the biceps and brachialis relieves the flexor spasm of the elbow, and prevents the ugly reflex flexion of the elbow which so often occurs during walking.

Most recovery will occur early, and deformities which are present at 3 months will usually persist. Indeed, many authorities believe that if there is no voluntary control at 3 weeks, there will be no useful recovery of function. Surgery can achieve permanent correction of such deformities, but is usually reserved for the younger hemiplegics whose clinical condition is unlikely to deteriorate.

SURGICAL INTERVENTION

Distinction must be made between spastic deformity and structural contracture. The spastic deformity disappears in sleep, and can be relieved by positioning or a slow passive stretch. Spastic deformity can be controlled by braces and splints, but no brace, whether static or dynamic, will control progressive spasticity. Surgical procedures aimed at rebalancing muscle power are equally doomed to failure. Infiltration of the muscle with local anaesthetics will enable the deformity to be analysed, and temporary reduction of spasticity by infiltration with 40–45 per cent alcohol can allow active rehabilitation to proceed. Non-progressive spasticity of fixed contractures is amenable to corrective surgery. Tendon lengthening, direct injection of the motor points or selective neurectomy are the procedures of choice. Achilles-tendon lengthening for the spastic drop-foot, associated with tenotomies of the flexors, if necessary, is often helpful. Split anterior-tibial transfer can compensate for lateral dorsiflexion. Hamstring release for knee flexion contractures is more successful than Eggars procedure. No surgical procedures will improve weak hip abduction, and no surgical procedures will restore normal gait, for hemiplegia is a disorder in which imperfect motor control is inherent and perfect co-ordination cannot be regained by surgical procedures. Thus, reconstructive procedures should aim at reducing deformity and improving standing and walking stability, rather than aiming at an unrealistic normality.

WHEELCHAIR USE

Some hemiplegics are so immobilized by the total effect of the stroke that they cannot walk and need to lead a wheelchair existence. Recovery is invariably greater in the leg than in the arm, and thus concentration on the walking re-education dominates the first phase of active rehabilitation. About 1 in 5 of survivors will not achieve independent walking and will require a wheelchair.

The provision of the most suitable wheelchair or wheelchairs for a hemiplegic patient is a matter which presents some difficulties.

Severely disabled The most severely disabled group of patients, e.g. those with dense hemiplegia or dementia, will be completely unable to propel a wheelchair, and for them a transit chair with 4 small wheels and a perambulator type handle is required. Unless seat height is critical, a 2-inch soft cushion, with or without a half sheepskin or other special cushions, should be supplied with this type of chair, since the patient sits in his chair throughout the day, and may well become sore. The chair is used to transport the patient about his home or residential institution.

Moderately disabled These patients are able to propel themselves with varying degrees of success. Some patients, in whom spasm is not severe, are able to propel themselves with both hands, provided sensation is adequate to prevent damage to the hands on the wheels. For them, the lightest, smallest standard wheelchairs with rear-wheel propulsion, which are consistent with comfort and stability, are indicated.

Patients in whom severe spasticity, or lack of sensation, prevents propulsion by the hemiplegic arm, have two alternative methods of propelling themselves. In the first, a lightweight standard chair is provided which a patient propels with the unaffected arm and one foot, or else with the unaffected arm and both feet. As the arm propels the large rear wheel on the unaffected side, the feet either 'walk' the chair along, or else the unaffected heel is dug into the ground and the chair approximates towards it. The foot or feet here act both as pivots and propelling agents, and prevent the chair from merely travelling the circular path along which one-armed propulsion directs it.

In the second, a single-armed propelling chair is provided, to be propelled by the unaffected arm. Although such a chair seems the obvious answer for a man with only one functional arm, it may in fact be of little use, particularly for a stiff, elderly person in whom there may be some intellectual deficit, since most available models are big, heavy and need a considerable space for manœuvring. Front-wheel propelling chairs are particularly suitable for a hemiplegic who has hemianopia, since the concentric steering rims are more easily kept within his field of vision while he is learning to manipulate them. The Ministry Standard Model 3 and Model 1 are both front-wheel propelling chairs which can be modified for one-armed control. The former chair is 4-wheeled and needs a large space to stand and turn; the latter is 3-wheeled and is easily manœuvrable indoors.

When hemiplegic patients are being taught to use their chairs, it is helpful to put them to practise in a gym or hall with a large full-length mirror at one end of it. They are urged to do some runs under direct visual control, watching their hands and feet as they operate the chair, and some under indirect control, checking the movements of the chair and their limbs in the mirror. This adds to the total sensory impact by which a hemiplegic must reorganize his damaged motor function, and it increases the facility with which he manages the chair.

Some younger hemiplegics can become very skilful with single-handed control chairs, used indoors, but few can achieve outdoor mobility involving any slopes or rough ground with this type of chair.

Most elderly hemiplegics are not going to achieve a high level of activity, and their interest will be best served by providing them with a wheelchair early in their disability. This enables them to attain some limited mobility and independence without much expenditure of effort either on the part of those giving care or of the patients themselves. It also enables friends and relatives to take them out into the community and maintain their morale.

RETURN TO WORK

For those who become hemiplegic before retirement age, return to work is of paramount importance in its economic, social and personal effects on the life of patients and families alike.

It is therefore necessary to ensure that this return is achieved smoothly. Often this can be done by direct arrangement between a patient and his employer, particularly if he has been known to them for a long time. Sometimes an appeal to the D.R.O. is necessary to ask the employers for minor structural alterations of equipment used at work to permit its use by a man with one normal arm and one spastic one. Often the best solution is the transfer of a patient from one department to another in which less manipulatory and/or ambulatory skill is required.

When a patient disabled by hemiplegia attempts to return to work in a place designed for the able-bodied, and at a process designed for bimanual participation, difficulties may occur. These may be difficulties of transport, entrance and egress to place of work, relationship of work surface to patient, relationship of patient with workmates from whom aphasia and the slowness of spastic movement now set him apart, in addition to the patient's inability to walk the distances between a work area and toilet, or work area and canteen, in the time allotted for this.

Hemianopia, partial sensory loss, memory defect and apraxia may also cause a loss of manipulative skill which bars a patient from the use of machinery.

The consideration of the possible difficulties before a return to work is attempted may avert embarrassments, frustration, loss of face and even loss of employment. A formal work assessment is helpful in indicating potential areas of difficulty, and such an assessment must include an estimation of mental, as well as physical, capabilities.

RESULTS OF REHABILITATION

In general terms, it seems likely that the best results following a stroke are to be achieved by intensive rehabilitation during the first 6 to 12 weeks after the cerebrovascular accident, during the phase of the greatest and fastest recovery. Thereafter, the patient's activities should be, as far as possible, self-determined and self-administered. The rehabilitation period therefore attempts to make regular performance of the more important exercises an unquestioned habit; so that a patient will carry on with shoulder, hand and finger exercises and walking, speech and writing practice, making them a part of his daily life, even when he no longer has the supervision of his therapists to encourage him to do so.

Not only his self-discipline but his own motivation must be stimulated so that formal exercises are supplemented by and incorporated into creative and social activities.

Active exercises to be performed almost indefinitely are frequently prescribed for the treatment of the paretic limbs after cerebrovascular accident, but their goal is more likely to be achieved through:

(1) Improvement and co-ordination.
(2) Prevention of contractures.

Many patients are unnecessarily attending physiotherapy departments when they could be better occupied attending social clubs and day centres where general activities would combine exercise with interest and entertainment.

Intensive rehabilitation can achieve improved function in the majority of patients surviving the first few months after the acute cerebrovascular episode. About two thirds of the patients should achieve personal independence and one third are likely to be fit for employment. For one patient, rehabilitation potential may mean a change from the bed-bound state to the ability to transfer to a wheelchair, and for another the ability to return to work in the community.

The end results of rehabilitation are influenced by many factors, some of which are related to the patient himself and some to the environment in which his rehabilitation occurs. Age, of course, has considerable influence on the end results which can be achieved in any particular patient, and the older patient, who has the greater chance of having associated disabilities, has the lower rehabilitation potential. Involvement of the dominant hand and the presence of severe speech defects are two other factors commonly associated with poor rehabilitation achievements.

Immediate surroundings, the therapists giving care and the rehabilitation regimes employed are all important factors in determining the end results. At one rehabilitation unit, less than 10 per cent of patients were able to walk independently on admission, but about 50–60 per cent had achieved some useful level of work or contribution to housework before discharge.

The average length of time patients stay in a rehabilitation unit in the United Kingdom is 6 weeks. These units have the advantage of providing comprehensive physiotherapy and realistic occupational therapy, together with speech therapy, psychiatric advice when necessary, and a close liaison with social workers to plan early return to home surroundings. They attempt to channel the rehabilitation activities of patients into normal activities as quickly as possible, since even the most enlightened occupational therapy and physiotherapy are not substitutes for the activities of daily living.

Attendance at a rehabilitation unit should be kept as short as possible, since the longer a patient is away from his usual routine the more difficult it will be for him to return to it. Therefore it is essential that the functional aims are realistic. Unrealistic optimism about a patient's performance and progress leads to an over-long admission in an effort to achieve an impossible degree of functional improvement which brings only discredit to the process of rehabilitation and its proponents.

SUMMARY

There is no better summary of rehabilitation of strokes than that in Bryan Mathews' book, *Practical Neurology* (1970).

> Treatment must still be based on the long recognised principles of mobilisation, proper hydration and feeding, and the prevention of infection. There is simply no virtue at all in the patient staying immobile in bed. From the onset he must be moved repeatedly in bed and at the very first opportunity he must be got out of bed into a chair for rapidly increasing periods. Formal physiotherapy must be given when available but a willing relative can soon learn to provide the essentials of repeated passive movement and attempted active movement. If there is any difficulty in swallowing a nasal tube should be passed as dehydration is

most harmful and inhalation of food even more so. Prophylactic penicillin should also be given if there is severe paralysis. An accurate prognosis is hard to give. Early return of movement is a good sign, while adverse signs are extensive sensory loss, prolonged flaccidity, and previous strokes. After a severe hemiplegia, useful recovery of the hand is unlikely, and the utmost attention should be paid to getting the patient back on his feet. Even if the leg is flaccid, some form of supported walking can be attained by the use of a caliper to hold the knee rigid. Dysphasia may prove a major disability even if good recovery from the paralysis has occurred, for even a mild degree will prevent employment in many otherwise suitable jobs. Patients certainly improve while having speech therapy, but as the natural tendency is to improvement it is difficult to be certain of any indisputable effect. The patient's attitude of mind will greatly affect the degree of functional recovery, but indifference is usually the result of repeated cerebral infarction and severe disability.

It is always necessary to remember that rehabilitation measures cannot succeed in those patients who are not motivated to improve, and persuasion, explanation and cajolery have little effect in such cases.

The management of stroke during the acute stage is concerned with the maintenance of the life processes, the prevention of deterioration of the locomotor system while its control is no longer properly co-ordinated, and the diagnosis of the causative lesion of the stroke itself.

Concurrently with such management, regular assessment of the clinical picture is necessary, so that the rate and pattern of progress may be perceived. Only through such assessment may the programme of rehabilitation be tailored to the individual abilities and disabilities of each patient. Such tailoring is particularly necessary for stroke patients, when the locomotor symptoms and signs actually manifest may be caused by such a wide variety of cerebral lesions.

Motor recovery and functional capability are the final yardsticks for judging the success of rehabilitation, but there are marked discrepancies between physical ability and functional independence. The major barrier will be any impairment of the patient's mental state.

The peculiarly fascinating yet exasperating quality about stroke rehabilitation is the large element which chance plays in its success. There is still no standardized, universally accepted form of progressive therapy. Encouraging results are obtained with patients treated at one centre which specializes in proprioceptive neuromuscular facilitation techniques; equally encouraging ones at another which follows the Bobath techniques. Some centres provide light and well-balanced splints and calipers which apparently stop flexion contractures and enhance the recovery of less spastic muscles; others forbid splints and calipers as pieces of equipment designed to reduce the proprioceptive sensory input of the joints and muscles which they stabilize. Some centres claim good results from routine use of speech therapy for their aphasic hemiplegics; others believe that speech therapists are useful in the diagnosis of aphasia but not in its treatment. Would a patient from one centre have recovered equally well in another? It is not only the treatment which varies, but the patient, the therapist, the associated features of the hemiplegia, and the atmosphere of the centre as a whole.

One of the few constant findings which can be extracted from the many reports and accounts of stroke therapy is that any treatment designed to increase the sensory input and facilitate motor output of the brain will benefit stroke patients. The degree of benefit will depend upon the expertise of the therapist in applying the treatment, the empathy which she can establish with the patients she treats, and the co-operation and motivation with which they are capable of responding.

There are almost certainly right and wrong methods of treatment for any particular state of recovery of any one patient. Equally certainly, therefore, there must be a correct pattern of treatment for each patient and it cannot be right to treat all patients by the same method. Principles of treatment hold constant, but not the treatment itself. The catalytic affect which enthusiasm and expertise in the application of any chosen technique has upon the recovery of patients makes it difficult to evaluate that technique in absolute terms. Yet it must eventually be possible to select the appropriate technique or combination of techniques which will assist the recovery of functional competence to the highest degree permitted by the absolute brain damage which has occurred in any particular patient. Until this time, we are still shooting in the dark. Until then, we should preface all advice on treatment of stroke with, 'We do not know, but we think that . . .'.

Little has yet been done to study and classify the behaviour patterns of patients during the stages of functional recovery. It is appreciated that the absolute motor paralysis following stroke corresponds to the size and site of the causative cerebral necrosis and the number and location of nerve cells and tracts thereby destroyed. It has long been appreciated also that areas of potential recovery exist in the brain immediately following infarction or haemorrhage, and that the final degree of destruction of brain tissue depends on the ability of the collateral circulation to compensate for the circulatory insufficiency caused by the initial vascular catastrophe. What has not yet been determined is how the actual pattern of recovery is related to the pathophysiology of the causative brain lesion.

It may be that when techniques for diagnosing the site and extent of the causative lesions of stroke are perfected, it will be possible to specify the pattern along which recovery will occur in any one patient, and to adjust the programme of rehabilitation accordingly.

BIBLIOGRAPHY AND REFERENCES

Adams, G. F. and Hurwitz, L. J. (1963). 'Mental barriers to recovery from stroke.' *Lancet* **2**, 533

Adler, E. (1969). *Stroke in Israel, 1957–1961.* Israel; Polypress

Carter, A. B. (1963). 'Strokes.' *Proc. R. Soc. Med.* **86**, 483

Harris, R., Bruk, M. I. and Copp, E. P. (1964). 'Rehabilitation and resettlement in hemiplegia.' *Ann. phys. Med.* **7**, 209

Hurwitz, L. J. (1969). 'Management of strokes.' *Br. med. J.* **3**, 699

Lenman, J. R. (1959). 'A clinical and experimental study of the effects of exercises in motor weakness in neurological disease.' *J. Neurol. Neurosurg. Psychiat.* **22**, 182

Matthews, W. B. (1970). *Practical Neurology.* London; Blackwell

Millard, J. B. (1966). 'Rehabilitation and the hemiplegic patient.' *Ann. phys. Med.* **8**, 244

Rushworth, G. (1964). 'Pathophysiology of spasticity.' *Proc. R. Soc. Med.* **57**, 29

Storey, P. B. (1968). 'Some psychological aspects of disability and resettlement.' *Physiotherapy* **54**, 54–57

Working Group on Strokes of Geriatric Committee, Royal College of Physicians (1974). 'Stroke disability in Great Britain.' London; Royal College of Physicians

Yates, G. (1968). 'A method for the provision of lightweight aesthetic orthopaedic appliances.' *Orthopaedics: Oxford* **1**, 153

Zankle, H. T. (1971). *Stroke Rehabilitation.* Illinois; Thomas

10—The Young Amputee

INTRODUCTION

There are in the United Kingdom about 90 000 amputees. Each year about 5000 new amputees present for provision with artificial limbs and for rehabilitation; of this total about one tenth is made up of upper limb amputees; and of the lower limb amputees three quarters are in the older age group (over 60 years of age) and come to amputation for peripheral vascular insufficiency.

The annual total for *young* amputees in the United Kingdom is made up of approximately:

150–200 congenital amputations and severe limb abnormalities.
200–300 upper limb amputations.
800–1000 lower limb amputations.

In this younger age group the major cause of amputation is trauma.

The problems of rehabilitation of the elderly lower limb amputee are so different from those of the younger patients that they are described separately (*see* Chapter 11).

LOWER LIMB AMPUTEES

Result of rehabilitation

The factors which determine the end result of rehabilitation of lower limb amputees are:

Patient's age and sex.

Social environment.
The level of the amputation.
The pathology leading to amputation.
The patient's physiological condition (closely allied to age).
The patient's mental state (also often related to age and educational level).
The patient's work status, stage of training, and suitability for re-employment as an amputee.
The design of the artificial legs.

Age

Patients adapt themselves to amputation with a facility which is in inverse proportion to their ages. Small children with a lower limb prosthesis—like small children learning to ski—quickly become proficient. The prosthetists' problem usually lies in constructing sufficiently durable prostheses quickly enough to keep up with the child's rate of growth and activity. It is important that children should be seen regularly, and often, at the local limb-fitting centre since during growth spurts they may need a new prosthesis as often as every 3 months. They seldom need formal walking training.

Social environment

The acceptance which friends and family show for a patient's amputation will have a profound effect upon the acceptance with which the patient himself views his disablement. The more educated the background from which the patient comes the more easily will he be reintegrated into it as an amputee. Work, hobbies and social activities are less likely to depend on hard physical work or exercise. The well-educated lower limb amputee can usually return to his own job or be easily directed into a similar one. Alternatively, he may be encouraged to take on further training or education aimed at eventual employment in a suitable occupation.

Lower limb amputees with a poor standard of education often have less incentive to restart work which may have demanded strenuous exertion, and will be even more onerous for an amputee to perform. Jobs entailing long periods of standing, or of driving or climbing ladders present particular difficulties for an amputee, particularly when the amputation is above the knee. Even so, many young amputees do undertake such occupations and make a great success of them although eventually they are especially prone to osteo-arthritis in the contralateral knee and in the lumbar spine. For this reason, if there is a chance of retraining for a less arduous occupation, a patient should be persuaded to take it although those patients with a poor level of education will be more limited in their choice.

Level of amputation

Other factors being equal, the lower the level of amputation the less the need for formal rehabilitation. The patient with a through-ankle or below-knee prosthesis usually walks home on his definitive limb as soon as the socket has been fashioned to fit the stump properly and the alignment and suspension of the prosthesis have been correctly adjusted. Young patients with amputations at these levels rarely require any form of walking aid or walking training. It is only when the amputation is associated with multiple injuries, scarring from burns or radiation therapy, or where convalescence has been prolonged and has delayed limb-fitting that rehabilitation is likely to be prolonged. Formal walking training provides a background for the prosthetist to undertake the difficult limb-fitting required in these cases.

Higher levels of above-knee amputation produce short stumps which tend to slip out of the prosthetic socket and become sore during the patient's attempts to use the prosthesis. Walking training for such patients is more difficult and walking distances eventually achieved may be limited.

Through-hip amputations or hemipelvectomies necessitate the prescription of prostheses with bulky wrap-around corsets of leather or plastic, often articulating with the prosthetic leg by a 'tilting-table' device. The prosthetic corset needs to be padded with meticulous accuracy to ensure proper fit and weight-bearing. Even when this has been done, women in particular need help and advice about personal care and activities of daily living. Women usually find that they have to remove the prosthetic corset to micturate and defaecate, and have difficulties during menstruation unless they use vaginal tampons. Most women with this type of amputation elect to spend part of the time wearing the prosthesis and part with it off, using a lightweight wheelchair from which they are able to continue with their household tasks. Men often fare better and frequently manage to return to a full day's work although they almost always elect to walk with a stiff knee and seldom manage any gait other than an abduction one.

Cushioning for a wheelchair for such a patient may need to be specially constructed from a block of foam (plastic or rubber) carved to accommodate for the loss of the amputated hip or hemipelvis and then covered in rexine or suitable plastic. Often a medical sheepskin provides added comfort.

Individual features which will lead to difficulties in fitting artificial limbs and learning how to use them are:

Contractures of the stump.
Extensive scarring.

Phantom limb pain.
Persistent stump oedema.
Obesity.

Immediate post-operative limb-fitting

Traditionally, the favoured levels for lower limb amputations are 10–12 in (25·4–30·5 cm) below the greater trochanter, and 5–6 in (12·5–15·0 cm) below the knee, and the favoured shape for stumps has been the blunt-ended cone. Recent trends have moved towards the provision of total surface contact sockets or suction sockets for above-knee amputations; the use of patellar-tendon bearing appliances for below-knee amputations; and towards early post-operative fitting. The surgical techniques used to provide the fleshy stumps suitable for such techniques and appliances involve long skin-flaps tailored to the requirements of the individual stump. The muscles are divided distally and overlapped; bone ends are covered with a periosteal flap; nerve trunks are divided well proximally and their ends buried in muscle. Meticulous haemostasis is essential.

Such techniques produce 'fleshy' stumps with less phantom pain and often better post-operative healing. They are also able to accept a rigid post-operative dressing to which a temporary walking appliance can be attached. The dressing is usually covered with plaster of paris and applied with a special cast into which attachments for a modular pylon can be incorporated. Patients for whom such techniques are used may be stood out of bed at 24 hours, providing end pressure is maintained, and the temporary pylon is then aligned. The first partial weight-bearing standing is introduced at about 3–4 days. By the time the sutures are ready for removal, the patient can be standing and walking short distances. At about 14 days post-operatively, the cast (rigid dressing) is removed, the stitches taken out, and a second rigid dressing (either plaster of paris or plastic) applied with a temporary pylon attached. Providing there are no other problems, the patient can be discharged from hospital about 28 days post-operatively, walking with his pylon.

Such techniques require very close collaboration between surgeon and prosthetists and can only be undertaken in centres which are staffed and equipped to undertake the complex techniques involved. Although widely used in some centres, this method of immediate post-operative fitting is seldom used in the United Kingdom. Early trials indicated that the advantages of *immediate* post-operative fitting over *early* post-operative fitting usually failed to justify the extra organizational complexities and the dangers involved in the former technique.

There are several ways of achieving early post-operative fitting.

With the availability of 'modular assembly' pylons, it is possible for the young amputee to walk, as soon post-operatively as the surgeon deems advisable, on a prosthesis with a corset top, side steels, short shin-piece and foot, assembled from standard parts by the physiotherapist at the hospital or the prosthetists at the Limb-Fitting Centre. Alternatively, he can be provided with a standard rocker pylon which can be constructed from pre-operative measurements and can be ready in 3–10 days post-operatively, final riveting being completed after one post-operative fitting. In some centres a modular assembly definitive prosthesis is now being issued as a preliminary limb, and the traditional pylon stage is being by-passed.

PHANTOM LIMB PAIN

Some degree of phantom limb pain is a feature of amputation in both young and old. The patient complains that he is acutely aware of the 'ghost' of his amputated limb at certain times of the day or night. He knows exactly what the limb is doing, where it is in space, and the position of its various parts. Phantom pain is initially painful, and a variable degree of such pain is almost inevitable in the early days after amputation. In most patients it gradually reduces to an itch then merely a sense of awareness. The 'ghost' limb gradually shortens and finally disappears. Cold, ischaemia, trauma or infection in the stump may summon it back again. Reassurance about the natural history and common occurrence of phantom pain prevents it from having more than a nuisance value in the majority of patients, but to some it presents a serious and continuing problem.

Much phantom pain can be prevented by adequate physical and psychological pre-operative preparation. Psychological preparation of the patient consists mainly in imparting realistic factual information and in outlining the positive aspect of amputation treatment—freedom from the pain of an ischaemic foot, the removal of a persistent source of infection, freedom from a long series of surgical procedures, the chance to regain full weight-bearing walking activity, whichever is appropriate.

Early post-operative mobilization and activity and the employment of myoplastic techniques of amputation and stump-shaping also contribute to the avoidance of phantom pain. However, even when adequate pre-operative explanations have been offered, and meticulous attention to surgical techniques has been given, severe phantom pain may still develop and persist in distressing intensity in some patients.

There appears to be no one constant factor which dictates the development of phantom pain of this character nor which explains the persistence long after most phantom pain disappears. Clinical impression is that patients who have had a prolonged period of severe pre-operative ischaemic pain, or who have experienced intense pain at the time of injury, or who have been left with stumps which are ischaemic, infected, heavily scarred, or with skin adherent to the underlying bone, are particularly prone to phantom pain. The one constant feature of all these conditions is excessive, afferent stimulation, whether this is pre-operative or post-operative in occurrence. A tender stump and stump pain may cause phantom pain but do not necessarily do so. The sensibility of the patient to pain and his underlying psychological condition, in addition to his pre-operative exposure to pain, are instrumental in determining whether or not the painful stump is interpreted as phantom pain.

Although the interrelationship between pain and handicap is unclear, it is essential for the therapist and prosthetist to attempt to analyse the possible causative factors in phantom pain and thus help the clinician clarify the objectives of treatment, since severe phantom pain can work greatly against successful rehabilitation and can cause insomnia and predispose to depression.

There is some evidence that pain patterns can be learned, and that there may be situations of a reduced threshold to pain or even 'reflex pain'. It is possible that amputees, if allowed to suffer pain unnecessarily during the post-operative period, may develop a pain reflex. There is a point of view which considers that such intervals of predictable pain as the post-operative recovery period after amputation, should *always* be adequately covered with intramuscular analgesics. This intramuscular coverage may be supplemented by a variable dosage of oral analgesics, which is left to the discretion of the nursing staff, who may be reluctant to use powerful drugs. It may be that administration of inadequate post-operative analgesics, although based upon the best of intentions, may be the cause of persisting handicap.

Even when all eradicable causes of stump pain have been removed, phantom pain may still persist. Analgesics and muscle relaxants may improve the patient's tolerance of the pain, but they seldom bring relief and should be avoided whenever possible.

Much work remains to be done on the control of phantom pain. Some behavioural psychologists recommend that the patient prove to his conscious mind that the phantom limb is only a phantom and must therefore be ignored. Thus, if the limb itches, he scratches the place in space where he feels the itching to be, meanwhile 'watching it', describing his actions to himself, and systematically combating any sensation of the 'limb' with visual, auditory, and proprioceptive sensations from other limbs which negate the presence of the amputated limb.

Other workers report some success with clinical hypnosis, and it is possible that this form of therapy, properly applied, may prove the most effective treatment yet available against phantom pain, particularly when the patient can learn sufficient self-hypnosis to boost the initial instructions of the hypnotist. It is an interesting fact that neither stump pain nor phantom pain occur as frequently or in as distressing an intensity in upper limb amputation stumps as in lower. The reason for this difference may provide the clue to the effective treatment of phantom pain in the future.

Treatment of sore stump

If the patient complains of a sore or painful stump, it is vital that the precipitating cause should be determined and eradicated early. Sepsis, ischaemia, failure to heal, undissolved sutures, infected sequestra or neuromata may all produce sore stumps before limb-fitting is commenced. Control of sepsis, re-shaping of the stump, or even re-amputation at a higher level with removal of dead bone; injection of the tender areas of the stump with lignocaine 2 per cent with or without hydrocortisone 25 mg/ml; use of ultrasonics; a mechanical or electrically operated vibrator—all these treatments, appropriately applied, may affect the control of stump pain.

Frequently, the cause of the pain cannot be found and eradicated. For such patients, satisfactory limb-fitting is particularly difficult, and walking distances are likely to be limited.

Designing artificial legs

There are many designs of artificial limbs. They depend particularly upon the culture and climate of the country concerned, the traditions of craftsmanship, the economy, and the educational and social environment. The trend towards early primary fitting is also having considerable impact upon design features. From the patient's point of view, comfort, stability, and cosmesis are the dominating features which should dictate design.

There are three main factors which determine the mechanical performance of a functional lower limb—dynamics, elevator control, and cadence control (knee mechanism)—but it is not part of this book to discuss them.

AIMS OF REHABILITATION

The three aims of immediate post-amputation rehabilitation are: (1) to promote stump healing; (2) to promote mobility and power in the stump; (3) to promote general clinical rehabilitation.

There is considerable evidence that persistent stump oedema delays healing and that correct stump bandaging has a part to play in preventing the post-operative oedema. Traditional conical stumps are difficult to bandage really well, and the bandaging may have to be continued for some weeks if the patient is unable to get up and use a walking pylon.

In general terms, it can be said to be more important to rehabilitate the patient than the stump. Early mobilization of the patient will ensure early activity of the stump and prevent contractures. Efficient stump bandaging and early fitting of a traditional pylon will speed the healing of the amputation wound and the absorption of stump oedema. There is usually no reason, other than administrative difficulties, why the young amputee should not be ambulant on a walking pylon 2–3 weeks after the amputation—even earlier if his general condition allows and pre-operative measurement has been possible or if a modular assembly pylon or limb is used.

In a well-organized centre the functional results and speed of rehabilitation are little different from those achieved by immediate post-operative fitting.

Rehabilitation of the young lower limb amputee

In general, the young amputee will welcome an energetic rehabilitation programme directed towards general physical fitness and based upon a mixture of individual and group exercises. Provided his general condition permits, he can walk with crutches a few days post-operatively.

As soon as his walking appliance, whether a pylon or a limb, is provided, he should be encouraged to undertake normal activities. The first week or two are often critical, and if this can be spent on full-time rehabilitation in close proximity to the limb-fitting centre, the artificial limb can be modified and altered as required without undue delays. Close collaboration between the prosthetist and the therapist is the most important feature in achieving acceptance of the artificial leg.

Once the initial walking training is completed and the limb is comfortable, a programme of active rehabilitation should be directed towards integrating the patient back into full, normal, social life. He may need to overcome a lack of confidence, and apart from direct practice at walking up and down slopes or walking over various types of ground surface, it is also necessary to encourage him to walk in crowds, cross busy roads, climb ladders and to get on and off public transport.

The appearance of the artificial limb is important; indeed, return to normal life is often inhibited while the patient is wearing a temporary rocker pylon. The definitive limb can be given an appropriate appearance; particularly for girls, it is important to model the shape and size of the artificial calf to match the remaining normal one.

Walking training for the young amputee

It is usually possible to achieve an almost perfect gait with the young amputee, and this should always be the aim of rehabilitation. The best gait is the one which is most relaxed and economical in terms of energy and avoids undue stress on any one part of the body.

Incorrect walking, or limping, has many possible physical causes which the good prosthetist and physiotherapist should be able to detect and eliminate. Unfortunately, bad walking techniques due to physical factors can quickly become bad walking habits which remain after the original cause has been eliminated, and such habits may be difficult to correct. Tilting over the artificial leg is one of the commonest limps. Many prosthetists make the artificial leg about $\frac{1}{2}$ in (1·25 cm) short to facilitate the swing-through, but a short prosthesis may easily cause a 'tilting' limp. A similar limp can occur in patients with above-knee amputations:

(1) If the socket is aligned in abduction.

(2) If there is an abduction contracture of the stump for which the socket must allow.

(3) If the patient holds the stump abducted. This often denotes a medial socket wall which is too high and is therefore exerting excessive pressure on the adductor tendon. The patient attempts to compensate for this by voluntary abduction.

(4) If the socket fails adequately to support a short or thin stump.

The so-called 'abduction' or 'circumduction gait' occurs when the prosthesis is too long, but can also be associated with a prosthesis which is aligned in too much abduction or in which the medial wall is too high. In this instance, instead of the patient lifting off the good leg and tilting over on to the abducted prosthesis, he tends to swing the prosthesis through into an abducted position. The 'circumduction gait' may also be used by the above-knee amputee who lacks confidence in walking with a 'free knee' and walks with the knee locked on a prosthesis in which knee flexion was intended to occur. Sometimes with a prosthesis that is too long, that has inadequate socket suspension, or with which there is considerable stump pain, the patient will develop a 'vaulting gait'.

In a prosthesis for an above-knee amputation, incorrect alignment of the lower part of the appliance, or of the foot, will give rise to a rotation of the foot at 'heel strike'. A similar, abnormal gait can arise from poor muscle control of an above-knee stump. Uneven pacing is a common walking fault and can arise from several possible faults in the appliance:

Improperly fitting socket.
Insufficient friction of an artificial knee joint.
Weak artificial knee extension aid.

A weak stump, poor balance or lack of confidence in the artificial limb will also lead to uneven pacing. Fixed flexion deformity of the above-knee stump will tend to cause the patient to take a longer step with the artificial leg than the normal. Other limps may be caused by excessive internal and external rotation, incorrect alignment at the prosthetic knee, or defects in the alignment of the prosthetic foot.

Thus, a non-perfect gait may arise from defects in the artificial limb, in the patient's stump, or in his management of his prosthesis. An experienced prosthetist or therapist will recognize many of these limps, and their correction will be accomplished by trial and error. Attempts are being made to analyse the gait of the amputee by mechanical means, but there is little evidence that the mechanical analysis can improve upon the eye of the experienced prosthetist.

Resettlement

The loss of a leg is often regarded as a tragedy, but with good physical rehabilitation, good prosthetics, and good counselling, the lower limb amputee need not be particularly handicapped. There are some jobs which are not suitable for an amputee, but with appropriate advice on the scope and availability of training and on possible entitlement to assistance with training and transport, most young amputees should be fully resettled into active work.

UPPER LIMB AMPUTEES

Any single centre for rehabilitation or prosthetic fitting tends to have only limited experience in the fitting of artificial arms, since the total number of upper limb amputees is relatively small. Furthermore, the majority of upper limb amputees are young men, and they rapidly adapt to a single-handed mode of life. When they eventually come to a limb-fitting centre, they often find that the artificial limb becomes a positive encumbrance, rather than a useful appliance. This situation is aggravated by the very nature of the disability and the method of controlling the appliance. The higher up the arm the amputation, the more difficult it is to replace the function of the arm and the less control the patient has of the appliance. It is the hand which is all-important, and no appliance can substitute for all the functions (including sensation) of a hand. The arm is mainly concerned with placing the hand in space, and thus achieving reach.

Types of artificial arm

Artificial arms are either passive (cosmetic) or functional, and are activated either by body movement or external power.

The majority (50–60 per cent) of all upper limb amputees have a below-elbow or through-wrist stump. About 40 per cent of arm amputees have above-elbow stumps and only a few (less than 5 per cent) have a shoulder disarticulation or forequarter amputation.

The forequarter amputations present many problems to the prosthetist. The artificial arm has to be supported by a cap fitting over the shoulder and held in position by restraining straps. The appliance tends to bear against the rib cage. Such appliances are rarely used for heavy work except by a few very well-built tough men.

The shoulder disarticulation amputations give rise to considerable fitting problems because of the sharp contour of the retained acromion process. Otherwise the appliance fitted is usually similar to the forequarter appliance—a friction joint at the shoulder, a manually operated elbow lock and a cord control for the terminal device.

Even when provided with a well-fitting, working prosthesis, patients with this type of amputation will often only use a cosmetic or dress arm, which can be made of lighter material and is therefore less cumbersome to wear.

Above-elbow amputees ideally have an 8 in (20·3 cm) stump (acromion to stump tip). 'Capping' and limb-fitting is easier for them than for patients with the higher level amputations. The available leverage is relatively poor if the stump is shorter, and if longer there is difficulty in getting the elbow mechanism into the remaining available space, while matching the elbow position with the remaining arm. Appliances can be fitted with a cord-operated elbow flexion and lock and a cord-operated terminal device.

Below-elbow amputation is ideally performed at 7 in (17·8 cm) below the olecranon process and allows for the fitting of an effective functional artificial arm. With the elbow joint preserved, the patient has virtually normal capability for positioning the 'hand' and for manipulating the cord-operated terminal devices.

A through-wrist amputation preserves pronation and supination but presents prosthetic difficulties in that it may not be possible to obtain equality in length of the arms if conventional sockets and terminal devices are prescribed.

Following *partial amputation of the hand* the stump can be fitted with a variety of devices, both cosmetic and functional. Preservation of the thumb is the key to the preservation of hand function. The design of the device can usually be specially tailored to suit both the disability and the employment of any particular patient.

Acceptance and rejection of artificial arms

Body-powered conventional artificial arms are provided for almost all upper limb amputees, but only about 1 out of every 3 patients wear their prostheses, and half of those who wear prostheses only wear them for appearance. The 'failure' rate is rarely publicly admitted by prosthetists or clinicians but is well known to those working in the field. Energetic pre-operative and post-operative management is necessary if this high level of rejection is to be reduced.

Although the design of the conventional artificial arm is easily criticized—for weight, for appearance, for cost, and for difficulties with fitting—it can be a spectacular success and many upper limb amputees use their artificial arms for most delicate and precise work or for heavy and stressful activities.

Much of the difficulty of getting the upper limb amputee to use his prosthetic arm is due to the delay between amputation and limb-fitting, and every delay works against acceptance of the artificial limb. The lower limb amputee can achieve an immediate obvious gain by using his artificial leg—even if it is an ugly, awkward pylon. It enables him to stand and walk on two legs again. The upper limb amputee has no such immediate functional gain. He has to carry an extra weight which is cumbersome, and wear a harness which is restricting, and often has to learn to do things in an awkward and roundabout fashion using his prosthesis, when he can achieve them more simply single-handed. If he had an arm injury prior to amputation (e.g. brachial plexus lesion), the chances are that he will have adapted to single-handed activity before the amputation and will be even less likely to accept the prosthesis.

The upper limb amputee will often become single-handed for all activities of daily living long before he is measured for his artificial arm by the prosthetist, since it is only a matter of days before he learns to cope with most normal activities. Even on returning home or restarting work, very few activities demand bimanual dexterity—most can be achieved one-handed, sometimes with some minimal assistance from a support or prop. It is the exceptional upper limb amputee whose need for proficiency with prosthetic usage will motivate him to persevere with his attempts to integrate his prosthesis into his body image and function.

In order to achieve acceptance of an artificial arm and to become skilled in its use, the patient must either want to use it for a specific purpose or he must be fitted almost immediately after amputation with a device which will enable him to maintain his bimanual activity patterns. Simple devices made from lightweight materials can be produced in most hospital occupational therapy departments, and their provision should be routine post-operative procedure. Pre-amputation or immediate post-amputation referral to the Limb-Fitting Centre further enables the prosthetist, occupational therapist and surgeon to phase amputation, prosthetic supply, and prosthetic training so as to produce a rehabilitation programme which is as expeditious and as rewarding as possible. Retraining for activities of daily living and the activities entailed in employment can follow the fitting of the definitive limb and are an important part of the rehabilitation of the upper limb amputee who intends to make use of his prosthesis.

Every attempt should be made to help the patient to understand that the use of the artificial limb has a prophylactic value against the development of osteo-arthrosis of the joints of the opposite arm through prolonged and repeated activity over the years, while the one arm is doing the work of two.

Often the introduction of one amputee to another who wears his prosthesis successfully will provide some incentive to persevere with prosthetic training. So, too, may the demonstration of the various devices which can be fitted to a working limb to enable it to be used for driving or for activities which need bimanual dexterity and were of particular interest to the patient before his amputation.

Some men who are particularly well built and powerful will use artificial arms for heavy work, but many amputees are unable or unwilling to continue with heavy manual activities. They can however be trained for less physically demanding jobs, such as clerical work, if their standard of education so permits. Failing this, there are many machines which can be effectively operated by one-arm control or by one normal arm and one prosthetic arm with hook attachment.

Any prosthesis, indeed any appliance, brings both benefits and problems to the user, and his acceptance or rejection of the device is dependent upon whether or not he considers that the advantages of using the prosthesis outweigh the disadvantages.

In making the decision whether or not to wear the prosthesis, the patient is concerned not only with the mechanical function of the design, but also with the whole situation in which he has to live. The benefits accruing from any device will vary with the situation in which it is worn, with the age of the user, and with the demands placed upon the appliance and the patient by family, work, leisure and domestic activities.

The mental effort and concentration needed to operate an upper limb prosthesis must be reduced to a minimum for child amputees. Functional scope must improve as the child grows and demands the means to take a full part in the work and play of his contemporaries. The complexity of control may need to be correspondingly increased to provide functional gain.

Design problems in artificial arms

Not only do sockets and harnesses provide support for the artificial arms they subtend, but they also impart the stability of the trunk to these appliances, and establish the areas of contact between patient and appliance through which a sensation of 'feel' is established.

To achieve these purposes, the total contact area needs to be large, although for each individual area of contact there is an optimal size beyond which any increase gives rise to sweating problems. A certain proportion of the total skin area must be left clear to allow adequate sweating and so avoid overheating.

Many materials have been tried for the construction of the cap or socket of the definitive artificial arm; most prosthetists still consider leather to be the one of choice. Even when leather is used, however, capping the shoulder after above-elbow and forequarter amputations presents considerable difficulties since the capping must be strong enough to carry the weight of the prosthetic arm while yet avoiding undue pressure and discomfort. The maintenance of prosthetic stability is a further problem encountered in the construction of appliances for below-elbow amputations. In order to hold the appliance on whilst giving stability to resist weight or pull, it is necessary to encroach upon the elbow and upper arm. There have been many attempts to achieve this without using an above-elbow socket or shoulder straps, but such attachments invariably entail some loss of elbow movement and risk being pulled off under working conditions.

Terminal devices

There are many terminal devices, both active and passive, which can be fitted to a prosthetic arm. The most important single terminal device is the split hook. Its choice as the main terminal hand-equivalent for a prosthetic arm is a logical one. Nevertheless, emotion often over-rides the obvious decision and persuades patients to decline the split-hook and wear instead a cosmetic hand. Some efficient arm users will accept both hook and hand, wearing the hook for the greater part of the day and changing to a cosmetic hand on social occasions. However, a really skilled split-hook user rarely bothers to change from his device of choice.

There is a considerable range of designs of split-hooks available, varying in the curvature of the hook, the shape of the hook tip, and the nature of the hook's covering (if any). The power of the grip is provided by external power (usually elastic), and body movement (shoulder shrug) is used to effect hook opening. Extent of grip is determined by the curvature of the hook tip itself. Since the elbow must be rigid (or locked for the above-elbow amputee) in order to transmit power from shoulder to hook, the adaptability of the arm is correspondingly limited. It is largely for this reason that an artificial arm is more likely to be used in a supportive role and the remaining normal arm with its greater manœuvrability will be the dominant arm. The transmission of body power from shoulder to hook is usually accomplished by steel cable. Teflon-lined housing for the cable reduces friction. Proprioception through the hook to the arm depends upon the cable having no elasticity, but also depends upon an optimal amount of friction. If all friction is eliminated, or if the cable stretches, the patient cannot learn to 'feel' the amount of opening of the hook and judge his 'grip'. To date there is no synthetic cable with negligible elasticity available, and steel cable remains the material of choice.

Thus, the total proprioceptive impression of his prosthetic arm which an amputee receives is derived from a combination of sensations originating from the socket, the harness and the power-transmitting cable. Until this substitute proprioception has been established, it is important that visual and auditory impressions should be deliberately employed to provide the afferent feedback necessary for the amputee to control his limb. During the training period, the supervising therist continually directs attention towards this alternative form of control. Eventually, a skilled patient develops an amazing facility in the manipulation of his prosthesis—for such a patient the individual features of prosthetic design are critical.

Early fitting of upper limb devices

Since neither the multiple problems of peripheral vascular disease nor the strain of weight-bearing complicate prosthetic fitting for the upper limb amputee, it should be much easier to achieve an early fitting of the prosthesis. Within days of his operation, he should be fitted with a temporary prosthesis made from plaster of paris or lightweight plastic (e.g. plastazote). On to this temporary prosthesis, a terminal device with conventional cable control may be added after a further 2–3 weeks. By 6–8 weeks post-operatively, he is ready to be fitted with the conventional arm for which he has been continually prepared by an unbroken pattern of bimanual activity since a few days post-operatively. It is the responsibility of the amputating surgeon to ensure that this sequence of events is initiated as early as possible after operation, or prepared for pre-operatively. This surgeon should accept that his obligations do not end with the removal of the limb but only with the successful reintegration of the amputee back into gainful employment in a comfortable and functional prosthesis.

Congenital upper limb amputees

Congenital absence of part of a limb is spoken of as 'congenital amputation' and the most commonly occurring form of congenital amputation of the upper limb is the below-elbow variety. This type of amputation is unlikely to be of great significance to the patient, either in childhood or adult life, but on the mother, who produces the child, and the father, the impact of such an abnormality is great. It is the mother's attitude which will largely determine that of the child, and therefore, for her sake and for that of the child, it is important that during the first stressful weeks she should be given all the supporting care she needs. To her, the birth of a deformed child is a catastrophe, for which she often feels a deep and unreasoning guilt. Early and competent family counselling is essential to help her over this time and to assist her to develop a healthy attitude to the limb and the child. Equally important is an early introduction to other mothers with a similar experience. The best encouragement for the mother of a newborn child with a congenital amputation is to see a child with a similar amputation who has achieved normal school life and has become well-adjusted to his amputation (with or without the use of an artificial limb).

There are two schools of thought about the fitting of artificial arms for these children. Some authorities fit artificial arms well before the child is a year old, on the ground that this early fitting is most likely to lead to acceptance of the use of an artificial arm. Other authorities leave fitting until much later, arguing that there is little real evidence of early fitting leading to better acceptance, although even this late fitting may be followed by rejection.

Fitting very young children with limbs is extremely difficult, partly because of their lack of understanding of the situation and partly because of the difficulty of achieving a good fit. It is probably more important for the limb-fitting service and the parent to have a mutual understanding and agreement that the centre will be prepared to provide an artificial arm at any stage of development at which the child or the parents wish, or seem prepared, to accept it. Under no circumstances should the centre impose the fitting upon an unwilling child, nor should the child or the parents be made to feel at all to blame or 'ungrateful' if the child rejects the prosthesis. The child may reject for a time and then be prepared to accept at a later date. Nothing can be more unhelpful than an autocratic attitude on the part of the limb-fitting team, and a failure to respond to changing attitudes of the child and family as the child grows.

As with any orthotic or prosthetic device, the most important factor in determining success or failure is the attitude of the patient, and in the case of young children, that attitude can be strongly influenced by the parents. The acceptance often depends mainly on whether or not the device gives the patient a distinct advantage in the kind of activities in which he is interested. Thus, with children, it is part of the training programme to seek activities which are essentially bimanual and can therefore be achieved using the artificial arm but not without. In the early stages, parental approbation may be a big enough incentive on its own. As the child develops, the activities in which he is interested will change, and at times, cosmesis will be more important than function. As far as the parents are concerned, cosmesis is very often a predominating factor influencing the wish for prosthetic fittings.

The thalidomide disaster triggered off a widespread interest in externally powered artificial arms, and many designs have flourished for a while to be superseded by new ones. Unfortunately, the engineering developments have not been able to keep pace with the development of the children concerned, and few children have persisted with powered devices. However, some designs seem to have a future, and undoubtedly as the power sources become more adaptable, the engineering more reliable and the hardware lighter to wear and easier to produce, there will clearly be a place for powered devices in general prosthetic care. Patients without any arms or with flail arms are likely to derive some benefit from powered prehension devices, but it may be that there will be other advantages for the less severely disabled. For this reason, it is also incumbent upon the limb-fitting centres to continue to monitor upper limb amputees, both children and adults, so that they can be continually reassessed in the light of current practice and future developments.

BIBLIOGRAPHY AND REFERENCES

Barber, L. M. and Nickel, V. L. (1969). 'Carbon dioxide powered arm and hand devices.' *Am. J. occup. Ther.* **23**, 215

British Medical Association Planning Unit Report No. 2 (1969). Aids for the Disabled. London; B.M.A.

British Orthopaedic Association (1973). Report of Committee on Prosthetic and Orthotic Services.

Brewerton, D. A. and Daniel, J. W. (1969). 'Return to work after injury.' *The Hand* **1**, 125

Brooks, M. and Shaperman, J. (1965). 'Infant prosthetic fitting.' *Am. J. occup. Ther.* **19**, 329

Carter, I., Torrance, W. N. and Merry, P. H. (1969). 'Functional results following amputation of the upper limb.' *Ann phys. Med.* **10**, 137

Fulford, G. E. and Hale, M. J. (1968). *Amputation and prostheses*. Bristol; Wright

Loughlin, E. (1968). 'Immediate post-surgical prosthetics fitting of bilateral below-elbow amputee: a report.' *Artif. Limbs* **12**, 17

Nickel, V. L. and Waring, W. (1965). 'Future developments in externally powered orthotic and prosthetic devices.' *J. Bone Jt Surg.* **47B**, 469

Proceedings of a Symposium on Basic Problems of Prehension, Movement and Control of Artificial Limbs (1969). London; The Institution of Mechanical Engineers

Sarmiento, A. (1968). 'Immediate post-surgical prosthetics fitting in the management of upper extremity amputees.' *Artif. Limbs* **12**, 14

Simpson, D. C. (1969). 'An externally powered prosthesis for the complete arm.' *Biomed. Eng.* **2**, 106

Series: 'Studies of the upper extremity amputee' (1958). *Artif. Limbs,* Vol. **5**, Nos. 1 and 2

— Peizer, E. E. 'Design and scope.' No. 1, 4

— Berger, N. 'The population.' No. 1, 57

— Springer, W. P. 'The treatment process.' No. 1, 73

— Fishman, S. 'Educative implications.' No. 1, 88

— Ford, E. R. and Lewis, E. R. 'The Armamentarium.' No. 2, 4

— Kay, H. W. and Peizer, E. 'Prosthetic usefulness and wearer performance.' No. 2, 31

— Silver, J. and Silverman, S. 'Psychological factors.' No. 2, 88

— Fishman, S. 'Research implications.' No. 2, 117

11—The Elderly Amputee

INTRODUCTION

The Limb-Fitting Service in the United Kingdom derives from an organization established to provide artificial limbs to otherwise fit young men wounded in battle.

The spectacular achievements of the young amputees have perhaps served to obscure the effect which amputation of one or both legs may have upon the older patient. Currently about 60 per cent of all amputations in the United Kingdom are lower limb amputations for vascular insufficiency in patients over 65 years old. Thus the major rehabilitation problems are those of the elderly lower limb amputee with impaired peripheral circulation. Many of the patients will have had a period of illness and hospitalization prior to amputation, and frequently the supply of the initial prosthesis may be delayed for one reason or another. Thus it becomes increasingly important that the limb-fitting and clinical rehabilitation are more closely integrated.

Experience demonstrates the value of an intensive period of rehabilitation coinciding with the supply of the first temporary pylon. It is during this initial period that close liaison and understanding between therapist and limb-fitter can make the acceptance and usage of an artificial limb a successful venture. Slow delivery, inadequate time for trial and fitting, and inadequate training all contribute to rejection of prostheses.

As the average age of amputees tends to rise, the number of elderly double amputees increases. Many centres tend to feel that these patients must go through the conventional routine of short- and intermediate-length pylons and make a serious attempt at walking in double, almost full-length prostheses. This is rarely a practical solution for the elderly, and guidance on establishing independence in a wheelchair, in preference to a frustrating struggle with artificial limbs, is sadly lacking in many hospitals where elderly patients have their amputations. When some walking within the house is desirable, for example to reach the bathroom or lavatory, provision of leather 'stump boots' enable the patient to walk in prostheses which are light to wear, comfortable to sit in, and easy to put on and take off.

Cosmetic limbs are sometimes issued to those who are unable to walk in definitive prostheses. If these are made with the knees fixed in flexion and are fitted on with gutter thigh-pieces on which the thigh stumps rest, there is little danger of the patient attempting to use them inadvertently to walk. Worn under trousers, and with normal shoes on the feet, they are comfortable to sit in and give the amputee a normal appearance which may be deeply satisfying to himself and his family.

It is often assumed that every patient who has a limb amputated will be fitted with an artificial leg, but there are, in fact, three main ways of achieving mobility for a patient with a lower limb amputation.

Crutch walking (three-point walking) for which a patient wears no prosthesis but walks on his contralateral leg and a pair of crutches or crutch equivalents.

Prosthetic walking in which a patient wears a prosthetic substitute for his amputated leg and walks on this and on his contralateral leg with or without the assistance of sticks, crutches, quadrupeds or frame.

Wheelchair mobility in which a patient does not ambulate, but is transported in a wheelchair which is propelled by himself or helper, or powered by a battery.

Whereas, for a young amputee, the course of events is customarily amputation—early prosthetic fitting—prosthetic ambulation, it cannot be assumed that this sequence will automatically occur in the case of the geriatric patient. Prosthetic fitting attempts to supply to the young amputee the mechanical means of achieving the necessary mobility to satisfy the demands of a healthy body. The supply of a mechanically efficient prosthesis to an elderly patient, whom disease or degeneration has rendered incapable of using it, may well increase his physical disability. For this reason, it is essential that the several ways of obtaining mobility for a geriatric patient undergoing amputation should be always kept in mind throughout his entire post-operative progress. Without the consideration of these alternatives by those responsible for his rehabilitation, such a patient may be automatically fed into the pipeline of prosthetic fitting and supply, whether or not he stands a reasonable chance of ultimate prosthetic ambulation.

The capability of a patient to become functionally proficient following the substitution of an artificial limb for the amputated limb depends upon a number of factors:

(1) His general physical condition.
(2) The state of the amputation stump.
(3) The degree of circulatory impairment in heart and brain, stump and contralateral leg.
(4) The patient's mental state (i.e. confused, depressed).
(5) His psychological status (i.e. intelligence, educational level).
(6) The state of the upper limbs (power, range, pain, sensation, co-ordination).
(7) Efficiency of special senses.

These factors may vary greatly throughout the patient's post-operative convalescence, and consequently, an elderly amputee needs careful supervision throughout the initial period of his rehabilitation programme so that his physical and mental reactions at any one stage may dictate the way in which further rehabilitation should proceed. Sufficient supervision is only feasible under in-patient conditions, and the admission of the geriatric amputee to a unit geared to his needs and closely associated with an Artificial Limb and Appliance Centre (A.L.A.C.) is therefore a prerequisite of successful independence training. Such admission may be advantageously organized to coincide with the fitting and issue of the temporary prosthesis or rocker pylon, which can be issued initially to many geriatric amputees within a month of amputation. Measurement for the prosthesis may be pre-operative in the ward, after operation if the prosthetist is readily available, or 2–3 weeks post-operatively when the patient is fit enough to visit the nearest A.L.A.C. by ambulance.

Although some hospitals make their own early walking aids using plastazote or leather for the sockets, most hospitals in the United Kingdom still refer their patients to their regional A.L.A.Cs where pylons can be made within 3–10 days of order.

A pylon, or temporary prosthesis, consists of an individually made metal cylinder or container which encloses the thigh and is ischial weight-bearing. The container is attached to a rocker foot by side-irons with locking hinges at the knee. During walking the knee is kept locked but can be bent during sitting and re-extended by striking the heel on the ground when the standing posture is regained. It is light, stable, and apart from the metal cylinder or socket, readily assembled from standard components.

Early walking aids are similar to the pylon in basic design with a few notable exceptions: the socket is corset-type and is made of foam-lined plastic or leather. It is therefore easily adjustable to the variations in stump size which occur during the early post-operative weeks. The terminal device is a foot, not a rocker, and is subtended by a shin-piece. The patient can therefore present a more normal appearance.

The use of a pylon or early walking aid means that the geriatric amputee can learn to walk again on a temporary prosthesis long before his stump has attained a steady state. Because it is cheap, the pylon can be used and discarded (although often its components can be used again). The manufacture of an expensive definitive limb demands a stable stump, and must therefore be postponed for several weeks, possibly months, post-operatively. Without the temporary use of a rocker pylon or early walking aid, the mobility of relatively able amputees during this waiting period would be drastically reduced.

The advantages of fitting a temporary prosthesis are:

(1) Quicker maturation of the stump, which allows earlier fitting of the permanent prosthesis.

(2) Early walking preserves muscle tone, prevents contractures and reduces the amount of physiotherapy required. The patient's psychological approach to the amputation is improved by early walking.

(3) The patient's ability to use a definitive prosthesis can be assessed. This is particularly important in the elderly patient and may prevent the manufacture of a permanent prosthesis which will never be used.

(4) The patient's prosthetic problems can be assessed. This ensures a more accurate prescription for the permanent prosthesis.

(5) Patients with a short expectation of life have rapid restoration of function.

(6) Gait training is facilitated because of early fitting.

(7) The cost of a temporary prosthesis is much less than that of a permanent prosthesis.

The advantages of pylon usage must raise the question of immediate post-operative fitting: if it is so beneficial to walk early post-operatively on a pylon, why is it not of even greater benefit to walk immediately post-operatively on a prosthesis incorporated in the operative dressing casing? However, organizing immediate post-operative fitting (I.P.O.F.) as a routine procedure has many practical difficulties and implies the:

(1) Need for special team of surgical, nursing and physiotherapy staff to be readily available.

(2) Need for availability of prosthetists.

(3) Need for adequate supervision of post-operative patients.

(4) Need for adequate facilities to train pre-operative patients.
(5) Danger of severe recurrent post-operative haemorrhage.
(6) Danger of undetected sepsis.

For a geriatric amputee there are particular contra-indications to this procedure:

(*a*) High incidence of arteriosclerosis and peripheral circulatory insufficiency increases the need to observe the stump for haemorrhage, sepsis and non-healing.

(*b*) Many elderly patients have been very ill and/or debilitated pre-operatively, and are, in addition, further debilitated by the amputation itself. They need time to recover before embarking upon a whole new territory of unknown procedures and exercises.

(*c*) The surgical wounds in geriatric patients, many of whom are diabetic and most of whom have peripheral vascular insufficiency, need longer to heal than those of younger patients and therefore benefit from a few days' respite before being subjected to the stresses and strains of prosthetic use.

(*d*) Many geriatric amputees are not physically fit enough to undergo walking training without adequate stump-strengthening exercises, spine-strengthening drill, and exercises to improve power and range of shoulders and hands. Successful prosthetic ambulation requires far more strength and co-ordination from the upper limbs than is generally appreciated, and 1–2 weeks post-operatively spent in strengthening appropriate muscles and establishing good balance represent time well spent in such patients.

Early fitting with a pylon or early walking aid and carefully supervised graduated rehabilitation are the most effective measures in reducing stump oedema and shaping the stump and are much more effective than classical stump bandaging. Indeed, *early* post-operative fitting is probably the most appropriate compromise between the traditional approach in which stump measurement and manufacture of a prosthesis are delayed until the stump is well-shaped by bandaging and the more exciting, but hazardous, technique of immediate post-operative fitting. When early post-operative fitting can be arranged under in-patient conditions, the 1–2 week interval necessary for this procedure constitutes a useful assessment period during which medical and paramedical staff are able to observe a patient's performance and reactions and decide whether he is able to cope with prosthetic walking of any kind. Such an assessment defines the following groups of patients:

(1) Patients capable of using a pylon so well that they are probable candidates for the provision of definitive limbs.

(2) Patients capable of using a pylon, but unlikely to manage a definitive limb. Such patients may wish to retain the pylon or have a geriatric pylon (i.e. a considerably more acceptable pylon with a foot/ankle attachment to replace the rocker end).

(3) Patients capable of a limited use of the pylon, i.e. for getting to and from the lavatory or for walking exercise only, but who will be, in the main, wheelchair-mobile.

(4) Patients incapable of using any prosthesis for walking and capable only of adopting a wheelchair existence.

When walking and independence training can be arranged on an in-patient basis, the patient is given the best chance of making good use of his prosthesis.

Permanent prosthesis or definitive limb

Whether or not a patient has been mobilized on a pylon or on an early walking aid, after he has used it for about a month in his own home, he is sent to the A.L.A.C. to decide:

(1) Whether or not he should use a prosthesis at all.

(2) Whether he should keep the preliminary prosthesis which he already has.

(3) Whether he should be measured for a definitive limb.

If he is thought to be suitable for a definitive limb, his measurements are taken and a cast is made of his below-knee (B.K.) stump, while an above-knee (A.K.) stump is remeasured. The positive is sent to the limb manufacturers to enable a socket to be individually made to his specifications and needs. This has been the customary procedure in this country for many years, but with the coming of the Modular Assembly Prosthesis (M.A.P.) limbs, limb-fitting may well be drastically altered in the near future.

Trials are currently in process to evaluate the use and effectiveness of this limb which can be assembled in a matter of hours from standard parts; the time may not be so far off when almost every amputee will be able to attend an A.L.A.C. one day for measurement for a prosthesis, return on the next day to have it fitted, and attend for final fitting and adjustment on the third day, walking out with the prosthesis in place.

PRE-OPERATIVE CARE

General

Geriatric patients are referred for amputation of the lower limb when evidence of its future death seems incontravertible, or when the continuation of its living presence as part of the body becomes too painful to be sustained. Some patients present with sudden coldness of the foot following embolism, others with chronic spreading ulceration, others with spreading gangrene of one or more toes, frequently associated with diabetes and often precipitated by minor trauma. Others present with a long history of intermittent claudication and the eventual development of intolerable rest-pain. Many have had arterial surgery which has failed or proved only partly or temporarily successful. Except where gangrene follows embolism, they have almost always experienced a gradual reduction in mobility as the circulation in their legs has become less and less able to cope with the demands of the rest of the body.

In many patients peripheral vascular insufficiency in the lower limbs is merely the presenting feature of a generalized dysfunction of the circulatory system as a whole. Cardiac and cerebral vascular accidents may have occurred or be about to occur. Patients may have diabetes which has until now been undetected.

Whenever possible, lower limb amputation is preceded by:

(1) Adequate discussion between surgeon and patient of the pros and cons of amputation.

(2) Specific psychological preparation of each patient for amputation by the medical and nursing staff concerned in his care.

In addition to this psychological preparation, attention is given to the general medical state of the patient. Diabetics whose diabetes has got out of hand, or who have not previously been diagnosed, may need some days before they can be stabilized. Patients who are fibrillating need digitalization, and those with respiratory infections need breathing exercises, postural drainage, assisted coughing and the administration of antibiotics.

A lumbar sympathectomy may precede amputation to ensure a good blood supply to the skin of the stump elect, and arterial surgery may be performed to improve the circulation of the stump as a whole.

If the temporary prosthesis is to be a pylon provided through the A.L.A.C. the pre-operative measurements should be made by or in collaboration with the prosthetist.

If the temporary prosthesis is to be an early walking aid the measurements must be communicated to the physiotherapist responsible for assembling the aid, so that it may be ready at the patient's bedside when he wakes from the anaesthetic.

Ideally, the surgeon should order a light, self-propelled wheelchair for the patient's immediate post-operative use. Pre-operative order by telephone to the nearest A.L.A.C. (followed by the customary form

AOF5G) should ensure the presence of the chair to assist early post-operative mobilization.

Adequate drug therapy needs to be arranged pre-operatively and since it is probable that the amputee will need regular and fairly heavy night sedation initially, together with analgesics, he will tend to become constipated. While it is essential that the doctor prescribes adequate medication to ensure pain relief, it is also essential that he prescribes some bulky mucilaginous compound to facilitate regular bowel action. Apart from contributing greatly to the patient's overall comfort, this may well assist in preventing the occurrence of deep-vein thrombosis in the contralateral leg or in the amputation stump.

Physiotherapy

It is vitally important that the physiotherapist in charge of the geriatric amputee's care should establish a good relationship with the patient before the operation. It is she who will spend most time with him, will help him to prepare himself for his prosthesis, instruct him in its use and assess his ability to use it. It is she who can inspire him with the feeling that he is having active treatment, with independent mobility as its aim and object. She should make the most of any pre-operative interval by giving the patient exercises in bed and as frequent sessions in the gymnasium or the physiotherapy departments as her time-table and the patient's condition will permit. His exercise regime would be designed to:

(1) Strengthen the contralateral leg, and the potential stump, for prosthetic walking.
(2) Strengthen the upper limbs for manipulation of walking aids.
(3) Improve balance, mobility and strength of the trunk.
(4) Increase the vital capacity and assist effective coughing.
(5) Provide practice in simulated prosthetic walking, with the leg to be amputated held flexed at the knee and resting on a platform or sling, while the patient assists weight-bearing with crutches or frame, preferably the latter.

In addition, the physiotherapist should check the order of a wheelchair for each patient from the A.L.A.C. and see that, if the proposed amputation is at below-knee level, a padded board is available to place partly under the chair cushion, with padded part projecting forwards so that it will support the below-knee stump. She should also check pre-operatively that a walking aid of the appropriate height for the patient is available, and if not, order one from the supplies department or from the A.L.A.C.

Walking training can often be adversely affected by a patient attempting to walk with his remaining foot in a loose slipper. Frequently this is the only footwear he possesses which is comfortable or able to fit on an ulcerated or oedematous foot. A lace-up felt boot with a firm sole with sheepskin lining if necessary over the pressure areas is an acceptable substitute for this slipper and will stand him in better stead during prosthetic training.

Nursing

An elderly patient awaiting lower limb amputation should be nursed on a bed with a firm base or with a board under the mattress to minimize the development of flexion contractures and to assist exercise regime. If his peripheral circulation is poor, and his buttocks and contralateral leg are at risk, he may need a medical sheepskin or a ripple (alternating pressure) mattress to sleep on. If the patient is incontinent, early trials indicate that a compartmentalized mattress or cushion filled with polystyrene granules is effective in preventing buttock ulceration. If pressure sores have developed a water-bed (or flotation-bed) may speed his recovery.

Usually it is sufficient to nurse him on a sheepskin with his contralateral leg and foot in another half-sheepskin, or with the foot partially enclosed in a plastic bootee with sheepskin lining or in a sheepskin bootee. Bootees need to be issued pre-operatively and not when ulceration of the heel and malleoli has occurred.

A strategically padded cradle should support the bed-clothes and prevent ulceration of the foot from over-zealous contact. A monkey pole at the head end of the bed will enable the patient to move himself up the bed by flexing his knee fully, pressing on the mattress with the sole of the foot and hauling and swinging simultaneously on the handgrip of the monkey pole. It is important that all potential amputees be instructed in this method of changing their positions, pre-operatively, since the alternative method of pushing with the heel assisted by a backward press-up by the arms is an effective contributory cause of ulceration of the heel.

POST-OPERATIVE CARE

Nursing and medical

Among a group of elderly patients who come to operation by virtue of a failing peripheral circulation and who are often suffering in addition from diabetes or chronic bronchitis as a result of habitual cigarette smoking, *post-operative complications* occur frequently. Such complications naturally lengthen convalescence and sabotage the main aims of post-operative care. These aims are:

(1) To produce a stump which is well-healed, strong and mobile, and of good shape, size and position for prosthetic bearing.

(2) To conserve and improve the strength and circulation of the contralateral leg and the strength of the trunk and upper limbs.

(3) To promote the general health of the patient and encourage his early remobilization.

Of these aims, early mobilization is vitally important in preventing the development of many post-operative complications, and it is essential to get geriatric amputees out of bed and into wheelchairs as early as the second post-operative day, whenever possible.

In all patients the presence of locomotor disease of the upper limbs, trunk or contralateral leg; of special sense defects; of circulatory insufficiency, whether cerebral, cardiac or peripheral; or of severe or uncontrolled diabetes will contribute towards the development of complications since they severely reduce the body's ability to adjust to the loss of one part by the compensatory action of its remaining parts.

Post-operative care and complications may be conveniently considered under: (1) stump; (2) contralateral leg; (3) circulatory system; (4) respiratory system; and (5) other.

Stump care

Until it is possible to assist stump shape and size by prosthetic walking, when muscle action and the support of a rigid socket combine to assist in the dispersal of oedema, the condition of the stump may be considerably influenced by exercise, position and external support. The performance of regular exercises and of regular periods of prone lying are supervised by the physiotherapist and the nursing staff who are also responsible for dressing and bandaging the stump if the surgeon so orders.

There are two schools of thought about stump bandaging. One advocates it and one forbids it. Certainly, firm bandaging by an experienced nurse or physiotherapist can reduce oedema and promote a good stump shape. But the view is becoming increasingly widely held that any bandaging of a stump of an elderly patient with vascular insufficiency is likely to contribute to, if not actually cause, delayed healing of the amputation wound. The decision to bandage or not to bandage lies with the amputating surgeon. Bandaging, when the bandage is wound round and round the stump and constricts the circulation, can produce severe stump deformity. Dumb-bell-shaped stumps, or stumps with a large pendulous mass of oedematous subcutaneous tissue hanging from them are frequently caused by constrictive, incorrect bandaging. *If bandaging is used,* two 6 in (15 cm) bandages should be used for above-knee stumps and one or two 4 in (10 cm) bandages for stumps which are below-knee. The bandaging must be taken above the joint proximal to the amputation level—therefore, around the waist for an above-knee amputation and around the thigh for a below-knee stump—and should be in oblique turns and figures of eight, not in circles. There are several different makes of stretch bandages available which are equally effective. If *bandaging is not used*, tubi grip attached by tapes to an elasticated waistband, or cotton net tubing similarly attached, are alternative methods of anchoring the dressing in place. Strips of adhesive plaster of any kind should never be used for this purpose, as allergic skin reactions and even ulceration result from their use in a high proportion of patients. Micropore tape is a permisible form of dressing retainer and apparently is unlikely to produce any skin irritation.

Stump complications

The two most frequently occurring complications in amputation stumps are delayed healing and flexion contractures.

Delayed healing

This may follow: (1) ischaemia; (2) operative or post-operative haematoma; (3) infection.

Ischaemia In the absence of infection and haematoma, failure to heal may be due to an inadequate blood supply. Depending on the age and condition of any one patient, it may be decided to re-amputate at a higher level or to accept a longer convalescence and healing by slow granulation.

Haematoma This may follow inadequate haemostasis at operation or trauma to the stump post-operatively. Very large haematomata may need aspiration or evacuation; smaller ones resolve with firm bandaging and exercise.

Infection Should infection of the amputation wound occur, systemic antibiotics and appropriate local treatment such as eusol or saline, with or without removal of undissolved stitches from stitch abscesses, may be sufficient to bring about healing. Persistent stump infection after adequate exhibition of antibiotics controlled by laboratory sensitivity tests will call for x-ray examination of the stump. Should necrotic bone be revealed, operative removal of the sequestrum is essential for healing, possibly followed by reamputation at a higher level.

Flexion contractures

The three chief factors contributing to the development of flexion contractures in the joint or joints proximal to the amputation level are: (1) pain; (2) spasm; (3) immobility and bad posture (in bed or chair).

Pain This can be very severe after amputation, both in the amputation stump and in the phantom limb. A well-constructed stump, fashioned by myoplastic or osteomyoplastic technique, with a clean, well-positioned scar, does much to prevent the development of both stump and phantom pain, but ischaemia, infection, haematomata or neuromata may nevertheless cause localized pain and tenderness in the stump. The experience of severe pre-operative pain, whether from trauma or ischaemia, may predispose to the development of post-operative phantom pain, to which one or more of the causes of stump tenderness may further contribute. Control of both types of pain may be difficult. Elimination of contributory causes must be combined with prescription of adequate analgesics, together with suitable anti-depressants.

Spasm Without analgesia and appropriate stump care, persistent pain in an amputation stump can cause spasm of the muscles flexing the joint or joints proximal to the amputation. If this persists, a flexion contracture can rapidly develop. A firm mattress, prone lying and extension exercises will be powerless to prevent such contractures unless local causes of pain are eliminated.

Repeated application of a mechanical vibrator to trigger points of local tenderness is sometimes effective in relieving stump and phantom pain. So too, is injection of these points with local anaesthetic. Occasionally, further operation is needed if intractable pain arises from adherence of the amputation scar to nerve or bony tissue.

Immobility Prolonged rest in bed or chair, post-operatively, without frequent changes of position and without exercise sessions, also tends to cause flexion contractures. Resting an above-knee stump on a pillow in bed, or hanging a below-knee stump over the seat-edge while sitting in a geriatric chair or wheelchair, are further encouragements to their development. As has been already stated, it is advised that a below-knee stump is supported on a foam-padded board with sheepskin cover, projecting from beneath the seat cushion, unless the prosthesis is being worn.

Contralateral leg

Care of the contralateral leg is a continuation of the pre-operative treatment already described. The three complications most often found in the contralateral leg are: (1) ulceration of the heel and/or malleoli; (2) oedema; (3) deep-vein thrombosis.

Ulceration

If inadequate prophylactic care is taken and ulceration develops, it should be treated quickly and adequately to prevent secondary infection. Appropriate local applications such as Aserbine lotion or gentian violet 1 per cent in aqueous solution, must be combined with: (1) removal of pressure from the ulceration area; (2) prevention of oedema.

Should secondary infection occur, administration of an antibiotic is indicated. If the infection becomes chronic, x-ray examination of the ulcerated area will exclude the presence of underlying osteomyelitis. Sometimes a lumbar sympathectomy may be indicated, to improve the blood supply to the skin of the ulcerated leg and to promote healing of a painful and indolent ulcer.

Oedema

The most frequent cause of oedema in the contralateral leg and foot of a geriatric amputee is the increased venous and lymphatic pressure which builds up when a patient sits for long periods with his leg dependent and inactive, and there is no muscle pump to assist lymphatic and venous return. Oedema of such origin may be treated by encouraging frequent short spells of walking, using a walking aid or crutches, even before a pylon or early walking aid is issued. Static contractions of the calf and foot muscles, while the patient is seated and wearing tubigrip or an elastic stocking, are also helpful.

Walking practice is not contra-indicated even in the presence of ulceration of the leg or foot, as long as it is not painful and does not exacerbate the condition of the ulcer. It is probable that early walking decreases the likelihood of such ulceration even occurring, and in its occurrence, promotes healing by improving both blood supply and tissue drainage of the surrounding tissues.

Oedema may, of course, be due to a deep-vein thrombosis which must always be excluded by appropriate physical, radiological or echo-scanning examination. General physical examination of each patient enables cardiac failure to be detected, and with specific pathological investigations, permits the exclusion of other causes.

Deep-vein thrombosis (D.V.T.)

Since it has been realized that D.V.T. in the calf frequently occurs during operation and the immediate post-operative recovery period, measures to combat thrombosis prophylactically are being urgently sought. Intravenous Dextran during and after operation is sometimes given for this purpose. The use of a sheepskin under the contralateral leg or of a ripple or polystyrene granule cushion and even movement of the leg mechanically or electrically stimulated while the patient is actually on the operating table and in the recovery room are other forms of possible preventative measures which have yet to be fully explored.

The use of a full sheepskin to lie on in his ward bed, and early mobilization of the patient, with frequent periods of exercise while in bed and chair, together with attendances in the gymnasium as soon as his condition allows, are vitally important in the prevention of D.V.T. for the elderly amputee. If thrombosis does occur, early detection by regular daily inspection of the contralateral leg, visually and by echo-scanner, gives the best hope of effective treatment.

Cardiovascular and respiratory post-operative complications

Elderly patients who have lower limb amputation may have had a previous hemiplegia or become hemiplegic during the post-operative period, and consequently rehabilitation is considerably prolonged and complicated by the residual weakness and spasticity and the possible accompanying sensory and intellectual deficit.

Cardiac infarction may also occur post-operatively, and pulmonary embolism, depending upon the degree and location of the pathological changes in the circulatory system. Anticoagulant therapy is used at the discretion of the supervising surgeon, who must take into consideration the age and general condition of the patient and the severity of the vascular accident. The usual respiratory complications which may follow any operation are increasingly likely to follow lower limb amputation in elderly patients because of their age and the fact that over 70 per cent of them are chronic, regular cigarette smokers. Thus collapsed lobes and bronchopneumonia may complicate the chronic bronchitis from which so many are already suffering pre-operatively and make rehabilitation longer and more difficult.

Diabetes and pre-diabetes

Frequently diabetes is not detected until the patient is admitted to hospital with gangrene or pregangrenous ischaemia of the leg, and there is little time for stabilization of his diabetes before amputation.

Alternatively, many patients spend some weeks undergoing conservative treatment for their peripheral ischaemia before amputation becomes inevitable. During this time they may require increasing amounts of hypoglycaemic agents, and some will require variable-dose insulin regimes. Control of the diabetes can necessitate increased quantities of hypoglycaemic agents until the amputation wound is healed.

Not only is the diabetes in a state of imbalance when the patient presents for limb-fitting and walking training, but also his activity level is changing and thus contributing further to the imbalance. Attendance at a rehabilitation unit or limb-fitting centre often involves an early ambulance trip, and although the patient usually receives his hypoglycaemics, he often fails to partake of an adequate breakfast.

Even in a residential rehabilitation unit, a patient often neglects to eat the full, balanced breakfast provided. The therapists concerned with diabetic amputees must learn to recognize the apparent confusion and lack of co-operation which may accompany the early stages of hypoglycaemia and have glucose tablets and appropriate drinks available in the gymnasium.

DIFFICULTIES DURING WALKING TRAINING

Six main factors have a powerful influence upon the outcome of limb-fitting and walking training: (1) state of the amputation stump; (2) condition of the contralateral leg; (3) general condition of the patient; (4) mental condition of the patient; (5) efficiency of the special senses; (6) home situation of the patient.

State of the amputation stump

Size

A short stump provides insufficient leverage to drive a prosthesis and tends to slip out of the socket. Fat or flabby stumps develop rolls or creases when inserted into prosthetic sockets, with resulting excoriation or discomfort. Thin stumps are more prone to develop pressure areas.

Stumps fluctuate in size from day to day, and an unused stump quickly becomes oedematous. Regular, frequent exercises and firm bandaging will help to preserve a stump's good shape if prosthetic wearing has to be abandoned for a time.

When prosthetic walking has been started almost all stumps shrink rapidly during the first few days of training, and it is necessary to add extra stump socks to ensure a good fit between stump and socket. If excessive shrinkage occurs, the inside measurements of the socket of the pylon may have to be reduced by lining and reshaping. If an early walking aid is being used the corset is merely pulled tighter.

Patients are supplied with a nylon undersock and woollen oversocks with their prosthesis and are taught how to adjust the fit of the socket by adding or discarding one or more socks. When three socks have been used, and the fit of a pylon socket is still not right, the socket needs structural alteration. Occasionally, the stump increases in size—either with brawny oedema or with extra muscle bulk—to such an extent that the pylon socket must be enlarged or even remade. The corset top of the early walking aid accommodates considerable stump expansion without needing structural alteration.

Position

It is possible to compensate for small flexion contractures in the stump by adjusting the angle or contour of the socket relative to the longitudinal axis of the prosthesis. In the case of a below-knee prosthesis such contractures can be accommodated in an increased anteroposterior diameter of the prosthetic calf. Larger contractures may entail the use of a 'kneeling' prosthesis, when the patient actually kneels on a weight-bearing pad. Flexion contracture of the hip increases the forward inclination of the trunk in the upright position and may affect the balance to such a degree that walking becomes impossible.

Strength

A debilitated patient, or a patient with an ipsilateral hemiparesis may have a weak stump and find it difficult to move a prosthesis, to control it, and to prevent it abducting.

Tenderness

Ischaemia, infection, haematoma, delayed healing, neuroma and adherent scar tissue may severally make a stump so tender that the presence of a prosthesis cannot be tolerated.

Condition of the contralateral leg

The health and strength of the contralateral leg is all important in limb-fitting and in walking training. Intermittent claudication in the contralateral leg may limit the duration and rate of walking. Measures for its earlier care have already been described and cannot be relaxed if the circulation to the foot is poor. Wherever possible damage to the skin of the foot must be avoided, not only by preventing heel and malleolar ulceration but also by avoiding infection from paronychia or blistered toes. Regular, careful chiropody for amputees and scrupulous cleansing of the feet is helpful; so too is the continued use of roomy, comfortable shoes, or of the felt boot previously described.

In maintaining the optimal condition of the contralateral leg, the avoidance of further cigarette smoking seems an obvious measure, which is seldom implemented. Recent surveys and research continue to incriminate smoking increasingly as a cause of peripheral vascular disease, and yet in the United Kingdom there is no deliberate campaign to deter single amputees from the habit.

When ulceration of the contralateral leg does occur, the presence of heel or malleolar pressure ulcers is not a contra-indication to continuing walking practice. Indeed, short periods of walking seem beneficial, if coupled with energetic measures to treat the ulcers. Paronychia or ulceration of the toes however need instant and careful treatment with the leg elevated, and walking training must be discontinued until healing has occurred.

General condition of the patient

Although any disability or illness must have an adverse effect on an amputee's efforts to learn to use his prosthesis, some conditions are particularly likely to prejudice his chance of success.

Cardiovascular disease

Many geriatric amputees have a considerably diminished cardiac efficiency. This may show itself by early fatigue on exercise, anginal pain, or the development of frank cardiac failure. Often a review of their medication may enable some change to be made which will improve their performance, e.g. digitalization, the addition of potassium supplements if diuretics are being taken, taking prophylactic coronary vasodilators before exercise. If it becomes obvious that despite such measures a patient is becoming consistently exhausted or distressed, then walking training should be stopped and a wheelchair life advocated.

Cerebral circulatory deficiency may manifest itself by drop attacks, hemiplegia, confusion or intellectual deterioration, and according to the severity of the defect, may make walking training difficult or impossible. Drop attacks are an absolute bar to prosthetic walking since the dangers of fracturing the stump or contralateral leg during a fall are so high.

Hemiplegia makes it difficult to hold crutches or a walking aid, and whether it is the contralateral leg or the stump which is affected, prosthetic walking becomes doubly difficult. The confusion caused by a poor cerebral circulation is usually associated with a poor memory for recent events, and in an otherwise physically competent patient, may make it impossible for instructions to be remembered from hour to hour. Walking training in such a patient has to be abandoned.

Respiratory disease

Although a high proportion of elderly amputees have coughs, their chronic bronchitis is seldom the factor which limits their walking training. However asthma, if it is controlled by steroids given in sufficient doses to cause fluid storage and weight gain, can be a very real impediment. Attempts to reduce the weight of the patient and the size of his stump by reducing the steroid intake may well precipitate asthmatic attacks and have to be abandoned.

Urinogenital system

Elderly male patients frequently have enlarged prostates and elderly female patients are often plagued with cystocoeles and uterine prolapse. Both tend to suffer from mild urinary incontinence, either by stress or leaking, and to become damp. Dampness leads to excoriation and ulceration of the thighs and buttocks by friction with the prosthetic socket. Prostatectomy, either shortly before or after an operation of a lower limb, is not infrequently a necessary procedure for men, while occasionally a pelvic floor repair is undertaken for women. It is essential to keep a patient dry, and if operation is contra-indicated, then the use of a condom and portable urinal type of incontinence device or an indwelling catheter is indicated for the male, and an indwelling catheter for the female.

Locomotor system

Patients with stiff, painful joints in the hands, arms, spine or contralateral lower limb may find it difficult or impossible to learn to use a prosthesis. If the pain is so severe as to prevent weight-bearing on the contralateral leg or to prevent the assistance of weight-bearing by gripping parallel bars, crutches or other walking aids, then walking training must be abandoned. This decision is particularly important in patients with rheumatoid arthritis when it is vital to preserve hand function, and patients should be actively discouraged from compensating for defective lower limb function by overuse of their upper limbs. For some of these patients, it is far more realistic to supply a powered wheelchair than a prosthesis, and this course of action should always be considered in patients for whom prosthetic walking can only be achieved with the expenditure of much painful effort of the upper limbs.

Speech defects

Aphasia and dysphasia may occur after accidents involving head injury, with trauma to the lower limb leading to amputation. They may also occur with hemiplegia following a cerebrovascular accident.

When a patient comprehends the spoken word but cannot express himself in speech, he may still be taught to walk with a prosthesis. He may find it difficult to do so, because he cannot ask questions or express his opinion, but his learning power is unimpeded. If his dysphasia or aphasia is one of comprehension, it is unlikely that he will be capable of mastering prosthetic walking.

Mental condition of the patient

Apart from the diminished intellectual capacity of the geriatric amputee with cerebral insufficiency, the presence of depression, apprehension, and confusion further mitigate against successful prosthetic training and usage.

Depression

Many lower limb amputees suffer from a reactive exogenous depression. Adequate pre-operative and post-operative discussions and explanation can do much to prepare a patient to accept amputation. A visit from an amputee who is managing to live an active prosthetic life should be contrived whenever possible. A wheelchair and a prosthesis awaiting a patient at his bedside can give him a sense of continuous process of organization directed towards his eventual independence and mobility and can provide a potent counteractive force to the development of depression. Nevertheless, if depression does develop, and it may manifest itself as undue apprehension or lack of co-operation, as well as the withdrawal from society and mood lability more commonly associated with its presence, then it must be treated rapidly and effectively.

Confusion

Many amputees are confused both pre-operatively and post-operatively, but as they recover from the combined effects of toxic absorption from an ischaemic limb, removal to strange surroundings and the hypoxia of a general anaesthetic, this confusion usually abates. Intermittent confusion, especially during the morning walking training session may herald hypoglycaemia. Persistent confusion may stem from cerebral ischaemia due to arteriosclerosis, or it may indicate a rising blood urea. It is important that all concerned with the patient's management report the presence of any confusion so that, whenever possible, its cause may be identified and treated.

Efficiency of the special senses

Visual defects

Blind people have difficulties of balance and posture. They cannot check the 'sit' of their limb visually. It is harder to put the limbs on and off and harder to monitor their possible rotation. If blind amputees use guide dogs or tapping sticks, then they cannot carry objects from place to place unless they can dispense with crutch or walking sticks. Walking with a guide dog is harder too, when the guided person is an amputee of uncertain balance.

Hearing defects

Deaf patients often do not hear instructions clearly or correctly but do not like to draw attention to their deafness by saying so. Nor can they hear the click when their pylon is locked for standing. It is well worth establishing the particular range of sounds which a deaf person can still hear, so that the voices of those who instruct him can be pitched accordingly.

Sensory loss

Associated with hemiplegia which frequently precedes or follows lower limb amputation, there may be a sensory loss involving the hemiplegic side. The patient may refuse to recognize the limb as part of him, and it is difficult to teach a man to wear a prosthesis, or to move so as to compensate for a prosthesis (depending on whether the hemiplegia is ipsilateral or contralateral to the amputated limb), when he considers the limb in question as an extraneous object.

Peripheral nerve lesions

Peripheral nerve lesions such as peripheral neuritis or diabetes may cause sensory loss and therefore lead to an increased likelihood of trauma to the insensitive part. Loss of sensation in the contralateral limb or stump itself predisposes to ulceration. These complications are much more likely to occur in a geriatric patient with amputation for peripheral vascular insufficiency than in a younger patient.

Home situation of the patient

Domestic resettlement of elderly patients is a problem for all who have to care for them. The geriatric services are usually well organized, with progressive care through the hospital wards, rehabilitation wards and day hospitals. Furthermore, they have a system of liaison between the social services and the hospital departments which is geared to smoothing the transition from hospital care to domestic independence or into appropriate residential care. For the elderly amputee it is often necessary to mobilize the full services of the geriatric rehabilitation programme, but often the patients are not transferred from acute surgical wards to the geriatric services, or the geriatric social workers are not integrated into the acute ward care.

Frequently the social and domestic situation has a direct bearing on the elderly amputee's response to rehabilitation. A patient with little will to get better does not learn to use his prosthesis quickly. If he is not wanted at home by his spouse or relations; if he is wanted by them but they do not have suitable accommodation for him; if they are too frail to cope with his care; or if he faces a life of loneliness—living alone and disabled—then he does not hurry to become so proficient that he must return to such a situation.

Thus it is essential that immediate liaison is established between those who deal with the rehabilitative treatment of the geriatric amputee and relatives, general practitioners and members of the social services, concerned with his further care after leaving hospital.

As soon as possible post-operatively the medical social worker at the hospital should investigate the domestic situation and obtain the clearest possible picture of the layout and dimensions of the patient's home, together with an accurate idea of available family help. Such information is essential if realistic assessment of a patient's capability to return home is to be made. Often minor adjustments, such as grab rails in the lavatory and bathroom and an extra banister rail at the stairs, and a ramp to allow entrance and egress from the front or the back door, will be sufficient to make it possible for a geriatric amputee to be able to live independently at home. Sometimes however inconveniently sited lavatories, lack of downstairs sleeping accommodation or insufficient floor space will necessitate rehousing in a disabled person's bungalow or downstairs flat, or even admission to Part III accommodation.

Whether a geriatric patient is cared for by an elderly spouse or a young family, amputation is often considered to increase his disability beyond the capabilities of whose who care for him. The provision of adequate home help and regular visits from his local social worker or health visitor will do much to ease the home situation. Too frequently the elderly amputee languishes in the acute ward of a busy hospital, occupying a bed which is needed for other acute surgical problems, and yet not obtaining the active rehabilitation programme he requires because his home is considered unsuitable and there is nowhere else to send him. The problems are usually not primarily medical, but social and administrative. With planning and collaboration between hospital and social services, many of those patients can be helped to continue living with some independence and dignity.

The elderly amputee is often well past retiring age and has lost much of the social support provided by work and family. Without regular follow-up by the health visitor or social worker, he may easily slip from the knife-edge of functional competence to which post-operative prosthetic and independence training has restored him. At best, the life of the elderly amputee is limited in scope and in duration. At worst, it degenerates into a miserable, lonely, handicapped existence. The use of public transport is rendered virtually impossible, and even the use of the footpath on wet and frosty days is extremely hazardous. For some of the more active amputees, a powered tricycle may provide some independence, and visits to day hospitals or occupational therapy centres will help to lessen the tedium for those who are unable to transport themselves from place to place.

Measures which are urgently needed to make the rehabilitation of geriatric amputees a realistic adjustment to active amputee life instead of an unpleasant phase in progressive disability, are:

The universal availability of a lightweight, easily fitted, easily adjustable early walking appliance.

The institution of earlier prosthetic fitting and earlier walking.

The elimination of the customary waiting period without any prosthesis while a conventional pylon is being made.

The adoption of either routine admission to special units for limb-fitting and walking training if the early walking appliance is not locally available, or of in-patient training in the parent hospital if it is.

The routine supply of a suitable wheelchair in the immediate post-amputation period.

The institution of a regular social follow-up to supplement the prosthetic and surgical follow up.

PROSTHETIC TRAINING

Pylons

Until recently, all amputees have followed the routine established for service personnel in the last war. At about 2 weeks post-operatively but often after a much longer interval, depending upon their general condition and on the state of the stump, they are referred to the Artificial Limb and Appliance Centre for their region. This referral is either made by a telephoned request for an appointment or else by an official form of referral (AOF3) despatched through the post (the latter procedure can delay limb-fitting by as much as a week). Unless severe oedema of the stump, whether from infection, haematoma or other reason, has prevented measurement, the stump is measured for the manufacture of the preliminary rocker pylon during the first attendance of the patient at the A.L.A.C. Very occasionally, if the peripheral circulation of the contralateral leg is very poor, measurement for the pylon is withheld until the fate of the other leg has become apparent. After measurement, patients usually return to their parent hospitals or to convalescent wards in those hospitals; to convalescent homes; or even to their own homes to await the arrival of the pylon.

About 2 weeks after their first attendance at the A.L.A.C., patients are recalled for a fitting, and after adjustment and riveting the pylons are delivered. If however there has been a great alteration in the size of the stump due to shrinkage or to the development of oedema, a pylon may be retained for a further 1–2 weeks for further alteration and possibly for the supply of a new metal socket. This rigid metal socket is therefore a potential disadvantage in the structure of the pylon because it is only capable of a moderate degree of alteration in diameter before riveting, and none afterwards, except by lining. At best, it usually takes 4–6 weeks after amputation before the pylon is delivered. At worst, it may take up to 6 months while the patient waits at home or in hospital without a prosthesis and often without even a wheelchair or walking aid.

Out-patient walking training has proved far from satisfactory. Patients, who are often diabetics, are brought long distances by ambulance after an early start and possibly a missed or scanty breakfast. There is often insufficient time to have the repeated short sessions of walking practice and exercise, interspersed with long rests, which are best suited to the physical condition of the average geriatric amputee; insufficient time to sort out the deficiencies of the pylon; insufficient time to make a reliable assessment of what any one patient's prosthetic capabilities under favourable conditions could really be; insufficient time to restore a patient to his maximal mobility or to discover and solve his problems of daily living.

Walking training for elderly amputees is best conducted on an in-patient basis, but few hospitals at present have sufficient beds at their disposal to enable them to admit geriatric amputees for the 5–6 weeks needed to complete their rehabilitation under the present arrangements for the provision of a prosthesis.

Early walking aids

There is an almost universal trend towards the use of a modular assembly technique for both definitive artificial legs and for early walking devices. This concept enables the prosthetist to assemble the appliance from standard component parts, which he marries to the socket which is specifically constructed for each patient. The initial modular prosthesis, or early walking aid, is very simple and may be assembled in a few hours by a prosthetist in the A.L.A.C. or by a physiotherapist in the physiotherapy department of a District General Hospital. It consists of a corset-type socket for the thigh made of plastic, leather or fibreglass, and sometimes lined with plastic foam; steel struts strengthen this socket, hinge at the knee and lead to a moulded shin-piece or foot. The limb is attached to a waist-band either by a single-hinged bar, or else by anterior and posterior suspensory straps. Pop-rivets attach the struts to the corset, which may be rolled to be partially ischial bearing. The foot is of the Sacke variety.

The advantages of such a prosthesis are:

(1) It is very light (about 4 lb or 1·8 kg) compared to the 7 lb (3·2 kg) of the rocker pylon and easier to put on and take off.

(2) Its corset top accommodates minor fluctuations of stump size and obviates the need to thrust through a rigid metal cylinder.

(3) Patients like the appearance of the foot and ankle and seem to find it no harder to walk on the prosthetic foot than on a rocker.

(4) If pre-operative measurements are taken the early walking aid can be ready at the patient's bed by the time of his recovery from the anaesthetic, to provide a great boost for his morale.

(5) Patients show less tendency to develop deep-vein thrombosis or pressure areas on the contralateral foot if they are walking a few days post-operatively.

(6) Each patient can *walk* bipedally, using the early walking aid from as early as 2 days post-operatively, depending on the wishes of the individual surgeon for the individual patient.

(7) A patient has his walking training at the same hospital as his amputation, and this provides a valuable feedback of information on the efficiency of any particular operative procedure to the surgeons concerned as well as a continuity of management which is beneficial to patients and staff.

(8) There is less chance of developing a flexion contracture at the joint proximal to amputation level if early walking is achieved.

(9) Patients who are ambulant are more easily able to attend physiotherapy and occupational therapy departments to give extra time to learning transfers and practising other daily living activities.

(10) Fitting the early walking aid does not add time to the patient's post-operative convalescence. In fact he often goes home earlier when he has walked a few days post-operatively with this appliance. Not only is he walking, but he is more competent to cope with domestic life because he does not have to hop behind a walking frame or stay confined in a wheelchair.

(11) The production of each prosthesis is an individual affair, in which the physiotherapist is with the patient at every stage of the proceedings, and the patient's every need can be considered.

Such devices however can only be regarded as short-term temporary aids to early walking and are no substitute for definitive artificial legs. Indeed, as newer techniques of manufacture and fitting of artificial legs become available, it may be that simpler aids become redundant because more effective, permanent, devices can be produced equally quickly.

Whenever possible, the first stages of walking training after lower limb amputation should be carried out with the amputee as an in-patient, in circumstances where the prosthetist and physiotherapist can collaborate. Walking training with a prosthesis will vary in detail depending on whether the rocker pylon, a modular assembly prosthesis or an early walking aid is used, but the essentials are the same.

(1) The patient is shown how to put on and then take off his prosthesis unaided.

(2) Initially, he is taught to get to his feet from a sitting position in either a chair or wheelchair placed between the parallel bars, emphasis being placed on the need to lock the knee of the prosthesis by striking the heel on the ground before a stable stance may be obtained.

(3) He then practises sitting down in the chair after unlocking the knee mechanism, while weight is taken on the contralateral leg.

(4) Increasing periods of standing between parallel bars are practised to improve balance. These culminate in gradually lengthening intervals of walking between the parallel bars.

(5) From parallel bars, patients progress to walking frame, elbow crutch walking and then to quadrupeds or sticks.

(6) Having mastered walking on a flat, smooth surface, the patient practises walking on carpet, rough ground and steps, together with getting in and out of a car, in and out of bed, and on and off the toilet.

(7) Joint sessions with physiotherapists and occupational therapists enable problems in daily living, such as dressing and undressing and personal care, and the management of domestic activities, to be rehearsed.

(8) When discomfort is experienced, the pylon or walking aid is carefully adjusted either by the limb-fitter or the physiotherapist.

(9) Regular periods of plinth-lying in the prone position are interspersed with exercise periods. In particular, a rest in the prone position after lunch each day is advised.

(10) Exercise periods are kept short and usually accompanied by music.

(11) The patient is encouraged to contract his thigh muscles with each step forwards of the prosthetic limb so that he actively participates in the prosthetic locomotion and is not merely a passenger of his artificial leg.

(12) He is taught to take short steps of equal length and to 'walk tall'.

(13) If his surgeon requests, he is instructed in stump bandaging.

BIBLIOGRAPHY AND REFERENCES

Chilvers, A. S. and Browse, N. L. (1971). 'The social fate of the amputee.' *Lancet* **2**, 1192

Clippinger, F. W. (1963). 'Use of temporary quadrilateral socket plaster pylon in the elderly amputee.' *Sth. med. J.* **56**, 588–92

Clippinger, F. W. (1965). 'Treatment of elderly amputee by temporary quadrilateral socket pylon prosthesis.' *Geriatrics* **20**, 683–7

Devas, M. B. (1971). 'Early walking of geriatric amputees.' *Br. med. J.* **1**, 394

Hamilton, E. A. and Nichols, P. J. R. (1972). 'Rehabilitation of the elderly amputee.' *Br. med. J.* **2**, 95

McKenzie, D. S. (1961). 'Prosthetic rehabilitation of aged in Great Britain.' In *Conference on Geriatric Amputees*. Washington; National Academy of Sciences, National Research Committee

Report of Committee on Prosthetic and Orthotic Services (1973). London; British Orthopaedic Association

Thompson, A. (1971). 'An early walking aid for geriatric amputees.' *Physiotherapy* **57**, 583

12—Rehabilitation after a Heart Attack

There is a high prevalence of coronary heart disease in the more developed countries; it has been estimated that 1 man in 5 in Great Britain is likely to have symptoms of coronary disease by the age of 65, and the incidence is increasing, especially in middle-aged and younger men. A reversal of attitudes to the treatment and long-term effects of heart disease has occurred in the last decade, which has resulted in more attention being given to rehabilitation of these patients.

The increasing frequency of myocardial infarction has led to the application of certain techniques already applied to the chronic, neuromuscular diseases. The World Health Organization has emphasized the complexity of cardiac rehabilitation, in their definition: 'the sum of activities required to ensure the best possible physical, mental and social conditions, so that patients may, by their own efforts, regain as normal as possible a place in the community and lead an active productive life'. Much cardiac rehabilitation is an extension of conventional clinical practice, and only in some late problem patients does it involve the special government-based rehabilitation centres.

A joint working-party of the Royal College of Physicians and the British Cardiac Society has now given guidelines for cardiac rehabilitation and also comments on the present position in Britain. It feels that insufficient attention is given to the psychological and social aspects of the illness and to the consequences for future employment; it points out that few hospitals have a rehabilitation service. Although there have been many recent advances in the management of patients with myocardial infarction, these have not always been paralleled by improvements in aftercare. Despite early mobilization in hospital a distressing number of postinfarction patients can be found leading a life of chronic invalidism not justified by their cardiac status. Whilst the overall requirement for supervised physical training remains uncertain, some cardiac patients undoubtedly need help of some kind, although much can be achieved by sensible counselling of patient and relatives.

The working-party emphasizes that cardiologists have tended to disagree on the need for rehabilitation, its value and the best means of achieving it. However, it concludes that cardiac rehabilitation is important, that conventional medical treatment is often insufficient to ensure a full active life, and that convalescence is often unduly prolonged because of ignorance and anxiety. The team feels that those that care for patients with heart attacks should have rehabilitation in mind from the beginning. It points out that further work and research are required and that the logistic problems are not small as the implementation of complex programmes will require more funds and personnel than are at present available.

The present team approach should be contrasted against the negative attitudes of the past, when it was believed that after a myocardial infarction a patient was not fit for any work involving any degree of physical or mental strain. In order to reduce the patient's insecurity or prevent its development, good coordination of the team is required but of greatest importance is good communication with the patient. The family doctor still has the key position of ensuring continuity.

The rehabilitation programme for the cardiac patient is an essential part of management and in most uncomplicated patients it is the only treatment one can offer. Myocardial damage does not usually impose long-term limitations to the physical capacity of the individual and the majority of patients are able to return to their previous work with little or no change in their routine. However, it is important to realize that each patient responds differently to the stress of a severe illness, which cuts abruptly across every aspect of his life, and it is the skill with which the rehabilitation programme is adapted to the patient's individual needs that will have far-reaching consequences, as this can profoundly affect the speed and completeness of recovery.

With increasing attention being paid to the acute coronary episode there is increasing likelihood that time is not spent in planning the long-term care of patients; the long-term aims are, of course, that the patient is restored to a useful and happy life within the limits of his physical capacity. The extent of rehabilitation depends on the individual's reaction to it; above all the patient should understand that the risk of succumbing to a heart attack is not much greater for him than for others of his own age group. Anxiety and depression about the initial illness are replaced by anxiety about future employment and finance. It is important in discussing the implications of the illness that the patient be allowed freedom to express his feelings on such diverse subjects as diet, leisure activities, change of employment and retirement.

Much anxiety and avoidable invalidism is due to the patient's ignorance of the disease in general and of his own state of health in particular. A careful, sympathetic and unhurried discussion with the patient and close family about the nature and implications of the illness is one of the first and most valuable aspects of rehabilitation and this should be carried out as soon as the clinical state allows. Further advice should be given as required; in this the nurse plays a most important role in the early stages of recovery by providing knowledge, support and encouragement. Simple factual information about the possible consequences of infarction is useful, not only in relieving anxiety, but also for its sedative and analgesic effect, as stress increases heart rate and blood pressure. The wife should be reassured before she reaches her husband's bedside, so that she does not transfer her own anxiety.

It is important not only to treat the physical symptoms, but also to pay attention to the psychological and social aspects of the individual, for the ultimate purpose of rehabilitation calls for a gradual withdrawal of help as self-confidence in both patient and spouse improve. This is a continuing process and the division of care into phases such as acute, convalescent and rehabilitative is not realistic. In fact, the lack of continuity in guidance of the patient throughout the whole rehabilitation period is a definite disadvantage.

Despite the increasing emphasis on early mobilization, many patients are not subsequently followed up after discharge from hospital and there is evidence that the family doctor and friends are over-cautious in their attitude to subsequent rehabilitation and return to work. Anxiety and depression are common in both patient and spouse following infarction and the psychological advantage of early mobilization in hospital will be lost if convalescence is prolonged. It has been suggested that there is increasing lack of self-confidence and an increasing chance of permanent unemployment if the patient is away from work more than 10 weeks. Any general discussion of rehabilitation is complicated by the variety of disability encountered. Differences in age, physique and personality, or in the kind of work to which the patient will return, all have to be taken into account.

HOSPITAL CARE

Physicians have always been very cautious in their management of patients with myocardial infarction but attitudes have become more dynamic. At one time 6 weeks' absolute bed rest was advised, for it was known that this was the time required for conversion of necrotic myocardium into scar tissue and it was suggested that exercise would increase the stress on the heart and would aggravate the risks of tissue hypoxia, leading to consequent arrhythmias and cardiac rupture. In the last decade there has been a progressive tendency towards earlier ambulation and return to work, due to the realization of the dangers of excessive bed rest and the discovery that the heart has remarkable recuperative powers. Apart from the psychological advantage of early mobilization there is less risk of thrombo-embolism, muscular wasting and loss of physical performance. Bed rest leads to a loss of normal postural vasomotor reflexes, so that the systolic blood pressure may fall by as much as 50 mmHg on standing. Recent studies have shown that early mobilization after 1 week is not detrimental and there is no increase in the incidence of heart failure, cardiac rupture or aneurysm formation. It is now common practice for patients suffering from an uncomplicated myocardial infarction to be walking after 1 week of bed rest and it may be that even this is too long. During this week bed rest need not be total except for patients in severe pain, in shock or with heart failure or severe arrhythmias. Leg exercises should be carried out daily and the patient can be allowed up for a commode as the physical efforts of defaecation are less on a commode than on a bed. Patients free from hypotension and chest pain can be nursed sitting out of bed from the second hospital day onwards. Those with a small uncomplicated infarct can increase their activity during the second week: they can sit up for increasing time, walk in the ward and bath themselves. If their progress is uneventful, patients are discharged inside 2 weeks, although there are still variations in duration of stay from one hospital to another. During the first few days both physiotherapists and nurses play an important part in ensuring that patients carry out active limb movements to a scheme that has been broadly indicated by the physician in charge.

DISCHARGE FROM HOSPITAL

Despite the increasing emphasis on early mobilization many patients are not given sufficient advice whilst in hospital. It is not sufficient to give vague advice such as 'take it easy for a while', or 'avoid excitement', both of which serve only to increase natural anxiety. Anxious doctors have anxious patients. Whenever possible, both the patient and spouse should be given exact guidelines; a heart attack is an extremely traumatic experience and patients are anxious and depressed, needing reassurance and clear advice. It is important that the spouse is present as there is often descrepancy between the physician's advice and what the spouse will permit. It is important that they are both told that a return to normal life is usual. It is also important that the convalescent phase not be prolonged, as patients become bored and worry about their ability to support their family.

During the first few weeks at home there is need for both physical and mental rest. The holiday atmosphere provides psychological benefit and graduated exercises result in improvement in exercise tolerance and an improvement in muscular weakness which has resulted from inactivity. Walking is the best form of exercise at this stage, but at first it is advisable to avoid hills and a cold wind. A rest at lunchtime and odd jobs around the house complete the day. Competitive games are best avoided in the initial stages, although swimming, cycling, horse riding and gardening all provide suitable recreation as long as chest pain and dyspnoea do not occur. Patients tire easily at this stage and the day should be planned so that fatigue is avoided. Much depends on the home circumstances and it may be necessary to change the bedroom temporarily, so that it is on the same floor as the lavatory.

Return to work is the most important milestone on the patient's way to full recovery, as he resumes his accustomed pattern of life and role in society. A sympathetic approach is required by employers. Initially a return to part-time employment is advisable, and this can usually be attempted within 6 weeks. It is much better to return to a familiar job than to go to work in a strange environment, but sometimes the work is unsuitable and certain occupations are barred for reasons of public safety. Sometimes a decision is difficult and the prospect of loss of income complicates advice. Retraining for a new occupation often proves to be a disappointment. Particularly in winter, the stress of travelling to work may be worse than the stress of work itself, and a shortened working day to avoid rush-hour travel is initially advisable. Often there is less stress involved when driving a car to work. Probably more errors are made on the side of caution than vice versa, for most patients can return to the level of physical and intellectual activity which they enjoyed before the attack. Any patient who has not returned to normal activity after 3 months requires assessment by a cardiologist.

About 85 per cent of patients return to work after a myocardial infarction and 65 per cent of these return to previous employment. This is without the help of specialized rehabilitation centres or a formal training programme. The length of time away from work can vary, with apparently little cause, from 6 weeks to more than a year, and unnecessary delay is common and encourages invalidism. Often the decision to return is based as much on psychological and social factors as on the fitness of the patient.

Of those who do not return to work, half are close to retirement or have been persuaded to retire by doctors, employers or friends. As would be expected, the highest return to work is found in patients who have stable sedentary employment. Neither the patient's age nor the presence of angina have any overall effect on return to work, but recurrent infarction and physical signs of severe cardiac damage are associated with invalidism. In large factories a rehabilitation workshop is useful, as patients returning to work who are uncertain of their capacity for their original job can increase their workload under medical supervision until they are employed within their capabilities.

Advice to change to a lighter occupation often leads to unemployment, sometimes permanently, and is damaging to morale even in a robust personality. Return to work is one of the most important outcomes of medical care but it is often delayed through lack of precise knowledge of the nature of the work involved and through lack of communication between the patient, the hospital and the family doctor and the patient's family and employer. It is these outside factors, such as a family doctor who tends to over-protect his patient, a reluctant employer, or a factory where the firm's doctor has to give his opinion, upon which return to work depends.

Although the quality of the patient's work is unimpaired, he tires easily and allowance must be made for this. Any general discussion of rehabilitation programmes is complicated by the extreme variation of different patients' needs. Allowance must be made for differences in physique and personality and in the kind of work to which the person will return. Outside factors such as family position and the attitude of employers and partners will often have to be taken into account.

Patients will wish to know whether they can drive a car again; usually there are no restrictions, except for those who drive public transport vehicles. Fatal road accidents as a consequence of cardiac crises are rare and there is no clear-cut evidence that driving heavy goods vehicles has proved hazardous to the owner or public. It is wise to avoid air travel for at least 3 months, despite the use of pressurized aircraft.

PSYCHOLOGICAL REHABILITATION

The ultimate purpose of rehabilitation calls for a gradual withdrawal of help from the patient as confidence of both the patient and his family improves. There is often marked anxiety and depression in both patient and spouse; the psychological strains are often considerable, sometimes outweighing the physical damage, and can be completely crippling. The importance of an early and detailed discussion with the patient by the medical staff has been emphasized, for the heart attack is often a terrifying experience. Often there is severe pain and a sense of impending death and the increasing role of the coronary care unit with its medical gadgetery and electronic monitoring systems only accentuates the patient's anxiety. It is important that at this stage the patient be strongly reassured. If this stage is mismanaged there can be far-reaching psychological consequences. The psychological stress that is inevitable can contribute materially to the disability. It is important to protect the patient as far as possible from mental trauma and it is important that there should be no sign of anxiety or confusion among the attendants.

The initial trauma of separation from home is replaced by anxiety and uncertainty about survival and the ability to support one's family. The need for mental rest after a heart attack is often overlooked, but it often happens that the attack occurs at a time of mental stress and physical exhaustion.

The patient is often middle-aged and has a number of financial and family commitments, and uncertainty about the future, in a patient who has often previously been healthy, provides a number of unfamiliar hurdles. It is often important for a patient's spouse or business partner to visit the patient so that business affairs can be tidied up, giving the patient peace of mind. Instillation of self-confidence can be given by medical and nursing ancillaries, but the attitude of the family and friends is important. It is difficult for a patient to make progress if he is surrounded by anxious people who impede every step forward in physical activity. Self-confidence slowly increases with the patient's increasing capacity.

DIET AND LEISURE

If a patient is overweight he should be encouraged to diet. Alcohol in large quantities has a cardiac depressant effect, but it also acts as a vasodilator and it is unnecessary to interfere with previous moderate habits. All patients should be advised to stop smoking, the only exception being elderly people to whom tobacco represents life's only pleasure. It is important to advise the patient to take at least a full hour's rest at lunchtime and also to avoid large meals as this increases the cardiac output and the gastric blood flow. In particular he should not exercise immediately after eating. It has been suggested that the stress of sexual intercourse on the cardiovascular system is no greater than many activities of daily living but it can be equivalent to running up two flights of stairs. It is wise to wait for 6 weeks after the acute attack. Occasionally trinitrin might be required prophylactically. If the patient does not ask about sexual life, it is the duty of the physician to broach the subject. Impotence from fear and anxiety or as a side-effect of drug therapy is fairly common. Many wives find satisfaction in playing a more active and dominant role during the initial weeks.

Adequate leisure is of great importance and activities involving gentle exercise—walking, light gardening, swimming, riding, carpentry—provide a wide choice of suitable occupations. Pursuits to be avoided if possible are those that combine emotional stimulation with physical inactivity, such as most spectator sports. Games such as golf, tennis and squash need not be permanently ruled out for patients previously accustomed to playing them, but energetic sports should not be resumed in an aggressively competitive manner. In all these activities the danger signal of excess is a sudden feeling of tiredness, dyspnoea or pain in the chest.

PHYSICAL TRAINING

Rehabilitation should not only be aimed at preventing reinfarction or death, but should be aimed at improving the quality of life by allowing more physical activity and a fuller social life. Therefore it follows that physical training is but part of the rehabilitation programme. A thorough assessment must be made prior to training and assessment of anxiety and mental attitude must be taken into account. It is important to know what the patient did before his illness and to understand what he will have to do on return to work; but it is more important to know what he wants to do, both at work and in his leisure activities.

There is increasing evidence that lack of physical activity may be a potent predisposing factor in the development of coronary artery disease. Bus conductors suffer less infarction than bus drivers and athletes who remain in training in middle age have a lower mortality from coronary disease. There is also much evidence that exercises after myocardial infarction can lead to psychological and physical improvement. Exercise programmes after myocardial infarction have been developed in many countries, particularly Europe and Scandinavia, and indeed, there are fewer facilities available in this country than in most other countries of the western world. Exercise is not a new therapy for ischaemic heart disease, for Heberden in 1802 described a patient with angina pectoris who noticed an improvement in symptoms after regular activity, and Stokes in 1854 used graduated exercise for cardiac patients.

Studies on the cardiovascular effects of physical training in healthy subjects of different ages have demonstrated the beneficial effects of exercise. There is increase in exercise tolerance and more work can be carried out for a longer time at less oxygen cost. The heart rate and blood pressure are reduced and there is an increased stroke volume and unchanged cardiac output at a submaximal work load. At maximal exercise, when oxygen uptake is higher, cardiac output and stroke volume are both increased. Training also leads to a change in the distribution of blood flow—there is an increase in splanchnic and renal blood flow and a reduction in muscle blood flow.

The physiological effects of training are not so clearly defined in patients after myocardial infarction and detailed haemodynamic studies have only been made in small groups of patients. Comparative studies have also been bedevilled by variations in the type and intensity of the physical training programmes. The considerable variations found in response to physical training probably depend on the functional state of the myocardium. With near-normal myocardial function, training can be carried out in much the same way and with similar effects as in normal subjects of the same age. However, when there is impairment of myocardial function, the stroke volume cannot increase with training and changes in the peripheral circulation predominate. Thus, training in these patients will also result in reduction of heart rate and blood pressure, but the reduction in the work of the heart is the result of an increased arteriovenous oxygen difference.

The increase of aerobic- or symptom-limited work capacity which occurs after 3 months of training is well documented. Thus patients with angina as a limiting symptom at a moderate work load are able to improve their exercise tolerance by about 50 per cent. This means that patients experiencing chest pain while walking upstairs will have no such limitation after training. Training also reduces the 'effort' of exercise and probably the reduction of fatigue and pain is the most reassuring and valuable result of these programmes.

Exercise produces changes in muscle metabolism; in particular, conditioned skeletal muscle is characterized by a higher oxidative capacity. This may be an important factor in the readjustment of the peripheral circulation. Also, regular training two or three times a week has been shown to reduce serum triglyceride and free fatty acid levels, although there is less effect on serum cholesterol. Both these effects may favourably influence pathogenetic processes in ischaemic heart disease.

Far less is known about the possible preventive effects of training regimes on reinfarction and death. This is because studies are based on randomly selected groups of patients and because many patients 'drop out' of long-term training programmes.

Thus, to summarize, exercise

(1) increases cardiovascular capacity, expressed as aerobic- or symptom-limited work capacity;

(2) lowers cost of physical activity by reduction in heart rate and blood pressure;

(3) changes muscle metabolism and reduces serum triglycerides and free fatty acids.

However, perhaps the most important gain is that of reduction in anxiety, and knowledge that physical effort does not cause harm, for patients tend to limit this once outside hospital.

An exercise programme is feasible in a district general hospital and interval training is the most suitable method of exercise. It is important that a thorough evaluation is made prior to entry into a training programme and assessment of anxiety and mental attitudes should be taken into account. Over-enthusiasm for physical training is no more to be encouraged than emotional scepticism and it should be understood that all programmes entail some risk. Therefore it should be undertaken by experienced physiotherapists under medical guidance with resuscitation equipment near at hand.

EXERCISE TESTING

Patients start an exercise course usually at about 6 weeks after discharge from hospital. A preliminary assessment of physical performance is often carried out in many European centres, although this does not have to be routine procedure. Exercise tests are usually carried out on a bicycle ergometer whilst measurements of heart rate, rhythm, blood pressure and oxygen uptake are made. Results give a good indication of the patient's capacity for work and help to determine the intensity of an individual exercise programme and to assess progress. Many patients are anxious on resuming exercise and this supervised test is a good indication of the degree of anxiety. Patients also tend to exercise to a greater extent if they are supervised and many gain confidence and are surprised at their good performance.

The risks of the test are small and well documented but facilities for resuscitation must be near at hand. There are several indications for terminating exercise, the most important being cardiac pain, ventricular extra-systoles and hypotension on increasing effort, the latter indicating impairment of left ventricular function. Patients with increasing angina or with signs and symptoms of deteriorating myocardial function should be excluded.

In most instances, it is the patient who determines termination of the test in that he develops angina or becomes dyspnoeic, or more commonly, complains of general or leg fatigue. But perhaps the commonest reason for stopping is fear.

EXERCISE PROGRAMME

Perhaps the most suitable method of supervision is to encourage attendance at hospital in the early stages of exercise training. Treatment can then take place in small groups and problems and anxieties can be discussed, if possible, with the spouse present. Although exercising in groups of about six is most suitable, it is important that the intensity of treatment is adapted to the individual and with this aim, initial training on a bicycle with medical supervision is essential, so that the intensity of treatment can be decided. Then exercise under the supervision of a physiotherapist is possible but medical and resuscitation facilities should be near at hand. The doctor must be aware and understand potential arrhythmias and have experience in dealing with these and cardiac arrest and resuscitation procedures. E.C.G. monitoring should be limited to avoid anxiety and the physiotherapist can use the heart rate to regulate the intensity of treatment. Isometric exercises should be avoided as they cause a marked increase in blood pressure and exercise should be preceded by a period of 'warming up' and followed by a period of 'cooling down'.

Exercises should consist of progressive circuit routines or interval training which should last for about 30 minutes. A combination of six to eight different exercises, which activate large muscle groups, should include a step test, 'Indian' walking, sitting from a supine position and throwing a medicine ball. At one stage of each training session patients should exercise on a bicycle ergometer at a known work load. This allows simple objective records of changes in physical working capacity and allows adjustments accordingly to the intensity of training. In addition the patient is encouraged by seeing signs of an improvement in his working performance. It is probably best if patients attend twice or three times a week for about 6 weeks, as longer may only lead to increased dependency and long-term programmes have resulted in a high default rate. It should be pointed out that the level, frequency and duration of training are largely empirical.

The amount of exercise can be increased at each session and this should be adjusted to the patient's capacity and previous performance. A training effect may be seen if the intensity is only moderate, and a practical objective is usually an intensity which corresponds to 60–80 per cent of the maximal working capacity. In middle-aged men, physical performance, as measured by maximal oxygen uptake, can be increased by 18 per cent.

Patients should be encouraged to continue their exercise routine after discharge but probably few do so, and attention should be given in future to improving motivation. It is not known whether home exercises are as effective as those carried out under hospital supervision. If possible, return to work should occur whilst treatment continues as problems often occur at this stage and can usually be easily resolved. Exercise programmes undoubtedly help patients gain reassurance and play a part in helping patients return to work but it is psychological and social factors, rather than the fitness of the patient, that figure most in this decision.

Exercise regimes are probably of most value to those in heavy employment, those with anxiety and those with relatively sedentary jobs who have a limited working capacity. At present, it is assumed that fairly strenuous short-term bouts of exercise which increase cardiac output and work are more suitable than sustained exercise over longer periods. However, it may be that exercise which leads to the most improvement in cardiac haemodynamic performance does not have the greatest therapeutic value. It may well be that sustained exercise has more pronounced metabolic effects. There are a number of questions which still need to be resolved. For instance, it is still not known when exercise should begin; it may be that light exercise whilst the patient is still in hospital are of most benefit. It is still not known whether training influences subsequent morbidity and mortality, nor whether it influences return to work.

Emphasis is placed in many centres on detailed measurements of cardiac performance, but we still do not know which parameters are most important. Perhaps patients benefit most from a lessening of anxiety and some workers have demonstrated equal subjective improvement to exercise regimes with relaxation techniques alone. Certainly, there is a need for further studies to determine whether less ambitious programmes with more emphasis on psychological aspects are of equal benefit. This is particularly important as to many patients and their families a myocardial infarction is still regarded as a disaster that is usually fatal, and the subsequent shock and anxiety are often far-reaching.

Although most patients can enter an exercise programme, some must be excluded because of medical contra-indication or mental attitudes and others rapidly resume their former position in society without help. The remainder form a heterogeneous group and each must be treated individually.

About one-quarter of patients are unable to attend hospital for training, some because of cardiac limitations or because of other medical disorders or simply because of difficulty in attendance. Joint and muscle stiffness are common with training, but it seems clear that, provided case selection is careful and medical supervision adequate, patients come to no harm. Patients who should probably be excluded are those with heart failure, those with hypertension requiring treatment, and those suffering from bronchitis with dyspnoea in mild exertion.

The aims of rehabilitation can be summarized as follows.

(1) To remove the deconditioning effect of the illness.
(2) To teach the patient prudent limits of activity.
(3) To remove the fear of exertion and improve morale.
(4) To increase cardiac function.
(5) To improve or relieve angina of effort.

It is suggested that formal cardiac rehabilitation units should be set up in district hospitals, as they have well-defined physiological and psychological benefits. In particular patients gain from the support that follows discharge from hospital.

CONCLUSIONS

The major cause of persisting disability is psychological, and there is no more upsetting sight than the post-coronary patient, devoid of organic symptoms, who is too frightened to work at his job or in his home surroundings. Having a coronary is alarming, and for the first time in his life the patient is confronted with the harsh reality that he is not immortal. If sympathetically questioned, many post-infarction patients will admit that for the first year they are frequently anxious.

Rehabilitation should start concurrently with the treatment of the acute episode. Patients are being mobilized and discharged home earlier than before. The family doctor plays a key part in deciding the patient's future rate of progress and liaison between hospital and family doctor is essential. Rehabilitation should be tailored to the patient's needs, giving consideration to age, sex, marital status, level of physical fitness and the nature of previous employment. Domestic, social, psychological and economic pressures dictate that patients should return as quickly as possible to a normal way of life.

Graded physical training that requires regular attendance at a hospital gymnasium is unlikely to gain widespread acceptance in Britain, since the cost to the N.H.S. and to the patients would be prohibitive, and supervised rehabilitation must, therefore, be reserved for selected patients who are not making satisfactory progress outside hospital.

Regular accepted exercise is safe for cardiac patients. Exercise does not necessarily hasten return to work, improve life expectancy or prevent further attacks, but the benefits to angina, morale and physical agility seem definite.

REFERENCE

Report of a Joint Working Party of the Royal College of Physicians of London and the British Cardiac Society (1975). *Cardiac Rehabilitation.*

13—Chronic Bronchitis

INTRODUCTION

The concept of a rehabilitative form of management of chronic bronchitis is one which has been developed comparatively recently, although the treatment of chronic bronchitis has challenged physicians since cigarette smoking and domestic and industrial processes provided sufficient pollution of the atmosphere to produce it.

Several forms of mainly symptomatic treatment have been traditionally employed, separately or synchronously—suppression of ineffective cough, promotion of expectoration, prevention of secondary infection and stimulation of bronchodilation. To such medical treatments, short-term because their effects last only as long as their term of employment, rehabilitative treatment attempts to graft a long-term, sustained improvement in respiratory function and exercise tolerance. This it tries to effect by careful physiotherapeutic training of the bronchitic patient in:

Breathing control.
Postural control.
Relaxation technique.
Diaphragmatic dominance in the pattern of respiration.
General physical fitness and the performance of regular daily exercise regimes demanding increasing effort.

When the patient can be persuaded to organize his remaining functional potential so that he aims at progressively increasing activity, instead of resigning himself to a life of progressively decreasing activity, rehabilitation is indeed taking place.

With the improvement in cardiovascular and respiratory efficiency resulting from this form of management, further intermittent improvement is effected by the occasional admission of the patient to hospital for mechanical assistance with breathing, or else by the provision of small portable respirators for use in the home.

By such measures, and by adaptations to home and place of work, and help with transport, it often becomes possible for the chronic bronchitic to plan for a resumption of gainful employment and the re-establishment of economic independence, rather than the alternative role of a chronic invalid, unemployed and housebound, maintained by Social Security, with the inevitable domestic stress and disharmony which results from such a situation.

AETIOLOGY AND PATHOLOGY

Chronic bronchitis is a disease of long chronicity, characterized by cough, sticky sputum, and gradually increasing dyspnoea. Pathologically, it is a non-infective condition of the mucosal cells lining the bronchi and bronchioles of the lungs, giving rise to progressive mucous gland hypertrophy, mucosal swelling and increased mucus secretion. This eventually produces diffuse airways obstruction and a decreased diameter of the tubes from which mucus clearance must occur. Active inspiration permits air to be drawn through narrowed airways, but during the passive deflation of expiration, the diminished diameter of these airways reduces expiratory airflow. Any active expiratory effort of coughing tends to cause increased intrathoracic, extrabronchial pressure, leading to further obstruction and collapse of the bronchi and bronchioles, and trapping of air in the periphery of the lungs.

A frequent accompaniment of this condition is the breakdown of intra-alveolar walls and the development of emphysema, although the precise nature of this process is not clearly understood. As a result, the areas of lung involved no longer take an effective part in respiration, since their component alveoli become over-distended and their mucosal lining is eventually replaced by relatively avascular fibrous tissue. Emphysematous areas produced in this manner have several adverse effects on the respiratory activity of the lungs: they reduce the volume of lung tissue in which effective gaseous exchange can occur, and they interfere with the normal mechanisms of respiration and sputum expulsion.

During the inspiratory phase of normal respiration the volume of the thoracic cage is increased by active muscular effort. Negative intrathoracic pressure is increased correspondingly, and the lungs increase in volume and draw in air. Gaseous exchange occurs in the alveoli, and expired air is extruded as the lungs passively deflate with the relaxation of the muscles of respiration and the decrease in volume of the thoracic cavity.

The extrusion of air in breathing during passive deflation of the lungs and the expulsion of sputum in coughing during active deflation of the lungs, both depend upon the effective transmission of changes in the thoracic pressure to the lungs themselves. When a significant part of the lung volume no longer reflects the pressure changes, the reaction of the lung as a whole is correspondingly diminished, the efficacy of the breathing and coughing mechanisms is reduced and the cycle of dysfunction and degeneration has been started.

It is difficult to separate physiotherapeutic from medical and social aspects of the management of chronic bronchitis, and they are all three considered as part of an integrated whole which is designed to fulfil certain specific aims.

THE AIMS OF REHABILITATION

All the various forms of treatment of chronic bronchitis are ultimately aimed at the reduction of dyspnoea and distress during rest, exercise and daily living activities, and at the overall improvement of the quality of life of the bronchitic patient.

Such treatment attempts to:

(1) Eliminate or reduce the primary causes of bronchial irritation.

(2) Reduce the degree of existing airways obstruction.

(3) Establish a more efficient respiratory pattern in a patient's everyday life by means of breathing training and a graduated exercise programme.

(4) Prevent and/or treat infective exacerbations.

(5) Integrate each patient into a scheme of management which has continuity and an understanding of the far-reaching consequences of this disease. Liaison between chest clinic, G.P., family and extramural services to obtain suitable work, suitable transport, and suitable housing conditions, and the institution of regular medical check-ups form an essential part of this.

How are these aims fulfilled?

Elimination or reduction of primary causes of bronchial irritation

Smoking

Smoking is the major cause of chronic bronchitis and the major factor which ensures its perpetuation and exacerbation. Unfortunately, the basic personality of the patient who initially felt the wish and then the need to smoke has seldom radically changed with age. Furthermore, as the addiction to nicotine or simply to the smoking habit becomes established over the years, it becomes harder to break. Yet unless smoking is abstained from altogether or substantially reduced, the effect of other rehabilitative measures is reduced or even negated.

Smog

Despite the dramatic reduction of smog since the institution of smoke-free zones and the enforcement of stricter regulations on industrial and domestic air pollution, there is still enough sulphur dioxide in the atmosphere to cause considerable bronchial irritation. Avoidance of a dust-charged or fume-polluted atmosphere is essential for the chronic bronchitic, and if necessary a change of occupation or a move to a better area should be urged.

Reduction of airways obstruction

As has been stated earlier, it is difficult to separate treatment from the rehabilitation of the chronic bronchitic patient. Both seek to re-establish a more normal pattern of breathing and a more normal existence and do so by endeavouring to train the patient to incorporate disciplines which have been learnt into a permanent way of life. There is no once-and-for-all cure, and no once-and-for-all rehabilitative process for chronic bronchitis. The patient can be helped, improved, but never completely cured.

Unless he stops smoking soon enough, he is caught in a self-perpetuating system of lung destruction, in which an increasing part of his lung tissue becomes almost non-contributory in ventilation, and the remaining part becomes progressively more difficult to use as an effective organ of respiration. As more and more bronchioles become obstructed, first by mucus and then by collapse, expiration becomes increasingly difficult and increasing muscular effort has to be utilized to achieve it.

Bronchodilation

Treatment is directed towards keeping as many bronchi and bronchioles patent as possible. One method of assisting this is by the administration of bronchodilator drugs, orally, parenterally and by inhalation.

Portable pocket bronchodilator inhalers are available, and inhalants are also used in conjunction with the larger respirators, such as the Bird Intermittent Positive Pressure Respirator, from which oxygen is delivered to the patient after humidification and enrichment with an appropriate bronchodilator aerosol.

The severely affected chronic bronchitic benefits greatly from periodic admissions to the chest ward of his nearest district general hospital for intensive physiotherapy and to use such a respirator. Alternatively, he is taught to use one of the several small machines now available for delivering oxygen on the Venturi principle. On these also there is a humidifier attachment by which moisture and a bronchodilator drug can be introduced into the inspired oxygen.

Bronchiolar Patency

Breathing exercises which deepen inspiration and avoid prolongation of expiration assist in maintaining bronchiolar patency by decreasing intrathoracic extrabronchial pressure and the resting respiratory level. During such exercises, patients are urged to breathe in a little more deeply, to avoid forced expiration, and to start breathing in again a little sooner than they usually do.

Establishment of a more efficient respiratory pattern

Therapists concentrate on retraining the diaphragmatic action of their patients to constitute the main muscular movement of the act of respiration. Diaphragmatic exercises are given against increased indirect resistance provided by pressure of the therapist's hand upon the abdomen, and control of rate and depth of breathing is also taught. The intercostal muscles in a bronchitic patient with an over-distended chest are working with the ribs in a position of mechanical disadvantage, and a minimum of ventilation is achieved for a maximum of effort. Thoracic respiration in this situation is inefficient. Unlike the intercostals, the diaphragm does not have to move a large mass of extraneous tissue, and small adjustments in the tone of the abdominal muscles accommodate its movements.

Advocates of this type of breathing exercise stress that diaphragmatic retraining is a part of a six-point programme involving instruction in:

(1) Breathing awareness.
(2) Increased inspiration with the diaphragm.
(3) Relaxed inspiration.
(4) Raising the respiratory level.
(5) Breathing control.
(6) Synchronization of daily activities with the breathing rhythm.

In all cases, the patient is taught to empty his chest by tipping, with or without 'clapping', before starting his exercises. Emphasis is placed on the importance of avoiding the patient's natural tendency to slow his respiratory rate while attempting to establish a new pattern. Initially, while the patient is at rest in the position of his own choice, and subsequently during exercise, always working on the inspiratory phase, the patient is taught to increase the rate and depth of breathing at will, later learning to reduce the rate and increase the depth in the same manner. By breathing in a little more deeply, and stopping breathing out a little sooner than normally, the 'level' of respiration is raised.

The greater the inflation of the lung, the greater the expiratory flow before the point of shutdown. By increasing the resting respiratory level, and so the inflation of the lung, controlled diaphragmatic breathing can produce increased lung inflation, increased intrabronchial pressure and an increased expiratory flow before bronchiolar shutdown occurs.

This patient-controlled method of increasing the resting respiratory level and bronchial patency is given an intermittent boost when the patient uses a positive pressure respirator, or when he breathes out with his lips pursed, so increasing the intrabronchial pressure and prolonging the interval of patency before extrabronchial pressure causes shutdown of some bronchi.

There are indications that using the diaphragm as the main muscular force in respiration promotes the optimal function of normal lung tissue (accommodates the tendency of emphysematous lung to act as a space-occupying lesion) and avoids increasing the ratio of emphysematous, low-ventilating lung tissue to normal high-ventilating lung tissue in the bronchitic emphysematous patient.

How much actual improvement can occur in the bronchitic patient treated by this method must depend upon the severity and duration of the airways obstruction already present. Some improvement inevitably occurs, and further conversion of normal lung tissue to emphysematous lung tissue is slowed or prevented.

When the control of breathing and the substitution of finely adjusted diaphragmatic respiration for thoracic respiration has been taught to a patient, his exercise tolerance may further be improved by sessions of general physical training. With such training, combined with new breathing patterns, the chronic bronchitic who is initially breathless on the mildest exertion may soon learn to think in terms of walking distances of hundreds of yards and eventually of several miles. His posture and his breathing pattern are steadily improved, and fatigue and respiratory distress are averted for increasing intervals. Such functional improvement occurs even in the absence of demonstrable improvement in the levels of oxygen and carbon dioxide in the blood.

The provision of a small portable respirator for use at home and at work may be very helpful. Housebound patients may sometimes benefit from a supply of oxygen at home to use before specific tasks, such as going upstairs, and a portable oxygen cylinder may occasionally enable a patient to get to work. A portable respirator may be attached to a walking frame or carried across the patient's shoulders. Regular use of oxygen at home, other than for specific tasks, is rarely useful or advisable.

Prevention of infective exacerbations

Continuous antibiotic therapy has been shown by extensive trials to be an unnecessary and expensive method of preventing infection in the chronic bronchitic. Instead, a patient is given a small store of broad spectrum antibiotic which he is instructed to take the moment his sputum becomes purulent. In this way, although the initial virus infection is not prevented, the damaging secondary bacterial infection is quickly controlled without the otherwise unavoidable delays in obtaining an antibiotic. Further supplies of antibiotic are obtained on request from the G.P. and are continued until the sputum has been clear for some days.

Expectoration may be assisted by administration of mucolytic expectorant—this is particularly valuable to patients with sticky sputum.

A variety of expectorants are still widely prescribed. All are best taken in very hot water, which is probably the effective agent in promoting expectoration.

When chronic bronchitis is complicated by bronchiectasis, regular postural drainage of the appropriate segments is taught, and the spouse or parent, or person giving care, is instructed in the 'clapping' or 'shaking' which supplements this. Often lying over the side of the bed or on a pile of pillows in the correct posture is sufficient, but some patients drain better when adequately positioned over a simple frame, easily made by the patient or a local handyman.

If the patient tends to suffer from sinusitis, he is further instructed in postural sinus drainage and in the art of washing out his sinuses without recourse to the E.N.T. department. Localized areas of bronchiectatic lung are resected as necessary. Annual inoculation with anti-influenza vaccine can provide valuable protection against the acute flare-up of respiratory infection which frequently follows an attack of influenza in a bronchitic patient. The inoculation is customarily given in the autumn.

Integrated management

The long-term rehabilitative care of the chronic bronchitic calls for the closest co-operation between the patients, their families, doctors, and paramedical workers. Conscientious attention to routine is demanded of the patient, often in vain, so that he has to be rehabilitated in spite of himself.

Abstention from smoking, regular performance of breathing exercises and regular medical supervision must be his life-long programme so that the needs occasioned by the deterioration in an inexorably progressive condition may be anticipated whenever possible.

He must accept that intermittent short admissions to hospital for boosting treatment will become necessary as his respiratory function diminishes. As an in-patient, intensive physiotherapy with intermittent positive pressure mechanical assistance to his breathing, and the exhibition of appropriate bronchodilators and antibiotics can combine to improve his respiratory status dramatically.

With a disease of such long chronicity, the social conditions of a patient's life assume a major importance, and his return home following in-patient treatment should be preluded by a visit from the domiciliary occupational therapist or social worker and the submission of a report on his home conditions to his medical advisers. Should his bronchitis be sufficiently severe, every effort is made to rehouse him in a ground-floor flat or disabled person's bungalow, rather than in a multi-storied house or a tower flat. If family or social considerations make it preferable that he remains in his present home, it may be sufficient merely for him to sleep downstairs, or he may be able to continue sleeping upstairs provided he has an electric heater for his room and has it switched on for at least half an hour before he retires to bed and then climbs the stairs very slowly. A night storage heater prevents the overall temperature of the house dropping too much during the night. Though local authorities are now encouraged by the Department of Health and Social Security (D.H.S.S.) to provide adequate heating where necessary, a patient may need financial assistance from some charitable fund to enable him to purchase adequate heating equipment or to install central heating.

The place and type of work of the chronic bronchitic both need careful consideration. Indoor work, sedentary if exercise tolerance is low, and in an atmosphere which is as free from fumes of industrial, fire or tobacco origin as possible, and is well-ventilated but yet of as constant a temperature as possible, is ideal. It is also difficult to obtain. Whenever possible, a patient should attempt to remain in his old place of employment for as long as possible, preferably keeping to his specific job, unless the conditions thereof are irritant to his bronchitis and dyspnoea. Liaison with his employer, or the personnel manager or medical officer of his place of work may enable some adaptations of working conditions to be made which enable him to continue at his job. If not, he must seek re-employment, or even retraining in an alternative trade.

Application to the Disablement Resettlement Officer for the district could lead to work assessment and formal retraining for a suitable occupation.

SOCIAL PROBLEMS

Transport

If the use of public transport to get to work entails one or more long walks, long periods of standing and then probably exposure to irritant tobacco smoke and to possible infection from fellow passengers, dyspnoea and further exacerbations of acute respiratory infection may result.

In this case the patient may be referred to his local D.H.S.S. Appliance Centre either by his chest physician or his general practitioner for consideration of his eligibility for assistance. If he is thought to be a respiratory cripple, whether or not he is at work, he becomes eligible for assistance. If not quite so disabled, but still needing personal transport to get him to work, he also becomes eligible and may be awarded either a Ministry three-wheeler car or tricycle, or else an allowance to maintain his own car for his own use (*see* Chapter 14).

The provision of a lightweight, folding, assistant-propelled wheelchair will enable the chronic bronchitic to be taken on visits and expeditions without having to walk distances which are beyond his capacity. Such chairs are particularly suitable for stowing in the boot of a car, and further enlarge the scope of a disabled person's activities, while the power-assisted attendant-operated outdoor chair enables the large patient with a small or unfit spouse to be also taken for walks, even in hilly areas.

Family care

Patients with chronic bronchitis may become depressed, and during acute episodes of respiratory infection or during the night hours when respiratory activity is normally diminished, they may also become hypoxic and confused. Families need a maximal amount of supportive care and explanation by medical and paramedical workers and need to be reassured, yet alerted to report such conditions, so that appropriate treatment may be instituted.

The continued presence of an unemployed and unemployable bronchitic in the home can also become irksome to the spouse who must give care, run the home, support the family, and possibly do a part-time job as well, particularly as the limited exercise tolerance of the bronchitic must also limit the amount of help which he can give with the household tasks.

Subsidized holidays in suitable homes where disabled people are catered for adequately, can be of inestimable use in keeping families together by occasionally making it possible for them to be apart.

CONCLUSION

Failure of the chronic bronchitic to accept the importance of his own responsibility for the success of his rehabilitative programme must doom it inevitably to failure. Thus the bronchitic who continues to smoke in the intervals between using his bronchodilator inhalant or his portable respirator is making a nonsense of his treatment. So too is the patient who attends the physiotherapy department religiously for exercises which he never incorporates into his daily life.

The rehabilitation of the chronic bronchitic is not a once and for all form of rehabilitation, but the establishment of a more effective method of breathing and of living and the acceptance of a recurrent process of modification and regulation of home life and working life, interspaced with short hospital admissions to boost respiratory efficiency.

BIBLIOGRAPHY AND REFERENCES

Fletcher, C. M., Elms, P. C., Fairburn, A. S. and Wood, C. H. (1959). 'The significance of respiratory symptoms and the diagnosis of chronic bronchitis in a working population.' *Br. med. J.* **2**, 257

Fletcher, C. M. (1959). 'Chronic bronchitis.' *Am. Rev. resp. Dis.* **80**, 483

Fletcher, C. M. (1965). 'Some recent advances in the prevention or treatment of chronic bronchitis and related disorders with special reference to the effects of cigarette smoking.' *Proc. R. Soc. Med.* **58**, 918

Fry, D. L. and Hyatt, R. E. (1960). 'Pulmonary mechanics: a unified analysis of the relationship between pressure, volume and gas flow of the lungs of normal and diseased human subjects.' *Am. J. Med.* **29**, 672

Gough, J., Fletcher, C. M., Gilson, J. C. and Oldham, P. D. (1952). 'Discussion on diagnosis of pulmonary emphysema.' *Proc R. Soc. Med.* **45**, 576

Grant, R. (1969). 'The physiological basis for increased exercise ability in patients with emphysema after breathing and exercise training (a review of the literature).' *Physiotherapy* **52**, 541

Harris, C. S. (1972). 'Chronic bronchitis.' *Br. J. hosp. Med.* **7**, 719

Innocenti, D. (1966). 'Breathing exercises in the treatment of emphysema.' *Physiotherapy* **52**, 437

14—Aids to Mobility

INTRODUCTION

An aid to mobility assists or substitutes for lower limb function in moving a patient bodily from place to place. The optimal aid to mobility is that aid which provides maximal assistance of the required kind for movement in space of any particular patient, with minimal adverse effects on future activity and minimal inconvenience to other people. In general, simple aids are best, calling for little manipulative skill, occupying the least space and proving to be the least prone to mechanical and other failures. There is a rational progression of aids of increasing complexity which provide an increasing degree of substitution for normal movement.

Partially weight-relieving (patient manipulation) sticks, crutches, walking frames.

Completely weight-relieving patient-propelled wheelchairs; attendant-propelled wheelchairs; powered wheelchair or outdoor vehicles.

PARTIAL WEIGHT-RELIEVING AIDS

Walking-sticks

The simplest partially weight-relieving aid is the walking-stick, whether of the classical wooden variety, or of the more modern tubular metal alloy construction. The walking-stick can be used to relieve weight by patients with unilateral lower limb disease when held in the contralateral hand, but this manner of weight relief often induces an unevenly paced gait. The use of *two* sticks enables the patient more efficiently to protect one leg by weight-bearing through the sticks, from 'heel strike' to 'toe off' of the involved leg and in this way to achieve considerable weight relief and an evenly paced walk.

Walking-sticks should always be of the correct height. The handle should be level with the greater trochanter when the patient is standing erect in shoes, or alternatively it should correspond in height with the lower end of the ulna when the arm hangs loosely at the side. The handle of a walking-stick should be chosen (or even designed) to suit the shape and strength of the hand of its user. A curved handle is preferred by some with normal strong hands, but many patients prefer a straight handle. Usually the elderly or arthritic are more comfortable when the handle is enlarged by being bound with sorbo rubber, plastic foam or felt. The most generally satisfactory diameter for 'grab rails' is about $1\frac{1}{4}$ in (3 cm), and this diameter is usually preferable for walking-stick handles.

There are some patients who prefer sticks with a moulded plastic handle whereas others (particularly those with rheumatoid arthritis) can only become really efficient with handles specially moulded to their own hands. Whichever type of stick is used, it should always be fitted with a large-based removable rubber or plastic ferrule, which should be replaced as soon as its tread becomes worn.

Greater support and stability may be provided by three-legged (tripod) or four-legged (quadruped) sticks. Some designs of tripod sticks are unstable in use, since the weight tends to be transferred medially to the triangular base, and thus qudruped sticks are usually preferable. There are many different designs, and it is usually wise for the therapist to instruct the patient in their use and to provide those walking aids which the patient can use most freely and with the greatest confidence and stability.

Crutches

Crutches of various types are suitable for different diseases and thus for different patients. The traditional under-arm crutch (axillary) is suitable only for short-term use, as a weight-relieving support to be used after trauma or operation until partial weight-bearing is permitted. It is contra-indicated for long-term and short-term use in the presence of joint disease of the upper limbs, since it imposes considerable strain on the joints and muscles of the upper limbs and on the shoulder joints in particular. The long-term use of axillary crutches is also contra-indicated following spinal cord injury with paraplegia or paraparesis of both lower limbs. However, for spina bifida patients or patients with cauda equina lesions or with flail or semi-flail legs, axillary crutches do provide an acceptable aid to three-point walking, both legs being swung together. This can become an efficient and stable form of progression for patients with normal arms and is quickly learned.

If prolonged use of crutches is needed, or if patients have joint disease, then elbow crutches are indicated. This type of crutch does not put as much strain on the joints and muscles of the arm as the axillary crutch and does not predispose to the development of osteoarthrosis in the shoulder joint or to brachial neuritis.

There are several different types of this crutch, not all of which are equally satisfactory. An elbow crutch is essentially a walking-stick with an extension to the vertical component, angled at about 30 degrees to the longitudinal (vertical) axis. At the upper end of this forearm extension is an arm clip usually made of spring steel, or of rigid padded or coated metal. This clip accommodates the upper forearm. Ideally, the length of both the walking-stick part and the forearm part of the crutch should be adjustable, so that the handgrip is at the level of the greater trochanter when the crutch is held beside the body, and the upper end of the arm grip is immediately distal to the head of the radius. In practice, however, it is usually more satisfactory for the physiotherapist to choose a pair of crutches of the correct size for a particular patient, since adjustable upper components are expensive to incorporate and often unstable to use.

It is also important that the arm grip is correctly aligned and well padded to avoid pressure of the edge over the ulna where there is little muscular protection. The handgrip is often too thin and is improved by padding with foam or leather. Some elbow crutches are now available with thicker, softer moulded plastic handgrips.

Correctly used, elbow crutches provide greater stability than walking-sticks. Not only do they stabilize the wrists, but they also spread the load of the bodyweight, since the forearms as well as the hands provide some weight relief. Significant flexion deformity of the elbows and poor hand function may make the use of these crutches difficult. If elbows and wrists are painful, the use of elbow crutches cannot be tolerated. A further disadvantage is that their long-term use, by placing additional strain on elbows, wrists and hands, not only exacerbates any arthritic pain but accelerates degenerative changes in the affected joints.

The alternative 'gutter crutch' demands less of the upper arm joints, as the patient rests the forearm in the gutter. This type of appliance is particularly suitable for patients with painful, weak hands and wrists. Its height should be adjustable to permit the forearm to rest comfortably in the horizontal gutter support when the patient is standing erect. The position and length of the gutter support, and the position, angle and width of the handgrip should also be adjusted to, or selected for, the patient's individual requirements. Usually some extra padding of foam or leather will be needed for the forearm gutter to overlap the metal edges. Leather or velcro straps fix the crutch to the forearm.

Walking frames

Even more support and stability can be provided by walking frames. These are usually wide based and particularly lightweight as they are commonly used for very elderly and frail patients, as well as for young ones with severe temporary disability. A great variety of walking frames exists, with different heights and widths. Some frames have two small wheels on the leading legs, or on all four legs. There are many different sorts of handgrips, or forearm gutter supports, or axillary supports. Some frames have hinged side-pieces (reciprocal walking frames). Most frames (other than the reciprocal walking frames) are rigid and take up a lot of room when standing free in the average house. However, their stability is often their most important characteristic, enabling patients to use them for getting in and out of a chair and on and off the toilet, as well as acting as an aid to ambulation.

Use of a multitiered trolley, if necessary with handgrips or forearm supports, may be a preferable solution for the disabled housewife who needs a support for walking about the house but finds herself unable to carry domestic objects from place to place while using a walking aid. The trolley provides both a walking support and a carrying surface.

The recently introduced portable parallel bars further increase the potential range of independent action of the elderly or frail patient. Designed to help the double amputee transfer from a sitting to a standing position, they are hinged to a standard walking frame and can be coupled to a standard wheelchair or to sockets fixed to an armchair, or to fitments on each side of the toilet pedestal.

WHEELCHAIRS

Historical background

In this country, the history of the design and development of wheelchairs really began with their free supply under the auspices of the Ministry of Pensions. When this Ministry was formed in 1917 some wheelchairs were already being provided for disabled servicemen by the Lord Kitchener Memorial Fund. In 1918 the Ministry of Pensions assumed the responsibility for providing wheelchairs to:

(1) Paraplegics.
(2) Double amputees, with one amputation above the knee.
(3) Double below-knee amputees (if the patient's general condition made the supply necessary).

In the light of current supplies this disability group is interesting, as it would nowadays represent about 10 per cent of the total supply. Hand-propelled tricycles were provided for non-pensioners to go to work; and from 1920 onwards some powered attachments were made available by the Red Cross, for severely disabled pensioners in hilly districts. It was not until 1945 that the Ministry of Pensions assumed responsibility for powered tricycles.

The National Health Service was inaugurated on 1 July 1948, when the Ministry of Health had the duty to promote the establishment of a comprehensive health service, including the provision of appliances. For organizational reasons the Ministry of Pensions continued to act for the Ministry of Health for the ordering, supply and repair of wheelchairs and tricycles. The Ministry of Health did not assume *direct* responsibility for these activities until 1953. Thus, prior to 1953 the general thinking behind the supply of wheelchairs was directed towards the needs of war pensioners. In the early days of the Health Service the usual wheelchair supplied was a rigid-framed chair designed for indoor use. During the first two years of the N.H.S. (1948–50), 9000 wheelchairs were supplied, mostly of this type.

Before the inception of the National Health Service there is little evidence of any serious work on design and development of wheelchairs; the social evolution which followed its inception had a direct and lasting effect on the production of wheelchairs and all other appliances. The wheelchairs currently available have thus evolved to fill a social need rather than as a response to a specific engineering project.

Part of the changing pattern of design has been due to the changing organization and control of supply. Before 1956 it was sufficient that a consultant informed the Medical Officer at the nearest Artificial Limb and Appliance Centre that the need for a chair existed. The patient was examined at the Centre and a chair ordered and provided. This meant that before a chair could be supplied, on each occasion the patient was seen by a general practitioner, a hospital consultant and an Appliance Medical Officer. (Such a system still exists today for the provision of powered outdoor and indoor transport.) After 1956 it was agreed that the hospital consultant could prescribe the particular wheelchair which he considered most suitable for his patient.

This closer involvement of the consultant with chair prescription unquestionably led to increasing interest in the design of wheelchairs, as doctors outside the D.H.S.S.'s own organization could now bring more interest and influence to bear upon the type of chair supplied to their patients. As, however, there was simultaneously an increasing supply of outdoor invalid transport there grew up an increasing demand for a simple wheelchair for use in combination with these vehicles. The simple transit chair which was originally produced for this purpose weighed about 30 lb (12 kg) and could fold flat to go into an invalid tricycle. It had fixed armrests, fixed footrests and a very short backrest. Although ideal for some patients, its small size and fixed arm- and footrests rendered it unsuitable for many others. But it was this chair which gradually developed into the general purpose indoor/outdoor chair for self-propulsion. By 1963 these general-purpose wheelchairs were being supplied at a rate of over 15 000 per year. At the same time there was increasing pressure for the supply of a comfortable wheelchair for the elderly disabled. This need was for an attendant-operated pushchair which was comfortable.

Now for the first time, general practitioners are being allowed to prescribe wheelchairs. Although they are only allowed to prescribe from a small range of 'standard' chairs, it is likely that this will bring further changes in the design and contribute to the evolution of the wheelchair.

The majority of the wheelchairs on issue by the Department of Health in England and Wales are of the type of general-purpose self-propelling wheelchair (Model 8 or variant). The increasing popularity of this type of chair may be attributable to the ease with which it may be folded for car transit and the provision which it makes for occupant/attendant propulsion. It has come to be used as an indoor/outdoor wheelchair because the disadvantages of 'tracking' castors and lack of suspension are mitigated by the obvious advantages of using only one wheelchair for both environments—namely not having to transfer the occupant unnecessarily and not having to create the extra storage space required for a second chair.

Design features and problems

In recent years there has been considerable interest in the design of the wheelchair, and several bodies have sponsored major research programmes. These programmes have been engendered by an increasingly large and loud voice of criticism coming from patients, patients' relatives, charitable organizations concerned with the welfare of the disabled, and clinicians, who note the effects of the chairs on the patients for whom they are prescribed.

The standard wheelchair is easy to criticize, particularly its appearance and its weight, but over the years, as the population of wheelchair users has grown, the Department of Health has gradually extended the range of features and alternatives available. It is the need to provide quickly and cheaply a wheelchair suitable for all patients which has led to the provision of a highly criticized chair of compromise design. Indeed the more that attempts are made to extend the range of the population accommodated by any particular type of chair, the more probable it is that irreconcilable criteria will occur and the resulting situation will be unsatisfactory to the broad mass of the population served.

The wheelchair user

A census of the physically disabled shows that there are over 3 million adults in the U.K. with a physical disability, and five sixths of these are of pensionable age.

The commonest disabilities are:

Arthritis (rheumatoid and degenerative).
Strokes.
Multiple sclerosis.
Amputation (of lower limb).
Cerebral palsy.
Spinal cord lesion (trauma and spina bifida).
Muscular dystrophy.
Degenerative neuromuscular disease.
Cardiovascular/respiratory disease.

It is these conditions which not unnaturally feature largely among the wheelchair users. Approximately 14 per cent of wheelchair users suffer from rheumatoid arthritis, 14 per cent from osteo-arthritis, 13 per cent from cerebrovascular lesions, 9 per cent from lower limb amputations, 8 per cent from cerebral palsy, and 7 per cent from spinal injury. The wheelchair population includes rather more women than men (men 44 per cent, women 56 per cent), and 60 per cent of wheelchair users are over 50 years of age.

It is clear that wheelchair mobility is mainly required in the immediate environment of the home and its neighbourhood. Wheelchair users, according to their handicap and capabilities, can be grouped as follows:

(1) Semi-ambulant.
(2) Non-ambulant.
    (*a*) Chairbound accompanied.
    (*b*) Chairbound independent.

The semi-ambulant group, requiring the wheelchair for assistance, particularly where distances or bad surfaces are involved, is large.

The majority of wheelchair users are severely disabled. One half to two thirds are *dependent* upon the wheelchair for mobility, requiring a chair for use both indoors and out of doors (wheelchair-bound). About one half can stand long enough to transfer from chair to chair, chair to bed, but only a very few can stand or walk without support of some kind. This means that the majority of chair users are not only dependent upon the wheelchair, but are also dependent upon relatives, friends and helpers of some kind. The one third to one half of users who are semi-ambulant tend only to use a wheelchair out of doors, and most of this group are elderly and frail. Indeed, one third to one half of the semi-ambulant need their wheelchair permanently for outdoor use. If they do not have a wheelchair they never go out of doors. The majority of wheelchair users do not drive and cannot fold their chair, nor lift it into a vehicle.

Thus the general design of the wheelchair is changing to accommodate the needs of those who use them. Both the age and the diagnosis of the patients concerned are important here.

Elderly users The large and increasing number of elderly users has affected one aspect of design. Elderly patients require chairs which are light, portable, shock absorbing, reliable, very manœuvrable and capable of easy transport. Their attendants are often also elderly, and this too needs consideration.

Young adult users The smaller number of young adult users has influenced another aspect. Younger patients demand and are more likely to achieve a greater degree of independence than the elderly. They require chairs which are strong enough and versatile enough to permit them to undertake a wide variety of activities. Traumatic paraplegic patients fall into this category. Usually young, well motivated, extrovert and with powerful upper limbs, they are able to lead their lives almost independent of assistance. Not all young patients achieve such independence, and some severely handicapped young adults need considerable assistance to enable them to maintain even a limited degree of independence.

Handicapped children Such users do not only need scaled-down models of adult chairs. In addition they need light, collapsible chairs in which they may be taken shopping, and which can be easily lifted on and off buses. They also need simple self-propelled chariots in which they can achieve mobility at the same stage of development as the able child.

Functional anthropometry of wheelchair occupants varies with both age and disease, age being the more important factor. It is reasonable to assume that *independent* chairbound wheelchair users are mainly young adults. The additional effects of disabilities of insidious onset and degenerative disorders are more commonly found in elderly users, who make up the majority of *accompanied* chairbound wheelchair users. But the distinction between independent and accompanied wheelchair users can never be precise, and a substantial proportion of all users suffer from weakness of grip, incoordination and stiffness, or other upper limb disability.

We thus see how the major types of wheelchair have arisen from these determining needs:

(1) A comfortable pushchair for the elderly and severely disabled.

(2) A strong versatile self-propelled chair for the largely independent young adult.

(3) A group of chairs to fulfil the needs of the completely dependent child who yet attempts to approximate to normal development.

Population studies indicate that the largest group of wheelchair users is made up of elderly patients, disabled by arthritis or stroke, of very limited independence, requiring help to get in and out of the chair, and needing to be pushed when out of doors. A third of all wheelchair users are incontinent, and this fact emphasizes the need for a full clinical assessment when deciding a patient's wheelchair requirements.

The care of incontinent patients places particular demands on their wheelchairs which must facilitate toileting and cleansing by the nursing staff, and resist possible recurrent wetting.

For outdoor use the increasing availability of the motor car, and the awkwardness of the average car boot, creates an overriding need for wheelchairs to be light and foldable. Such is the pressure that the conventional standard chairs are rapidly giving way in popularity to similar but light-weight models with detachable armrests and legrests, reducing the main chassis and wheels to about 36 lb weight (16·4 kg). When the chair is to be attendant-pushed, the large propelling wheels can be replaced by smaller ones, thus reducing weight and overall size.

Design features of available wheelchairs

The main design features of a wheelchair are wheels (castors), footrests, seat and backrest, brakes, armrests, extras. These can be considered under three groupings:

Wheels and propulsion techniques.
Seat, backrest/armrests and the chair's comfort factor.
General construction: materials, weight, foldability and appearance.

Methods of propulsion

Although the majority of wheelchair users propel themselves with their hands on the wheels, there are other techniques of propulsion. Two sticks can be used to 'punt' the chair along, or the patient can 'walk' the chair. Some patients with rheumatoid arthritis find such modes of propulsion particularly suitable for use with a chair on four small universal castors.

Single-arm control

Although specially designed chairs are available which can be propelled by one hand operating one wheel, these chairs are very difficult to control. Not only do they demand considerable co-ordination of thought and action from the patient attempting to use them, but they are virtually impossible to propel on sloping or rough ground. Usually they will prove unsuitable for the elderly hemiplegic.

Wheels

One of the problems with the *pram-type of pushchair* is the difficulty of manœuvring a four-wheeled chair in a small space when all turning must be achieved by the pusher tilting the chair on the backwheels. Some *pushchairs* are therefore fitted with one or more 'castor' wheels and this makes manœuvring easier. There may be three wheels, with two for propulsion and one trailing castor, or there may be four wheels, with two castors in either the trailing or leading position.

In *self-propelled* chairs, the size and position of the wheels are both important. Large propelling wheels at the front of the chair allow easy manœuvring but not easy tilting to go up kerbs; they also interfere with sideways transfers, and prevent footrests being swung out of the way or detached easily for forward standing transfers. Increasing the diameter of the wheels makes for easier propulsion, but also produces chairs which are correspondingly bulkier and heavier for transit in cars. The usual compromise is to use 22 in (56 cm) propelling wheels, with 20 in (51 cm) or 24 in (61 cm) ones available as alternatives.

It is regrettable that the use of the tyres for gripping inevitably makes the hands of the patient who propels in this manner extremely dirty. Not only the size but also the surface of the tyre makes it suitable for hand propulsion. Even a weak hand with limited power can obtain a purchase on the tread of a wheelchair tyre, the most comfortable grip size of the tube for the average patient being about 1–1¼ in (25–30 cm) diameter. Hand-rims are less easily used for propulsion. Whether wooden, chromium-plated metal or nylon-coated steel, they are less suitable than tyres both in size and surface. The use of capstans or rubber strips bound round the hand-rims at intervals to make cog-like protuberances may improve their manipulation in some instances. Most hand-rims now are plastic, and do not splinter, flake or feel cold to the touch; but many tetraplegics will prefer to continue using the tyres to propel their chairs, wearing pads on their hands to protect the skin of their palms.

Castors should be as large as is practicable, in order to keep the effort required for propulsion as low as possible and to assist in negotiating thresholds, rugs and other obstacles. A reasonable compromise is to standardize on a 7 in (18 cm) diameter castor running on ball or needle roller-bearings which should be reasonably well sealed to exclude grit etc. Tyres may be solid rubber or pneumatic and should be easy to replace. Pneumatic tyres on the large wheels save about 5 lb (2 kg) of weight.

Footrests

Because of the need to maintain a high degree of manœuvrability in the majority of wheelchairs, the footrest is usually mounted in front of the castors. This means that it becomes the limiting factor on the turning radius of the chair, and should, therefore, be kept to minimum length. To enable the user to enter the wheelchair, the footrest must fold out of the way. It is common practice to divide the footrest and fold it upwards. Another method is to swing each section outwards, which has the advantage of reducing overall length. Fixed footrests should no longer be tolerated—they add unnecessary length to the chair, they are a nuisance to helpers getting patients in and out of the chair, and they are an unnecessary hazard to the patient who stands for transferring. The swinging, detachable footrest has become a standard feature on most D.H.S.S. wheelchairs and it is designed to provide a useful hand-hold in case the occupant has to be lifted when in the wheelchair, as well as being easy to swing away and detach. Any D.H.S.S. wheelchair can be supplied with such a footrest if this is requested on the order form (AOF5G).

In children's chairs it is customary to have the castor wheels fitted in front of the footrests to give added stability. This restricts the positioning of the feet and is a feature seldom used in wheelchairs for adult usage.

Seats, backrests and cushioning

For many patients the most important feature of a wheelchair is its seating comfort. Here again there are many factors which will often necessitate compromise, for much will depend upon the amount of movement which the patient can achieve within the chair and whether he is in the chair for short or long periods.

The simplest and most commonly prescribed form of *seating* used for folding wheelchairs is of the hammock type which does not interfere with the folding action. The original material used was canvas and this has been superseded by plastic-covered canvas material that can be supplied in a wide variety of colours. Seat materials must be very strong and the rate of sag should be kept to a minimum. The aim should be to provide materials which can be easily cleaned but have an ability to 'breathe' so that they do not become too sticky in hot weather. These two requirements are difficult to achieve simultaneously, and the problem of how to do so has not yet been solved—even in car seats. Ideally the seat and backrest should be easily removable for cleaning. This type of hammock seat is not entirely satisfactory in providing adequate comfort for those who need to use the wheelchair over long periods. For such patients, cushions need to be provided which can be removed when the wheelchair is folded. This cannot be regarded as an entirely satisfactory solution, and, ideally, the wheelchair should be foldable without removing any of its components.

Cushions are a subject on their own. Surprisingly the softest and thickest are usually the least comfortable, for they are readily compressed and also lead to sweatiness in the perineum and anal cleft. For many patients a cushion with a hard base is the most suitable, and this type of cushion can more easily be shaped to allow for the use of a urinal in the chair.

Cushions can make or mar comfort. It is a fairly safe maxim that the more cushions a patient uses in a wheelchair the more uncomfortable it becomes, and the more likely it is that the wrong style of chair has been provided. Extra cushions inserted behind the back will push the patient forward and create difficulties and discomfort with the knees and footrests. Extra cushions laid on the seat will often lift the patient too high and create discomfort for back and shoulders. Furthermore, adding cushions restricts mobility in the chair, prevents the patient from adjusting his position and easing pressure areas and often from achieving transfers easily.

For some patients, sheepskin covers or alternating pressure cushions are available, or cushions which are subdivided and filled with polystyrene granules. These cushions are usually prescribed for patients who are likely to develop pressure sores or in whom such sores have already occurred.

Patients with severe spinal deformity may need additional side cushioning; the use of removable side pads is often preferred by a patient with a collapsing scoliosis to the provision of a spinal brace; a sculptured back cushion with an appropriately sited groove may relieve the pressure on the apex of curvature of the spine of a patient with severe kyphosis.

Occasionally, spinal deformity is so great that cushioning cannot achieve comfort, and then it may become necessary to mould the entire seat and back of the wheelchair to the patient, using either plaster of paris or a vacuum pack to construct the initial negative cast.

Cushioning and support for the head may be provided by prescription of a *headrest*, which is an extra and detachable fitment available for most chairs. For such a headrest, the addition of side wings may be requested, or a carved foam cushion may be added by the therapist giving care.

The angle or rake of the *back* of a wheelchair is vitally important to the comfort of the patient who uses it. Most chairs have their backrests angled at about 5–20 degrees to their seats. For a severely disabled patient this is often not sufficient, and for him it may be essential to prescribe a non-standard chair with an adjustable or fully reclining backrest.

Brakes

It is essential that brakes are provided to prevent the wheelchair 'running away' when the patient is getting in or out. Both large wheels should be braked to prevent the wheelchair turning during this manœuvre.

Brakes have to be effective and they are often 'hard' to put on. Extension pieces may make them easier to reach, and, by giving greater leverage, easier to manipulate. In some early versions of the Model 8 chair, both brakes were operated by one lever, but the Bowden cable and linkage always stretched unevenly. As so many wheelchair users are elderly or arthritic, or both, it is not surprising that many have considerable difficulty in manipulating the brakes—a considerable hazard.

With solid tyres the brakes become ineffective as soon as the tread begins to wear. There is sometimes a need for a unidirectional brake to prevent the chair running backwards on a slope while the wheelchair user opens a door, or for patients who cannot get enough momentum to get up a slope.

Armrests

In addition to their primary function, armrests are used to:

(1) Assist in retaining the occupant in the seat.
(2) Keep the occupant's clothes clear of the wheels.
(3) Support a feeding or working tray.
(4) Support the occupant during entry and egress.

To enable the occupant to transfer sideways from the wheelchair it is often necessary to make the armrests removable. This presents problems because attendants are inclined to lift the folded wheelchair by the armrests, and so it is the usual practice to fit locking catches. This again leads to further problems, since many wheelchair users have weak grips or difficulty in manipulating small stiff springs, and they and their companions often find the locking devices usually supplied with detachable armrests of little help, or indeed a positive nuisance.

Armrests can be made of different heights and with or without padding. Their front portions may have a cut-out to permit the wheelchair to be drawn close to a working surface—these are known as desk arms or domestic arms. The overall height and distance apart of the armrests is important to the ease with which a patient can propel, and frequently a compromise must be accepted among the optimal dimensions required for the armrests to fulfil their separate functions.

The standard chair

The following standard types of wheelchair are supplied by the D.H.S.S.:

Folding pushchairs for outdoor use.
Rigid wheelchairs for indoor use.
Folding wheelchairs for occupant or attendant propulsion.
Electrically propelled wheelchairs for the severely disabled.

We have now arrived at a situation where the standard compromise indoor/outdoor chair can be provided with a series of alternatives and extras:

Propelling wheels at the front instead of at the rear.
Backrest set back 20 or 25 degrees.
20 in (51 cm), 22 in (56 cm) or 24 in (61 cm) diameter wheels.
Alternative seat sizes.
One-arm control.
Extension to footrests.
Domestic armrests.
Gantry for arm sling.
Detachable tray.
Latex foam cushions.
Backrest or headrest extension.

Furthermore, the basic design of wheelchair can be provided in three sizes—child, junior and standard—and nowadays many models are available in 'light-weight' versions (overall weight of basic chair about 37 lb (15 kg) compared with 56 lb (22 kg). These versions have been achieved by gradual evolution in response to demand over 10–15 years.

The paradox of personality

'Ideally,' say the patients, 'a wheelchair should be as similar as possible in appearance to other "normal" chairs in the user's home.' Wheelchairs are often referred to as 'clinical', thus reminding the patient that he is a 'patient'. But these attitudes, if understandable, are irrational. Who crosses a road in an armchair? This attitude is self-defeating. Acceptability comes from skill, skill from practice and practice from understanding and deliberate effort to overcome disability.

Architectural and geographical constraints

It is often architectural and geographical constraints which determine our selection of an appropriate wheelchair. Living from a wheelchair restricts the ability to reach and the ability to obtain access. Critical dimensions are interrelated, and frequently it is turning area and approach rather than the width of the doorway which restricts access. Inevitably space is critical, and usually the disabled, whether semi-ambulant or wheelchair-bound, need *more* space for manœuvring than the able-bodied.

These social factors are frequently the unyielding ones which determine whether or not rehabilitation will be successful. With modern legislation many barriers are being reduced, but many will remain with us for a number of generations yet.

Ergonomics and design

There are a number of theoretical features which should determine the design of wheelchairs for the future.

First, there are the general characteristics by which the patient (user) and the supplier should judge the design.

Comfort

Comfort is obviously of primary importance, but there will always be a compromise between the needs of the user in this and the requirements of stability, manœuvrability, weight and foldability. The most common method of meeting all these requirements has been to provide a flexible (canvas) seat and backrest and to supply separate removable latex foam cushions for those who need a higher degree of comfort. Other approaches have been made, such as to provide a separate folding seat unit, but this has the disadvantage of requiring a separate module which has to be folded and stowed separately on each occasion that it is necessary to fold the wheelchair. The availability of new materials and techniques is likely to offer solutions to these problems in the future, but material and design research are time-consuming and expensive, and many patients are very conventional in their attitudes.

Simplicity

It is implicit in good design that it should be as simple as the functional requirements will allow. It is likely to engender confidence in the occupant if he can see and know what his wheelchair is doing. The wheelchair should be easy to clean and to maintain. Faults and defects should be readily observed so that they can be removed before they let the user down in critical circumstances. It need hardly be mentioned that simplicity, reliability and low cost go hand-in-hand.

Reliability

Ideally wheelchairs should require no attention during their service life. Maintenance and the need for adjustments must be kept to a minimum because service instructions are often ignored. The user can rarely do the maintenance himself, and suitable labour is not often available these days. Failures can be dangerous and cases are known of users being injured as a result of breakdowns.

Stability

Manœuvrability and overall dimensions (e.g. to enable the wheelchair to pass through doorways) limit the extent to which stability can be provided. Present-day wheelchairs are relatively stable providing the occupant knows what he is doing and appreciates the limits to which he can go. In the prescription of a wheelchair, adequate stability must always be an important consideration, although it becomes increasingly difficult to achieve as progressively more compact chairs are demanded. Where there is an increased risk of instability on slopes—as in the case of bilateral lower limb amputees who may be sitting in their chairs without wearing their prostheses—compensatory stability is achieved by setting the rear wheels back 3 in (7·6 cm) from the normal position. This may be prescribed for any standard chair which is required.

Manœuvrability

It is essential that the wheelchair should be able to negotiate confined spaces and pass easily through doorways and around the home and workplace. There will always be a conflict between the user's personal requirements and the need to fit the wheelchair into an everyday environment. There is little object in giving him a wheelchair which cannot be taken into all the places he will want to visit.

Small bulk and weight

The overall dimensions must be as small as possible for a given seat size. The average doorway is 28 in (71·1 cm) wide. With a seat width of 17 in (43·2 cm) and an overall width of 25 in (63·5 cm) there is only a clearance of $1\frac{1}{2}$ in (3·75 cm) on each side of the wheelchair. Most doors open on to narrow passageways and so the turning radius must be kept to a minimum. The wheelchair must fold so that it can be stowed in an invalid vehicle and the D.H.S.S. specifies a maximum of 10 in (25 cm) width when folded. It must also fit between the front and rear seats of motor cars so that a user can enter the vehicle and stow the wheelchair unaided. The height and length should also be such that they permit it to be stowed in a car luggage space. All this manhandling requires that the weight should be kept to a minimum. Probably a minimum weight of 36 lb (15 kg) can be achieved for a light-weight wheelchair without sacrificing strength.

Good appearance

It is not possible to disguise two large wheels and two castors without adding weight and complexity. A wheelchair must be functional, but appearance can be improved by the use of tube work having flowing lines rather than being a mass of straight fabrications. The use of aesthetically more attractive materials, such as plastics, is now being considered, and may effect a radical change in design.

Low cost

This is obviously an important factor, particularly where large quantities are involved, and it is worthwhile noting that the D.H.S.S. is currently spending about £1 000 000 annually on new wheelchairs. Cost is allied to production rates, and these are adversely affected if special features are specified on a bespoke basis. What may not be so readily appreciated is the value of interchangeability as a derivative of standardization. It is well worth considering that it might be better to give the user a wheelchair which does not meet his exact requirements rather than to fit him up with something which is very special and cannot be replaced at short notice if it breaks down or needs to be withdrawn for repairing. There are obviously limits to which such a policy can be taken. There will always be a small percentage of users who have special needs and require custom-built wheelchairs which cannot be used by others.

The prescription and supply of self-propelled and attendant-propelled wheelchairs will continue to be an exercise in compromise until simple, safe modular assemblies are available, all architectural barriers are eliminated, and patients and relatives understand and accept certain restrictions and limitations for wheelchair users.

Powered indoor chairs are not discussed in this book as they are a provision for the more severely disabled.

Outside transport

The whole question of transport for the disabled is a vexed one. It is clear from the steady stream of major and minor injuries incurred during the use of public transport that it is hard enough for the able-bodied to use this form of travelling from place to place, let alone the disabled. If unable to use public transport then the disabled person must turn to private transport, whether this is provided for him or is of his own provision.

With physical disablement comes simultaneous loss of easy mobility, both within the home and often, more significantly, outside the home. Often a disabled man could return to work if he could get there and back, and often a family could be kept intact if the disabled mother had her own transport to do the shopping and take the children to and from school. Though the density and speed of traffic is rising, an ever-increasing number of disabled people venture on the roads. There is little evidence that, as a group, they are any more accident prone than their more able-bodied fellows. Indeed, the trend seems to be in the opposite direction. However, the combination of physical disability and inappropriate transport may well constitute a considerable danger to drivers and to other road users.

Despite the fact that an increasing number of disabled people are being provided with specially designed invalid tricycles (three-wheelers), an increasing number of specially adapted motor cars are being provided for particular categories of disabled patients, and more people are receiving financial grants towards the maintenance of their own cars, the disabled say that insufficient help is being given to an insufficient number of people.

The provision of an 'invalid car' has now been the practice for many years, but increasing pressure has persuaded successive governments that there is a case for providing the more disabled with specially adapted conventional motor cars. The provision of financial assistance in kind or cash which allows a disabled person to drive, provides him with the single escape route from the restrictions of his physical disability and may keep a family socially and economically independent.

Many doctors, however, think that it is more realistic to give the disabled a financial subsidy to keep off the roads rather than to encourage them to get on them. They maintain also that, although it is through their health (their physical disability) that patients qualify for assistance with transport, it is illogical that the supply of vehicles or monetary grants towards the conversion and upkeep of private cars should be the province of the D.H.S.S.

The present situation is that any doctor in the National Health Service can nominate a patient for consideration of his eligibility for D.H.S.S. assistance with outside transport. Referred to his regional Artificial Limb and Appliance Centre, he is examined by an Appliance Medical Officer. From an interview, a physical examination, a vision test and a test of walking ability, an estimation is made of the degree to which a patient satisfies the criteria upon which eligibility for assistance is decided. A further estimation is made of the patient's fitness to control a powered vehicle on the public highway under present motoring conditions.

If the patient is requesting assistance in the form of a Ministry three-wheeler or four-wheeler car, he is tested in the use of one or more appropriate models by D.H.S.S. Technical Officers. His ability to enter and leave the car independently is noted and also his ability to reach and handle the various controls, and his need for any structural modifications.

Actual eligibility is then conceded, or not, by the decision of a panel of lay members of the Civil Service and a single medical adviser at the D.H.S.S. This panel bases its decision on the medical report submitted by the examining Appliance Medical Officer and the technical report of the Technical Officer, which enumerates difficulties encountered with entry and egress, specifies the selection of the various standard controls which are necessary to enable the patient to control a vehicle with maximal ease and safety, and suggests the most suitable vehicle incorporating these.

Clear guidelines are laid down by the D.H.S.S. for the determination of eligibility of the disabled for assistance with powered transport.

> As part of the National Health Service, the Department of Health and Social Security can help those disabled persons who have a permanent disability and who qualify in one of the categories outlined below:
>
> (1) Those with amputations of both legs, one being above or through the knee.
>
> (2) Those with a defect of the locomotor system or with a severe chronic lung or heart condition who to all intents and purposes are unable to walk.
>
> (3) Those slightly less severely disabled, with a very limited walking ability, who, because of this, need personal transport to get to and from work. (Work in this context means full-time or almost full-time remunerative employment.) Eligibility depends on the extent to which the walking ability is limited; inadequacy or absence of public transport cannot be accepted as a determining factor.

Those who are found eligible for help may be provided with either a 'private car allowance' or a powered, three-wheeler vehicle. The private car allowance is (in 1974) usually £100 per annum paid quarterly in advance. Recipients are exempted from payment of vehicle excise duty, but receive no additional payment towards purchase or modification of their car.

The powered three-wheelers may be petrol or electrically driven. They are maintained and insured against third party risks by the D.H.S.S. and are replaced free of charge (except when the replacement is necessitated by the user's negligence).

In recent years cars have been provided and modified in place of a three-wheeler for certain categories of patient:

(1) Jointly for two such persons (i.e. persons so disabled as to be independently eligible for Ministry assistance) who are relatives and who live in the same household, provided that one at least will be able to drive.

(2) For an eligible disabled parent, able to drive, who for a substantial part of the day is in sole charge of his/her young child.

(3) For an eligible disabled person, able to drive, who lives with a blind relative.

(4) For an eligible disabled person suffering from severe haemophilia.

A disabled person may be entitled to a certificate enabling him to claim exemption from payment of vehicle excise duty (providing that he would be eligible for a three-wheeler invalid tricycle were he able to drive himself) if he needs to be driven and cared for by a full-time constant attendant and has a car which is registered in his name and which has been conspicuously and permanently adapted to make it suitable for his transport.

This system of providing outdoor transport for the disabled is not ideal as it is selective, and the selection may at times be unfair. Merely because a patient has a current driving licence and a motor car at the time he becomes disabled, he may, if his disablement is sufficiently great, be granted eligibility for a 'private car maintenance allowance' of £100 per annum. Yet a patient with a precisely similar disablement who has not got a current driving licence and does not own a car will *not* be granted an allowance, even though his family possesses a car and needs help to keep it running. Such a patient is compelled to apply for an invalid tricycle if he wants any sort of assistance with personal transport. This forces one more disabled driver on to the already overcrowded roads who could have been more safely and comfortably transported in the family car, driven by an able-bodied driver.

The disadvantages of the three-wheeler vehicle itself are many. First, it further isolates the disabled driver. He is not allowed to transport a passenger, and thus can never drive out with his wife and family. Nor has he any help to hand if he should get into difficulties. As a corollary to this disadvantage many disabled drivers complain that invalid tricycles make them conspicuous, and they wish to avoid this situation, desiring to be regarded as 'normal' people. The contrary view is that disabled drivers *should* be conspicuous and that the low accident record of invalid tricycles is in part due to the fact that other road users recognize them for what they are. If disabled drivers are to be provided with faster and larger vehicles, and to be allowed to drive passengers in their cars, then it could be argued that they should accept some form of ready identification.

Second, their design has been much criticized. They are frequently said to be relatively unstable, and because of their size and power, a hazard to both driver and other road users. Their controls are also criticized as requiring considerable strength and manipulative skill to handle. Recent impartial and expert testing has given these criticisms unqualified support and has requested the complete withdrawal of both the electric and petrol driven three-wheeler vehicles from use at the earliest possible moment. Further enquiries continue.

Third, unconventional aspects of these vehicles present certain problems. Few garages are prepared to attempt emergency repairs, and a disabled driver may well be stranded because of a minor mechanical fault. The servicing of these vehicles is dependent upon an organization of 'approved repairers', but these are few and far between.

As an alternative, adapted conventional cars are more stable, more readily serviced in an emergency, and the disabled person may travel with the companion of his choice.

Another alternative view is that a considerable sum of money is already spent in putting disabled drivers on the road, maintaining and repairing their cars, without charge, when they are worn and damaged, and financing the organization to support this service. The availability of the private car maintenance allowance under present regulations is seen as matching the financial resources of this aspect of the service, and further extension of the categories of patients eligible for assistance would be an unwarranted burden upon available resources.

It must however be pointed out that there are advantages to be accrued from continuing the provision of three-wheeler invalid carriages. They are adaptable and have been converted for use for many very severely disabled people. Indeed, there are a number of users who would be very unhappy at any suggestion of exchanging their tricycle for a car.

Recently, a new automatic transmission three-wheeler (Model 70) has been made available. This vehicle is capable of great versatility, and brakes, steering and throttle may be varied in type, position and method of manipulation in the standard model. Many modifications may be made to the fitments if found necessary. It is generally felt that a patient who cannot drive a Model 70 should not be driving at all. Even with this new and highly adaptable vehicle available, there are many who feel that the regulations should be redrafted so as to decrease the number of disabled people who are driving. A more freely available monetary grant, available either for private car maintenance or to cover the costs of hired transport, or hired driver, would facilitate this adjustment. Such a grant should depend upon the clinical need and the social handicap involved.

If transport is to be provided, the general view now seems to be that the vehicles should be appropriately adapted commercial saloon cars, and not three-wheelers. If the three-wheeler is to remain part of the provision for the disabled, then patients should be given much more adequate instruction and practice in driving them, and the vehicles themselves should be made more distinctive, so that they are instantly recognized for what they are, and drastically modified to improve their stability, safety and comfort.

Many of the disabled who at present apply for powered vehicles to enable them to go shopping might be better served by powered wheelchairs, operated by the patient, or attendant, as appropriate, and designed for outside use. As patient-operated, electrically powered wheelchairs become more freely available, some alteration of existing kerbs and crossings will be necessary and some definitive ruling as to place and manner of road crossing will need to be formulated.

BIBLIOGRAPHY AND REFERENCES

British Orthopaedic Association (1973). Report of Committee on Prosthetic and Orthotic Services. London; B.O.A.

Department of Health and Social Security (1970). *The Handbook of Invalid Chairs and Hand-propelled Tricycles* (MHM 408). London; H.M.S.O.

Hamilton, E. A., Molden, F. R. and Nichols, P. J. R. (1973). 'Portable parallel bars.' *Rheum. Rehab.* **12**, 100

Harris, A. I. (1971). *Handicapped and Impaired in Great Britain.* London; H.M.S.O.

Jolly, D. W. (Ed.) (1964). 'A symposium on the wheelchair.' *Paraplegia* **2**, 20

Kamenetz, H. H. (1969). *The Wheelchair Book.* U.S.A.; Thomas

Nichols, P. J. R. and Mowat, A. G. (1972). 'Splints, walking aids and appliances for the arthritic patient.' In *Reports on Rheumatic Diseases, No. 48*. London; Arthritis and Rheumatism Council

Nichols, P. J. R., Morgan, R. H. and Goble, R. E. A. (1966). 'Wheelchair users—a study in variation of disability.' *Ergonomics* **9**, 131

Platts, E. (1971). 'Characteristics and requirements of wheelchair users' (M.Phil. thesis). Loughborough University of Technology

Sharp, Lady (1974). *A Report on Mobility for Physically Disabled People.* London; H.M.S.O.

Wilshere, E. R., Hollings, E. M. and Nichols, P. J. R. (1972). *Equipment for the Disabled* (3rd edn). Horsham, Sussex; National Fund for Research into Crippling Diseases

Index